UPDATE IN INTENSIVE CARE MEDICINE

Series Editor: Jean-Louis Vincent

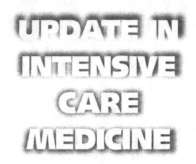

UPDATE IN INTENSIVE CARE MEDICINE

Springer
New York
Berlin
Heidelberg
Barcelona
Hong Kong
London
Milan
Paris
Tokyo

TISSUE OXYGENATION IN ACUTE MEDICINE

Volume Editors:

William J. Sibbald, MD, FRCPC, FCCHSE
Professor of Medicine, Critical Care
University of Toronto
and
Physician-in-Chief, Department
of Medicine
Sunnybrook and Women's College
Health Sciences Centre
Toronto, Ontario, Canada

Konrad F.W. Messmer, MD
Professor of Experimental Surgery
Director
Institute for Surgical Research
Ludwig-Maximilians-University
of Munich
Munich, Bavaria, Germany

Mitchell P. Fink, MD
Chief and Watson Professor of Surgery
Division of Critical Care Medicine
University of Pittsburgh Medical Center
Pittsburgh, Pennsylvania, USA

Series Editor:

Jean-Louis Vincent, MD, PhD, FCCM, FCCP
Head, Department of Intensive Care
Erasme University Hospital
Brussels, Belgium

With 76 Figures and 25 Tables

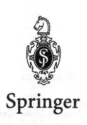

Springer

William J. Sibbald, MD, FRCPC, FCCHSE
Professor of Medicine, Critical Care
University of Toronto
and
Physician-in-Chief, Department
    of Medicine
Sunnybrook and Women's College
    Health Sciences Centre
Toronto, Ontario M4N 3M5
Canada

Mitchell P. Fink, MD
Chief and Watson Professor of Surgery
Division of Critical Care Medicine
University of Pittsburgh Medical Center
Pittsburgh, PA 15260
USA

Konrad F.W. Messmer, MD
Professor of Experimental Surgery
Director, Institute for Surgical Research
Ludwig-Maximilians-University
    of Munich
D-81377 Munich, Bavaria
Germany

Series Editor:
Jean-Louis Vincent, MD, PhD, FCCM, FCCP
Head, Department of Intensive Care
Erasme University Hospital
Route de Lennik 808
B-1070 Brussels
Belgium

Library of Congress Cataloging-in-Publication Data applied for.

Printed on acid-free paper.

Hardcover edition © 1998 Springer-Verlag Berlin Heidelberg.

Softcover edition © 2002 Springer-Verlag Berlin Heidelberg.

Production managed by PRO EDIT GmbH, Heidelberg, Germany.
Typeset and printed by Zechnersche Buchdruckerei, Speyer, Germany.
Bound by J. Schäffer, Grünstadt, Germany.
Printed in Germany.

9 8 7 6 5 4 3 2 1

ISSN 0933-6788
ISBN 3-540-42595-0   SPIN 10851584

Springer-Verlag New York Berlin Heidelberg
A member of BertelsmannSpringer Science+Business Media GmbH

Contents

Measuring Tissue Oxygenation

Blood and Blood Substitutes as Oxygen Carriers

List of Contributors

N.S. Chandel
Department of Medicine
University of Chicago
Chicago, Illinois
USA

G. Deby-Dupont
Department of Anesthesiology
and Intensive Care
University Hospital
Liège
Belgium

L. Einck
Sequella, Inc.
Rockville, Maryland
USA

C.G. Ellis
Department of Medical Biophysics
University of Western Ontario
London, Ontario
Canada

T.W. Evans
Department of Critical Care
Royal Brompton Hospital
London
UK

M.P. Fink
Division of Critical Care Medicine
University of Pittsburgh Medical Center
Pittsburgh, Pennsylvania
USA

A. Görlach
Institute for Physiology
Zurich
Switzerland

A. Gulati
Departments of Pharmaceutics and
Pharmodynamics
The University of Illinois at Chicago
Health Sciences Center
Chicago, Illinois
USA

O. Habler
Institute for Surgical Research
University of Munich
Munich
Germany

A.P. Halestrap
Department of Biochemistry and
Bristol Heart Institute
University of Bristol
Bristol
UK

J.W. Holaday
Entremed, Inc.
Rockville, Maryland
USA

C. Ince
Department of Anesthesiology
Academic Medical Center
Amsterdam
The Netherlands

M. Intaglietta
Department of Bioengineering
University of California, San Diego
La Jolla, California
USA

G. Kemming
Institute for Surgical Research
University of Munich
Munich
Germany

H. Kerger
Institute for Anesthesiology and
Operative Intensive Care Medicine
University of Heidelberg
Mannheim
Germany

M. Lamy
Department of Anesthesiology and Intensive
Care
University Hospital
Liège
Belgium

J.M. Marshall
Department of Physiology
The Medical School
University of Birmingham
Birmingham
UK

M. Mathy-Hartert
Centre for Biochemistry
Institute of Chemistry
Domaine Universitaire
Liège
Belgium

K. Messmer
Institute for Surgical Research
University of Munich
Munich
Germany

M.R. Pinsky
Department of Anesthesiology and Critical
Care Medicine
University of Pittsburgh
Pittsburgh, Pennsylvania
USA

R.N. Pittman
Department of Physiology
Medical College of Virginia Campus
Virginia Commonwealth University
Richmond, Virginia
USA

M. Sair
Department of Critical Care
Royal Brompton Hospital
London
UK

A.L. Salzman
Inotek Corporation
Beverly, Massachusetts
USA

P.T. Schumacker
Department of Medicine
The University of Chicago
Chicago, Illinois
USA

W.J. Sibbald
Department of Medicine
University of Toronto
and
Department of Medicine
Sunnybrook and Women's College
Health Sciences Centre
Toronto, Ontario
Canada

M. Siegemund
Department of Anesthesiology
Laboratory for Experimental Anesthesiology
Academic Medical Center
University of Amsterdam
Amsterdam
The Netherlands

A. Sielenkämper
Klinik und Poliklinik für Anaesthesiologie und
Operative Intensivmedizin
Westfälische Wilhelms-Universität
Münster
Germany

D.R. Spahn
Institute of Anesthesiology
University Hospital
Zurich
Switzerland

K.J. Tracey
Department of Surgery
North Shore University Hospital
and
The Picower Institute for
Medical Research
Manhasset, New York
USA

A.G. Tsai
Department of Bioengineering
University of California, San Diego
La Jolla, California
USA

J.H.G.M. van Beek
Laboratory for Physiology
Faculty of Medicine
Amsterdam
The Netherlands

P. Van der Linden
Department of Anesthesiology
Erasme University Hospital
Brussels
Belgium

M. van Iterson
Department of Anesthesiology
Laboratory for Experimental Anesthesiology
Academic Medical Center
University of Amsterdam
Amsterdam
The Netherlands

J.L. Vincent
Head, Department of Intensive Care
Erasme University Hospital
Brussels
Belgium

K. Walley
McDonald Research Laboratory
University of British Columbia
St. Paul's Hospital
Vancouver, British Columbia
Canada

C.P. Winlove
Physiological Flow Studies Unit
Imperial College School of Medicine
Royal Brompton Hospital
London
UK

Abbreviations

ALI	Acute lung injury
ARDS	Acute respiratory distress syndrome
ATP	Adenosine triphosphate
CaO_2	Arterial oxygen content
CO	Cardiac output
CO_2	Carbon dioxide
DCLHb	Diaspirin crosslinked hemoglobin
DO_2	Oxygen Delivery
DNA	Deoxyribonucleic acid
2,3-DPG	2,3-diphophoglycerate
Hb	Hemoglobin
HBOC	Hemoglobin-based oxygen carrier
Hct	Hematocrit
HIV	Human immunodeficiency virus
IHP	Inositol hexaphosphate
IL	Interleukin
ITP	Intrathoracic pressure
MAP	Mean arterial pressure
MPT	Mitochondrial permeability transition
MRI	Magnetic resonance imaging
NAD	Nicotinamide adenine dinucleotide
NF-κB	Nuclear factor kappa B
NMR	Nuclear magnetic resonance
NO	Nitric oxide
O_2	Oxygen
O_2ER	Oxygen extraction ratio
PARS	Poly (ADP-ribose) synthetase
PEEP	Positive end-expiratory pressure
PET	Positron emission tomography
PFC	Perflourocarbon
pHi	Gastric intramucosal pH
PO_2	Oxygen tension/partial pressure
RBC	Red blood cell
RNA	Ribonucleic acid
ROS	Reactive oxygen species

SO_2 Oxygen saturation
SvO_2 Mixed venous oxygen saturation
TNF   Tumor necrosis factor
VO_2 Oxygen uptake/consumption

Physiology of Oxygen Delivery

Role of the Cardiorespiratory System in Delivering Oxygen

M. R. Pinsky

Introduction

Clearly the primary role of the cardiorespiratory system is to meet the steady state demands of the body by delivering adequate amounts of oxygen (O_2) to meet the metabolic requirements, to sustain aerobic respiration in the tissues and to remove excess carbon dioxide (CO_2). Under normal conditions both ventilation and cardiac output (CO) are tightly coupled to these goals, with minute ventilation varying linearly with CO_2 production and CO varying linearly with O_2 consumption (VO_2). The controllers of these two systems are different. Since the focus of this book is on O_2 delivery (DO_2), issues of ventilatory drive will not be discussed. The controlling factors determining the hemodynamic response of CO to exercise are numerous and the exact process by which the two are linked has escaped definition for the last 150 years. Although these aspects of the circulation are discussed in the subsequent chapters, herein, we shall explore the global relations between ventilation and CO. Importantly, both spontaneous ventilatory efforts and artificial ventilation can profoundly alter both steady state CO and gas exchange efficiency in the lungs, stressing or supporting the peripheral circulation in its role of supplying O_2 to the metabolizing tissues.

Acute respiratory failure can directly alter cardiovascular function in a large number of seemingly unrelated ways. Importantly, the respiratory system and the cardiovascular system are not separate but tightly integrated. The ultimate cardiovascular response to acute respiratory failure is dependent on both the basal cardiovascular status of the subject, the type of respiratory dysfunction present and the ventilatory pattern. For example, both spontaneous inspiratory efforts during acute bronchospasm (increased airway resistance) and acute lung injury (ALI decreased lung compliance) will induce markedly negative swings in intrathoracic pressure (ITP). Similarly, both lung under-inflation and lung hyperinflation will alter pulmonary vascular resistance and heart-lung interactions, and increased work of breathing will stress the cardiovascular response to maintain and increase CO to meet the increased O_2 demand. Lung hyperinflation may also alter blood flow distribution by increasing hepatic outflow resistance. Furthermore, artificial ventilatory support will increase ITP during inspiration in contradistinction to spontaneous ventilation that will decrease ITP for the same tidal breath. Given this litany of hemodynamic effects, it may seem impossible to ascertain the exact heart-lung interaction balance present in a given critically ill patient. However, since heart-lung interactions involve only a few basic processes, the primary determinants of the hemodynamic state and its subsequent response to either changes in ventilatory support or hemodynamic challenges can usually be defined. The four basic hemodynamic concepts relating cardiovascular performance to ventilation are: inspiration increases lung volume above end-expiratory volume; spontaneous inspiration decreases ITP; positive-pressure ventilation increases ITP; and ventilation is exercise, it consumes O_2 and produces CO_2. These processes are summarized in Table 1.

Changes in Lung Volume

Lung inflation alters many processes that directly and indirectly impact on cardiovascular function. Inflation alters autonomic tone [1-4], pulmonary vascular resistance and, at high lung volumes, compresses both the heart in the cardiac fossa limiting absolute cardiac volumes, and the liver below the diaphragm increasing hepatic outflow resistance [5]. The associated diaphragmatic dissent also increases abdominal pressure and compresses the liver, markedly altering the intra-abdominal flow characteristics of venous return [6-8]. Each of these processes may predominate in determining the final cardiovascular state. Small

Table 1. Check list of heart-lung interactions

Venous Return	Left Ventricular Ejection
Impairment:	**Impairment:**
Lung Inflation	**Lung Inflation**
Increasing Pra by:	*By decreasing LV end-diastolic volume:*
Increasing pulmonary vascular resistance	RV dilation (ventricular interdependence)
Compressing the right ventricle	Compressing the left ventricle
Increasing the resistance for venous return by:	
Increasing hepatic outflow resistance	
ITP	**ITP**
Increases in ITP (increasing Pra)	Decreases in ITP (increasing LV afterload)
	Exercise
	Excessive workload for cardiovascular system to sustain
Augmentation:	**Augmentation:**
Lung Inflation	**Lung Inflation**
Increasing intra-abdominal pressure	Increasing LV ejection synchrony (?)
ITP	**ITP**
Decreases in ITP (decreasing Pra)	Increases in ITP (decreasing LV afterload)
Exercise	
Decreased transient time for blood flow	
Diaphragmatic contraction augment venous pressure	

tidal volumes (< 10 ml/kg) increase heart rate by vagal withdrawal called respiratory sinus arrhythmia [2–4], whereas larger tidal volumes (> 15 ml/kg) decrease heart rate, arterial tone and cardiac contractility by sympathetic withdrawal [1, 9–11]. These effects are probably only relevant in the diagnosis of dysautonomia [12] and in the care of neonatal subjects where autonomic tone is high.

However, the primary determinants of the hemodynamic response to increases in lung volume tend to be mechanical in nature [9] Lung inflation, independent of changes in ITP, primarily affects cardiac function and CO by altering right ventricular (RV) preload and afterload and left ventricular (LV) preload. First, inspiration induces diaphragmatic descent that may alter venous return. As originally described by Guyton et al. [13], venous return is a function of the ratio of the pressure difference between the right atrium and the systemic venous reservoirs, and the resistance to venous return. Since a large proportion of the venous blood volume is in the abdomen, increases in intra-abdominal pressure will increase the venous pressure in this vascular space, augmenting venous blood flow [14]. However, diaphragmatic descent will also compress the liver increasing hepatic outflow resistance and decreasing flow from the splanchnic venous reservoirs to the right heart. Complicating this further, inspiration will shift venous flow from high resistance splanchnic circuits, which must drain through the liver, to low resistance systemic venous circuits, making flow greater for the same driving pressure [15–17]. Thus, inspiration may increase, decrease or not alter venous return depending on which of these factors are predominant [18]. In subjects with ascities, increasing lung volume will not impair venous return as much as it will in normal subjects or those with their abdomens open, as during abdominal surgery. Inspiration will increase venous return in volume overloaded states, whereas in hypovolemic states and with hepatic cirrhosis, venous return will decrease.

The RV is not able to develop systolic arterial pressures equal to that of the left ventricle. Thus, RV output is sensitive to changes in pulmonary outflow resistance. Alveolar collapse often occurs in ALI states and is associated with increases in pulmonary vasomotor tone via hypoxic pulmonary vasoconstriction [19–23]. Alveolar recruitment by restoring end-expiratory lung volume back to functional residual capacity (FRC) often reverses this process. Increasing lung volume above FRC also increases RV outflow resistance [9, 24]. However, this is due to progressive increases in transpulmonary pressure (airway pressure relative to ITP) associated with increasing lung volume. Since the heart and great vessels exist in the thorax and sense ITP as their surrounding pressure, increases in transpulmonary pressure will induce pulmonary vascular collapse as transpulmonary pressure approaches pulmonary artery pressure [9, 25]. Hyperinflation increases pulmonary artery pressure and reversing hyperinflation, by prolonging expiration, reducing levels of positive-end expiratory pressure (PEEP) or tidal volumes, and bronchodilation, may all decrease pulmonary arterial pressure improving RV ejection.

LV end-diastolic volume (preload) can be altered by changes in lung volume in any of three ways. First, since the RV and LV outputs are in series, changes in RV preload must eventually alter LV preload in the same direction. Second, by ventricular interdependence, changes in RV end-diastolic volume inversely change

LV diastolic compliance [26,27]. Ventricular interdependence plays a major role in synchronously decreasing LV output during spontaneous inspiration because of the associated rapid and transient increase in RV end-diastolic volume induced by the increased venous return. As either tidal volumes or the swings in the venous flow rate increase, these inspiratory to expiratory differences in LV output also vary. Third, increasing lung volume restricts absolute cardiac volume by direct compression of the heart [9, 28]. As the lungs expand, the heart is compressed in the cardiac fossa and absolute bi-ventricular volume is limited in a fashion analogous to cardiac tamponade [29–31]. This process is thought to be very important in limiting LV output in patients with profound hyperinflation, such as asthma and chronic obstructive lung disease, during episodes of acute respiratory failure.

Changes in Intrathoracic Pressure

Since the heart lives within the thorax, it can be considered to be a pressure chamber within a pressure chamber. Therefore, changes in ITP will affect the pressure gradients for both systemic venous return to the RV and systemic outflow from the LV, independent of the heart itself [24, 32]. Increases in ITP, by both increasing right atrial pressure and decreasing transmural LV systolic pressure, will reduce these pressure gradients, thereby decreasing intrathoracic blood volume. Since intrathoracic blood volume best reflects cardiovascular preload [33], positive pressure ventilation is usually associated with a lower CO than spontaneous ventilation. This difference in CO is greatest in subjects who are preload dependent such as normal and hypovolemic subjects. However, decreases in ITP will augment venous return and impede LV ejection, thus increasing intrathoracic blood volume. Clearly, variations in right atrial pressure represent the major factor determining the fluctuation in pressure gradient for systemic venous return during ventilation [14]. Increases in ITP, as seen with positive-pressure ventilation, a Valsalva maneuver or during hyperinflation during spontaneous ventilation, decrease venous return [34], whereas decreases in ITP, as seen with spontaneous inspiration, increases venous return. Positive pressure ventilation only increases ITP in proportion to the increase in lung volume [35–38]. Differences do exist between regions of the lung, based on physical considerations of chest wall, diaphragm and cardiac fossa [39], as well as the distribution of aerated lung units within the lung in patients with ALI [40].

Spontaneous inspiratory efforts decrease ITP [41]. If airway obstruction is not present, then ITP decreases as lung volume increases. This has the effect of accelerating blood flow into the right ventricle by the associated decreasing right atrial pressure [32, 42]. Thus pulmonary blood flow increases on the subsequent beat [43, 44]. Accordingly, normal respiration-associated hemodynamic changes maximize ventilation-perfusion temporal matching because the spontaneous inspiration matches an increase in alveolar O_2 flux with an increase in pulmonary capillary flow [45]. However, the amount to which venous return can be augmented by decreasing right atrial pressure is profoundly limited. As intrathoracic systemic venous circuits enter the thorax from the rest of the body their surrounding pressure decreases from a positive value, as seen in the abdomen, or a zero value, as seen in the rest of the body, to a negative value (relative to atmospheric pressure). As ITP decreases to less than the intralumenal venous pressure, these large systemic veins collapse as they enter the thorax, limiting maximal venous flow [3].

This "flow-limitation" of venous return is useful in preventing RV over-distention. Negative swings in ITP can be of very great magnitude during inspiratory efforts in the setting of airway obstruction [46]. If the increase in venous blood flow were unlimited, the RV could easily become overdistended, profoundly limiting LV end-diastolic volume and markedly increasing its own wall stress. Such a circulatory system could easily fail. Since neither RV overdistention nor LV underdistention are events that the circulation would prefer to endure in cardiovascular stress states, flow limitation of venous return plays a useful role in the spontaneously breathing subject with lung disease.

LV afterload is a difficult parameter to define. In general it varies with maximal or mean systolic wall tension. Since, by the law of LaPlace, tension is proportional to the product of the transmural pressure and radius of curvature of a sphere, LV wall tension is proportional to the product of transmural LV pressure and LV volume, with maximal tension usually present at the moment of aortic value opening. Thus, increases in LV end-diastolic volume for a constant ejection pressure must also increase LV wall tension [47]. One can readily see from this construct that LV preload and afterload are tightly coupled. Since increasing ITP will mechanically decrease transmural LV pressure if arterial pressure is constant, increases in ITP unload the LV, whereas decreases in ITP have the opposite effect [32]. Thus, in ventricular failure states associated with fluid resuscitation, increases in ITP increase CO [24, 32].

Accordingly, spontaneous ventilatory efforts performed against a resistive (bronchospasm) or elastic (ALI) load, decrease LV stroke volume [48, 49]. The processes involved are multiple and often inter-related. Collectively, these processes are referred to as pulsus paradoxus [50–54]. Firstly, transient intraventricular septal shift from the RV lumen into the LV lumen occurs as the RV end-diastolic volume rapidly increases during negative ITP inspiration. This RV dilation, in combination with absolute pericardial volume restraint, limits absolute LV end-diastolic volume [9, 26, 55]. Thus, either volume overload, pericardial disease or RV failure can all accentuate pulsus paradoxus. Furthermore, increases in LV afterload (LV pressure minus ITP) by impeding LV emptying will increase LV end-systolic volume making LV stroke volume even less [32].

Importantly, how and for how long changes in ITP occur, impacts on the subsequent hemodynamic response [56, 57]. For example, sudden increases in ITP increase arterial pressure to an amount equal to the increase in ITP without changing aortic blood flow. This increase in arterial pressure is not associated with any change in ejection pressure. In heart failure states, this positive pressure inspiration associated increase in arterial pressure has been referred to as "reverse pulsus paradoxus." If the increase in ITP is sustained, however, then the ITP-induced decrease in systemic venous return will eventually decrease LV output, thus decreasing arterial pressure [34, 58]. In the steady state, because of baroreceptor mechanisms tending to keep carotid perfusion pressure constant, changes in ITP that result in altered arterial pressure will also reciprocally alter peripheral vasomotor tone. Baroreceptor reflexes tend to keep systemic pressure (arterial pressure) and flow (CO) constant. Accordingly, increased ITP-induced increased arterial pressure will induce vasodilation, decreasing LV afterload for a constant arterial pressure [59]. The initial increase in arterial pressure induced by the increase in ITP will not be associated with any change in transmural arterial pressure. However, reflect vasodilation would ensue to maintain a constant extrathoracic arterial pressure-flow relation [24]. Unfortunately, there are several down sides to this ITP induced decrease in LV afterload. Firstly, the improvement in LV ejection is very limited, because LV end-systolic volume can only decrease so much before it reaches a minimal volume, and no further. Second, the coronary circulation is not helped by this vasodilation-induced decrease in arterial pressure. Since coronary perfusion pressure is not increased by ITP-induced increases in arterial pressure, whereas mechanical constraint from the expanding lungs may obstruct coronary blood flow, coronary hypoperfusion from a combined coronary compression and a decrease in coronary perfusion pressure are potential complications of increased ITP [60, 61]. Finally, although increases in ITP should augment LV ejection by decreasing LV afterload. this effect should have limited therapeutic potential, because LV end-systolic volume can only decrease so much, and the obligatory decrease in venous return can induce a more important decrease in LV end-diastolic volume. Accordingly, the potential augmentation of LV ejection by increasing ITP is limited under most conditions because increasing ITP, by reducing LV ejection pressure, can only decrease LV end-systolic volume so much. Since end-systolic volume is usually already small and cannot decrease much more, CO usually decreases or remains constant as ITP increases. The exception to this observation is logically under conditions of fluid resuscitation (loss of preload responsiveness) heart failure (afterload dependent) states. Accordingly, in subjects with markedly dilated cardiomyopathies, increasing ITP can selectively augment LV ejection [62, 63, 64]. However, in the remainder of subjects, the associated decrease in venous return can profoundly decrease venous blood flow and thus CO.

There is still a very important aspect of this ITP-induced decrease in afterload that is highly relevant clinically. Mechanically speaking, there is no difference between increasing ITP from a basal end-expiratory level, and eliminating negative end-inspiratory ITP swings seen in spontaneous ventilation. Removing negative swings in ITP should be more clinically relevant than increasing ITP for many reasons. First, many pulmonary diseases are associated with either partial airway obstruction or stiff lungs necessitating exaggerated negative swings in ITP during inspiration. In patients with either interstitial fibrosis or acute hypoxemic respiratory failure, ITP must decrease greatly to generate a large enough transpulmonary pressure to ventilate the alveoli. Similarly, in obstructive diseases, such as upper airway obstruction or asthma, large decreases in ITP occur owing to increased resistance to inspiratory airflow. Thus, the potential exists for large negative swings in ITP as a common process seen in spontaneously breathing subjects with lung disease. Second, exaggerated decreases in ITP require increased respiratory efforts that increase the work of breathing. Such an increased metabolic demand requires increased CO to balance its O_2 requirements. Finally, the exaggerated decreases in ITP will also increase venous return. Recall that maximal venous return during negative swings in ITP is limited by vascular collapse. The level to which ITP must decrease to induce this vascular collapse venous flow-limitation is different in different circulatory conditions but occurs in most patients below an ITP of -10 cm H_2O [9]. Accordingly, if the negative swings in ITP exceed this threshold then all the further pressure drop will only influence LV afterload and the energy requirement to create it. Thus, further decreases in ITP will further increase only LV afterload without increasing venous return. Numerous studies have demonstrated that spontaneous ventilation in the setting of myocardial ischemia only increases the ischemic injury more, whereas removing the negative swings in ITP protects the ischemic myocardium from injury. Accordingly, abolishing these markedly negative swings in ITP should disproportionally reduce LV afterload more than venous return (LV preload). Using this logic, endotracheal intubation and ventilating, by abolishing negative swings in ITP should selectively remove excess negative swings in ITP reducing both LV afterload and myocardial O_2 requirements. These interactions have important implications in the decision to both institute and withdraw mechanical ventilatory support, as will be discussed elsewhere in this volume.

Work of Breathing

Spontaneous ventilatory efforts require muscular activity with all its associated metabolic demands. Ventilatory effort consumes O_2, produces CO_2, and requires an increased regional blood flow. Thus, for all practical purposes ventilatory effort represents a metabolic load on the cardiovascular system. Normally, spontaneous ventilation requires less than 5% of total DO_2 to meet its demand making little difference to the overall metabolic needs of the body [65]. In lung disease states, however, the work of breathing can be markedly increased, either due to increased stiffness of the lungs (such as pulmonary edema), increased airway resistance to airflow (such as bronchospasm), or decreased respiratory muscle contraction efficiency (such as in hyperinflation). Accordingly, the requirements for O_2 may increase to 25% or more of total DO_2 in patients with ALI [66]. Finally, if CO is also limited by disease then this level of metabolic activity (spontaneous ventilation) may not be possible even with additional cardiovascular support. This line of reasoning has important clinical applications. First, the introduction of mechanical ventilatory support for ventilatory and hypoxemic respiratory failure will reduce both the metabolic demand on the stressed cardiovascular system and myocardial O_2 requirements, if patient effort is also reduced [67]. Thus, mixed venous O_2 saturation (SvO_2) should also increase for a constant CO and arterial O_2 content (CaO_2). Given a fixed shunt fraction (Qs/Qt) the obligatory increase in SvO_2 will result in an increase in the PaO_2, despite no change in the ratio of shunt blood flow to CO. Similarly, if prior levels of blood flow were inadequate to meet basal metabolic demands, as may be the case in cardiogenic shock, then the institution of mechanical ventilation, should decrease the work of breathing, resulting in increased DO_2 to other vital organs and decreased serum lactic acid levels.

Finally, weaning from mechanical ventilatory support can be considered a cardiovascular stress test. Perhaps the poor predictive value of present day weaning indices may reflect the total exclusion of hemodynamic status in their development. Clearly, numerous clinical studies and case reports have documented that decreasing artificial ventilatory support induces cardiovascular stress, myocardial ischemia and cardiogenic pulmonary edema [68-75]. However, the extent to which weaning indices can be made more accurate by including assessment of hemodynamic status, and which specific parameters of hemodynamic status need to be measured, remains to be defined.

Conclusion

Heart-lung interactions are complex but can be broken down in the clinical setting into those that alter venous return, LV afterload, work of breathing, and hyperinflation. To the extent that these processes can be considered separately, reasonable predictions of the hemodynamic response to any form of ventilation is possible, assuming one knows the associated basal cardiovascular state of the patient. Potentially, because the hemodynamic response to specific forms of ventilation should be predictable based on the basal cardiovascular status, then the hemodynamic response to ventilation could be used as a diagnostic test to define the underlying cardiovascular state of a subject. This application of heart-lung interaction remains to be explored.

References

1. Glick G, Wechsler AS, Epstein DE (1969) Reflex cardiovascular depression produced by stimulation of pulmonary stretch receptors in the dog. J Clin Invest 48:467-472
2. Painal AS (1973) Vagal sensory receptors and their reflex effects. Physiol Rev 53:59-88
3. Anrep GV, Pascual W, Rossler R (1936) Respiratory variations in the heart rate. I The reflex mechanism of the respiratory arrhythmia. Proc R Soc Lond B Biol Sci 119:191-217
4. Taha BH, Simon PM, Dempsey JA, Skatrud JB, Iber C (1995) Respiratory sinus arrhythmia in humans: an obligatory role for vagal feedback from the lungs. J Appl Physiol 78:638-645
5. Matuschak GM, Pinsky MR, Rogers RM (1987) Effects of positive end-expiratory pressure on hepatic blood flow and hepatic performance. J Appl Physiol 62:1377-1383
6. Chihara E, Hasimoto S, Kinoshita T, Hirpose M, Tanaka Y, Morimoto T (1992) Elevated mean systemic filling pressure due to intermittent positive-pressure ventilation. Am J Physiol 262: H1116-H1121
7. Takata M, Wise RA, Robotham JL (1990) Effects of abdominal pressure on venous return: abdominal vascular zone conditions. J Appl Physiol 69:1961-1972
8. Barnes GE, Laine GA, Giam PY, Smith EE, Granger HJ (1985) Cardiovascular responses to elevation of intra-abdominal hydrostatic pressure. Am J Physiol 248:R208-R213
9. Butler, J (1983) The heart is in good hands. Circulation 67:1163-1168
10. Persson MG, Lonnqvist PA, Gustafsson LE (1995) Positive end-expiratory pressure ventilation elicits increases in endogenously formed nitric oxide as detected in air exhaled by rabbits. Anesthesiology 82:969-974

11. Daly MB, Hazzledine JL, Ungar A (1967) The reflex effects of alterations in lung volume on systemic vascular resistance in the dog. J Physiol 188:331–351
12. Bernardi L, Calciati A, Gratarola A, Battistin I, Fratino P, Finardi G (1986) Heart rate-respiration relationship: computerized method for early detection of cardiac autonomic damage in diabetic patients. Acta Cardiol 41:197–206
13. Guyton AC, Lindsey AW, Abernathy B, et al (1957) Venous return at various right atrial pressures and the normal venous return curve. Am J Physiol 189:609–615
14. Fessler HE, Brower RG, Wise RA, Permutt S (1992) Effects of positive end-expiratory pressure on the canine venous return curve. Am Rev Respir Dis 146:4–10
15. Brienza N, Revelly JP, Ayuse T, Robotham JL (1995) Effect of PEEP on liver arterial and venous blood flows. Am J Respir Crit Care Med 152:504–510
16. Sha M, Saito Y, Yokoyama K, Sawa T, Amaha K (1987) Effects of continuous positive-pressure ventilation on hepatic blood flow and intrahepatic oxygen delivery in dogs. Crit Care Med 15:1040–1043
17. Richard C, Berdeaux A, Delion F, et al (1986) Effect of mechanical ventilation on hepatic drug pharmacokinetics. Chest 90:837–842
18. Dorinsky PM, Hamlin RL, Gadek JE (1987) Alterations in regional blood flow during positive end-expiratory pressure ventilation. Crit Care Med 15:106–115
19. Hakim TS, Michel RP, Minami H, Chang K (1983) Site of pulmonary hypoxic vasoconstriction studied with arterial and venous occlusion. J Appl Physiol 54:1298–1302
20. Marshall BE, Marshall C (1988) A model for hypoxic constriction of the pulmonary circulation. J Appl Physiol 64:68–77
21. Marshall BE, Marshall C (1980) Continuity of response to hypoxic pulmonary vasoconstriction. J Appl Physiol 49:189–196
22. Dawson CA, Grimm DJ, Linehan JH (1979) Lung inflation and longitudinal distribution of pulmonary vascular resistance during hypoxia. J Appl Physiol 47:532–536
23. Hakim TS, Michel RP, Chang HK (1982) Effect of lung inflation on pulmonary vascular resistance by arterial and venous occlusion. J Appl Physiol 53:1110–1115
24. Pinsky MR, Matuschak GM, Klain M (1985) Determinants of cardiac augmentation by increases in intrathoracic pressure. J Appl Physiol 58:1189–1198
25. Howell JBL, Permutt S, Proctor DF, et al (1961) Effect of inflation of the lung on different parts of the pulmonary vascular bed. J Appl Physiol 16:71–76
26. Taylor RR, Covell JW, Sonnenblick EH, Ross J Jr (1967) Dependence of ventricular distensibility on filling the opposite ventricle. Am J Physiol 213:711–718
27. Brinker JA, Weiss I, Lappe DL, et al (1980) Leftward septal displacement during right ventricular loading in man. Circulation 61:626–633
28. Marini JJ, Culver BN, Butler J (1980) Mechanical effect of lung distention with positive pressure on cardiac function. Am Rev Resp Dis 124:382–386
29. Janicki JS, Weber KT (1980) The pericardium and ventricular interaction, distensibility and function. Am J Physiol 238:H494–H503
30. Olsen CO, Tyson GS, Maier GW, et al (1983) Dynamic ventricular interaction in the conscious dog. Circ Res 52:85–104
31. Bell RC, Robotham JL, Badke FR, Little WC, Kindred MK (1987) Left ventricular geometry during intermittent positive pressure ventilation in dogs. J Crit Care 2:230–244
32. Buda AJ, Pinsky MR, Ingels NB, et al (1979) Effect of intrathoracic pressure on left ventricular performance. N Engl J Med 301:453–459
33. Lichtwarck-Aschoff M, Zeravik J, Pfeiffer UJ (1992) Intrathoracic blood volume accurately reflects circulatory volume status in critically ill patients with mechanical ventilation. Intensive Care Med 18:142–147
34. Sharpey-Schaffer EP (1955) Effects of Valsalva maneuver on the normal and failing circulation. Br Med J 1:693–699
35. Romand JA, Shi W, Pinsky MR (1995) Cardiopulmonary effects of positive pressure ventilation during acute lung injury. Chest 108:1041–1048
36. O'Quinn RJ, Marini JJ, Culver BH, et al (1985) Transmission of airway pressure to pleural pressure during lung edema and chest wall restriction. J Appl Physiol 59:1171–1177

37. Pinsky, MR, Guimond JG (1991) The effects of positive end-expiratory pressure on heart-lung interactions. J Crit Care 6:1–11
38. Scharf SM, Ingram RH Jr (1977) Effects of decreasing lung compliance with oleic acid on the cardiovascular response to PEEP. Am J Physiol 233:H635–H641
39. Novak RA, Matuschak GM, Pinsky MR (1988) Effect of ventilatory frequency on regional pleural pressure. J Appl Physiol 65:1314–1323
40. Gattinoni L, Mascheroni D, Torresin A, et al (1986) Morphological response to positive end-expiratory pressure in acute respiratory failure. Intensive Care Med 12:137–142
41. Tarasiuk A, Scharf SM (1993) Effects of periodic obstructive apneas on venous return in closed-chest dogs. Am Rev Respir Dis 148:323–329
42. Pinsky MR (1984) Instantaneous venous return curves in an intact canine preparation. J Appl Physiol 56:765–771
43. Brecher GA, Hubay CA (1955) Pulmonary blood flow and venous return during spontaneous respiration. Circ Res 3:40–214
44. Pinsky MR (1984) Determinants of pulmonary arterial flow variation during respiration. J Appl Physiol 56:1237–1245
45. Jayaweera AR, Ehrlich W (1987) Changes of phasic pleural pressure in awake dogs during exercise: potential effects on cardiac output. Ann Biomed Eng 15:311–318
46. Stalcup SA, Mellins RB (1977) Mechanical forces producing pulmonary edema in acute asthma. N Engl J Med 297:592–596
47. Wise RA, Robotham JL, Summer WR (1981) Effects of spontaneous ventilation on the circulation. Lung 159:175–186
48. Morgan BC, Abel FL, Mullins GL, et al (1966) Flow patterns in cavae, pulmonary artery, pulmonary vein and aorta in intact dogs. Am J Physiol 210:903–909
49. Scharf SM, Brown R, Saunders N, et al (1979) Effects of normal and loaded spontaneous inspiration on cardiovascular function. J Appl Physiol 47:582–590
50. Guntheroth WG, Morgan BC, Mullins GL (1967) Effect of respiration on venous return and stroke volume in cardiac tamponade. Mechanism of pulsus paradoxus. Circ Res 20:381–390
51. Blaustein AS, Risser TA, Weiss JW, Parker JA, Holman L, McFadden ER (1986) Mechanisms of pulsus paradoxus during resistive respiratory loading and asthma. J Am Coll Cardiol 8:529–536
52. Strohl KP, Scharf SM, Brown R, Ingram RH Jr (1987) Cardiovascular performance during bronchospasm in dogs. Respiration 51:39–48
53. Scharf SM, Graver LM, Balaban K (1992) Cardiovascular effects of periodic occlusions of the upper airways in dogs. Am Rev Respir Dis 146:321–329
54. Viola AR, Puy RJM, Goldman E (1990) Mechanisms of pulsus paradoxus in airway obstruction. J Appl Physiol 68:1927–1931
55. Holt JP (1944) The effect of positive and negative intrathoracic pressure on cardiac output and venous return in the dog. Am J Physiol 142:594–603
56. Cournaud A, Motley HL, Werko L, et al (1948) Physiologic studies of the effect of intermittent positive pressure breathing on cardiac output in man. Am J Physiol 152:162–174
57. Harken AH, Brennan MF, Smith N, Barsamian EM (1974) The hemodynamic response to positive end-expiratory ventilation in hypovolemic patients. Surgery 76:786–793
58. Jardin FF, Farcot JC, Gueret P, Prost JF, Ozier Y, Bourdarias JP (1984) Echocardiographic evaluation of ventricles during continuous positive pressure breathing. J Appl Physiol 56:619–627
59. Fessler HE, Brower RG, Wise RA, Permutt S (1988) Mechanism of reduced LV afterload by systolic and diastolic pleural pressure. J Appl Physiol 65:1244–1250
60. Khilnani S, Graver LM, Balaban K, Scharf SM (1992) Effects of inspiratory loading on left ventricular myocardial blood flow and metabolism. J Appl Physiol 72:1488–1492
61. Satoh S, Watanabe J, Keitoku M, Itoh N, Maruyama Y, Takishima T (1988) Influences of pressure surrounding the heart and intracardiac pressure on the diastolic coronary pressure-flow relation in excised canine heart. Circ Res 63:788–797
62. Pinsky MR, Summer WR, Wise RA, Permutt S, Bromberger-Barnea B (1983) Augmentation of cardiac function by elevation of intrathoracic pressure. J Appl Physiol 54:950–955
63. Pinsky MR, Summer WR (1983) Cardiac augmentation by phasic high intrathoracic support (PHIPS) in man. Chest 84:370–375

64. Pinsky MR, Marquez J, Martin D, Klain M (1987) Ventricular assist by cardiac cycle-specific increases in intrathoracic pressure. Chest 91:709–715
65. Roussos C, Macklem PT (1982) The respiratory muscles. N Engl J Med 307:786–797
66. Stock MC, David DW, Manning JW, Ryan ML (1992) Lung mechanics and oxygen consumption during spontaneous ventilation and severe heart failure. Chest 102:279–283
67. Marini JJ, Rodriguez RM, Lamb V (1986) The inspiratory workload of patient-initiated mechanical ventilation. Am Rev Respir Dis 134:902–909
68. Rasanen J, Nikki P, Heikkila J (1984) Acute myocardial infarction complicated by respiratory failure. The effects of mechanical ventilation. Chest 85:21–28
69. Rasanen J, Vaisanen IT, Heikkila J, et al (1985) Acute myocardial infarction complicated by left ventricular dysfunction and respiratory failure. The effects of continuous positive airway pressure. Chest 87:158–162
70. Beach T, Millen E, Grenvik (1973) Hemodynamic response to discontinuance of mechanical ventilation. Crit Care Med 1:85–90
71. Lemaire F, Teboul JL, Cinoti L, et al (1988) Acute left ventricular dysfunction during unsuccessful weaning from mechanical ventilation. Anesthesiology 69:171–179
72. Calvin JE, Driedger AA, Sibbald WJ (1981) Positive end-expiratory pressure (PEEP) does not depress left ventricular function in patients with pulmonary edema. Am Rev Resp Dis 124:121–128
73. Rasanen J (1988) Respiratory failure in acute myocardial infarction. Appl Cardiopulm Pathophysiol 2:271–279
74. DeHoyos A, Liu PP, Benard DC, Bradley TD (1995) Haemodynamic effects of continuous positive airway pressure in humans with normal and impaired left ventricular function. Clin Sci 88:173–178
75. Naughton MT, Rahman MA, Hara K, Flora JS, Bradley TD (1995) Effect of continuous positive airway pressure on intrathoracic and left ventricular transmural pressures in patients with congestive heart failure. Circulation 91:1725–1731

Intraorgan Heterogeneity of Blood Flow, Oxygen Consumption and Tissue Oxygenation

J. H. G. M. van Beek

Introduction

The tissue blood flow inside organs is often not distributed homogeneously. The heart muscle is, for instance, perfused very heterogeneously, even in the healthy state without coronary stenosis [1, 2]. Ischemia is accompanied by increased mismatch between metabolism and perfusion. In the heart this may lead to heterogeneous tissue infarction. The heterogeneity of myocardial perfusion in the normal heart is surprising because there is no obvious anatomical distinction between low- and high-blood flow regions. In the brain, perfusion with blood is also heterogeneous, but this is not surprising given the distinct anatomical and functional features of regions inside the brain and of the nuclei and tracts within these regions. Even in skeletal muscle at rest, distinct flow heterogeneity is found [3, 4]. Perfusion is also very heterogeneous in the lung. The flow heterogeneity is partly based on the gravity-dependent zonation of the lung, but even greater flow heterogeneity may exist within each zone [5, 6].

Due to the greater subendocardial vulnerability to infarction, differences in blood flow transmurally across the left ventricular wall of the heart were investigated, but average blood flow measured in inner and outer muscle layers was found to differ usually less than 10–20%. Strikingly, flow differs much more amongst small regions within the same transmural layer, deviating by more than 50% from average in regions of 0.1–1 g wet weight. It follows from the high average oxygen (O_2) extraction in the coronary circulation, which may approach 70%, that local myocardial oxygen consumption (VO_2) cannot be homogeneous given the large range of local blood flow. In the regions with the lowest flow, O_2 would then be completely extracted and VO_2 would be limited by hypoxia. If, on the other hand, local energy turnover and VO_2 were proportional, then the O_2 extraction fraction, equaling VO_2/(blood flow × arterial O_2 concentration (CaO_2)), would be homogeneous and local tissue hypoxia is avoided. Therefore, whether local VO_2 and perfusion are matched to each other in the healthy state, and whether this matching is lost under pathologic conditions are important questions. Problems are caused by mismatch of perfusion and metabolism, not by perfusion heterogeneity *per se*. It is not a trivial question whether all regions in the heterogeneously perfused heart are sufficiently supplied with O_2. Heterogeneous local metabolism-perfusion mismatch during ischemia may lead to organ dysfunction and tissue damage. In the heart such heterogeneity might cause arrhythmias.

In this chapter we will mainly consider the heart, an organ with high blood flow and high energy turnover. First, we will discuss the situation in the normal heart, as a background for pathologic conditions where metabolism-perfusion mismatch develops. Coronary stenosis leads for instance to a smaller spread of absolute local blood flow values in the ischemic region, but leads to a much greater heterogeneity of the metabolism-perfusion ratio. The myocardial blood flow distribution after endotoxin shock is heterogeneous, to a similar extent as in controls, but the blood flow is completely redistributed during shock [7]. We will consider whether the development of metabolism/perfusion mismatch may sometimes constitute a defense mechanism to maintain organ function as well as possible under the circumstances, or whether a uniform and matched decrease of blood flow and metabolism is the best mechanism for survival of the organ.

Intraorgan Heterogeneity of Blood Flow

Based on biophysical models of cardiac contraction, a homogeneous work performance and energy turnover is expected throughout the myocardium [8]. One would then also expect homogeneous perfusion and O_2 delivery (DO_2) in the tissue. However, measurements of local myocardial blood flow with radioactively labeled microspheres revealed substantial heterogeneity of blood flow in the heart of dogs, baboon, sheep, rabbits and pigs, in the absence of coronary disease [1, 9–11]. The histogram of the blood flow distribution was quite broad (Fig. 1A). The spatial distribution was considerably broader than expected based on micro-

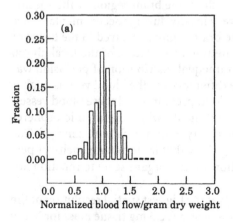
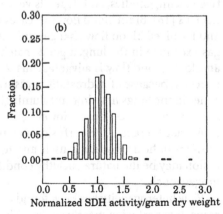

Fig. 1. Blood flow and mitochondrial enzyme distribution in the left ventricle of the porcine heart in regions of about 0.9 gram wet weight (a) Histogram of local blood flow (ml/min/g dry weight) and (b) of succinate dehydrogenase (SDH) activity, normalized for the mean value in each pig. The average left ventricular blood flow is 0.88 ml g^{-1} wet weight min^{-1}. The average SDH activity is 1.46 µmol g^{-1} wet weight min^{-1}. Based on 566 tissue samples from seven porcine left ventricles. (From [11] with permission)

sphere measurement error, and reflected true spatial heterogeneity. There was some concern that the distribution of the labeled microspheres would reflect the mechanics of the distribution of the relatively bulky microspheres, of about 15 μm diameter, but measurements with a molecule, desmethylimipramine, which could be used as a flow indicator because it was almost 100% extracted, revealed the same distribution as the microspheres. For the blood flow measurements the number of microspheres deposited in a tissue sample excised out of the organ is measured by measuring radioactivity of the sample. The spatial resolution of this method is in the range 0.1–1 g. The samples are internally heterogeneous, which explains why flow is dispersed over a broader range when a higher spatial resolution is attained with X-ray fluorescent microspheres [12].

The heterogeneity of myocardial flow is not only found in open-chest animals, but was also found by measurements of the local transit time of X-ray contrast agents using high-time resolution computed tomography [13] in closed-chest pigs. Very recently, heterogeneity of myocardial blood flow was reported using $^{13}NH_3$ as a flow tracer for positron emission tomography (PET) measurements in healthy human subjects [2]. A flow distribution over at least a sixfold range exists in normal heart muscle. DO_2 is therefore also rather heterogeneous. When cardiac work is increased, for instance by infusion of glucose-insulin-potassium solution, there tends to be an increase in blood flow proportional to local blood flow and heterogeneity is maintained [14]. In contrast, during pharmacological vasodilation or during asphyxia (high CO_2, low CaO_2) there is no relation between resting and maximal blood flow [15].

Not only in the continuously beating heart, but also in resting and contracting skeletal muscle a very heterogeneous blood flow distribution is found in experimental animals [3] but also with PET measurements in resting muscle of healthy volunteers [4]. For brain, the flow distribution has been measured with radioactive labeling studies, and depends very much on the brain region or the specific nucleus [16]. Brain blood flow increases very locally during specific mental tasks, and localized blood flow changes indicate brain regions involved in the task. For gas exchange in the lung, a good match between ventilation of the local alveoli and local blood flow is advantageous. An unequal distribution of perfusion was expected because of hydrostatic pressure differences in the blood vessels: higher zones in the lungs have low intraluminal blood pressures and these blood vessels are expected to collapse. However, measurements with labeled microspheres show that there is large perfusion heterogeneity within each lung zone [6]. The findings in heart, skeletal muscle and lung show that large heterogeneity of perfusion may be the natural, healthy condition, even if organs seem to function homogeneously.

Flow heterogeneity has been found even at the highest spatial resolution of the respective perfusion measurements. This is at about 2.5 mg tissue mass for X-ray fluorescent microspheres. Using autoradiography of the molecular flow marker 2-iododesmethylimipramine flow heterogeneity was found at the microscopic level [17]. Measurements of red blood cell flux show differences in perfusion even between adjacent capillaries in frog muscle [18]. Flow heterogeneity is therefore found at all spatial scales. Because measurements were originally made at more limited spatial resolution and because flow heterogeneity is found at all spatial resolutions a practical problem arises: measurements at different spatial resolution made in different laboratories must be compared.

To understand this problem and describe these heterogeneous spatial patterns, use is made of fractal geometry, a relatively recent mathematical discovery. Fractals are complex structures beyond simple regular geometrical structures such as squares and triangles [19]. Yet, while complex to the eye these fractal structures are simple at another level: they can be generated by repetitively applying simple rules, which is usually done on the computer. The recipe may be to take a picture at a low magnification, reduce its size, and paste it many times into the object (Fig. 2). This generates self-similar structures in which the structure of a part is a downscaled copy of the whole, and this self-similarity is repeated at progressively smaller scales (Fig. 3). This recipe may be repeated many times at ever smaller scales and generates objects with similar irregularity as found often in natural objects such as coastlines, clouds, plants, trees, etc. According to such mathematical rules crude models of self-similar bronchial and vascular trees have been constructed (Fig. 2). The heterogeneity of the bronchial tree has been analyzed with fractal techniques. At higher spatial resolution progressively more heterogeneity is found (Fig. 3). It was shown that the relative dispersion (= the standard deviation/mean) of the histogram of the myocardial blood flow distribution increases with the inverse of the spatial resolution of the measurement to the power of D-1. D is for instance about 1.2 for myocardial perfusion and turns out to have the mathematical properties of a dimension [9], which does not have the integer value of the classical one-, two- or three-dimensional spaces and is

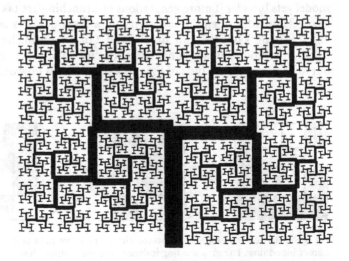

Fig. 2. A mathematical model of a repetitively dividing self-similar tree. Note that the same pattern is found at progressively smaller spatial scales. The finer details in the figure are smaller copies of the larger details, which reflects the property of self-similarity. This space-filling self-similar tree is a crude model of the bronchial or coronary trees filling the lung and heart muscle, respectively. (From [19] with permission)

called the fractal dimension [19]. This simple power law relation is the hallmark of fractal structures and is useful to predict flow heterogeneity at different scales. The success of the fractal analysis has a very important practical consequence: flow heterogeneity is equally important at all spatial scales. Indeed flow heterogeneity is more or less similar at all spatial scales so far measured, and exists for instance between regions with linear dimensions of 1 cm and 1 mm, and even within regions of 1 mm size additional flow heterogeneity is present [17, 18, 20].

The fractal point of view has one further corollary: the distribution of myocardial blood flow is not without structure, because a fractal dimension of about 1.2 means that there is a relatively high correlation between adjacent regions [21, 22]. The correlation coefficient r can be calculated from the fractal dimension according to the relation $r = 2^{3-2D} - 1$ which was derived by van Beek et al. [21]. For $D = 1.2$ the correlation coefficient is 0.52. This means that in a statistical sense high flow regions tend to have high flow regions as neighbors, and low flow regions tend to be close to low flow regions. Despite the fact that there is no consistent relation between low- and high-flow regions and anatomical position in the heart [Bassingthwaighte, personal communication], the heterogeneous flow distribution does not reflect white noise, but shows a spatial correlation structure.

An even simpler fractal model than the power law discussed above is the fractal bifurcating network (Fig. 4). Blood flow is distributed to the tissue via an asymmetrically branching network of blood vessels [21–26]. At each branch point, flow is distributed unevenly: a fraction γ (not equal to 0.5) of the blood flow goes into one daughter vessel at a branch, the remainder $(1 - \gamma)$ goes into the other daughter vessel. Thus the blood flow is distributed unevenly at successive bifurcations into progressively smaller blood vessels. This fractal process progressively generates a self-similar pattern of blood flow distribution at ever smaller scales. The histogram of the flow distribution calculated from this simple model gets broader if more generations of branching are taken into account, and also gets broader when the assymetry parameter deviates farther from 0.5 (Fig. 4b). It is remarkable that this simple model of generating heterogeneity played a role in the fundamental mathematical discipline of topology [19, 21], but turns out to be useful for analysis of the myocardial blood flow distribution.

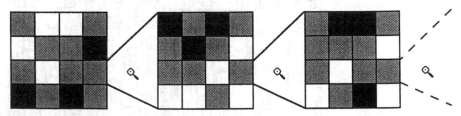

Fig. 3. Repetitively increasing spatial resolution of measurement of the heterogeneous distribution of blood flow. The grey shading indicates the local blood flow. Measurement resolution is improved repeatedly, symbolized by the small magnifying glass which reveals the internal structure of the sub-squares. Going from left to right, flow heterogeneity at finer scales is revealed. (From [23] with permission)

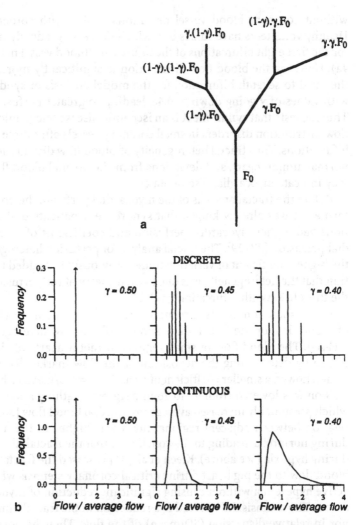

Fig. 4. a Branching network of blood vessels with asymmetric distribution of blood flow. Flow F_0 enters the blood vessel tree. At each bifurcation a fraction γ of the blood flow in the mother vessel enters one daughter branch, the remaining fraction $(1 - \gamma)$ enters the other daughter branch. The parameter γ may vary with the branching generation. Only two generations of branching are shown, but this pattern of asymmetric flow distribution is repeated many times to generate flow heterogeneity at progressively finer spatial resolution. **b** The flow histograms generated by the branching vessel network model of Fig. 4a after 8 generations of branching. The model yields discrete flows, but an approximating continuous flow distribution is also plotted. The farther the asymmetry parameter deviates from 0.5, the broader the flow distribution becomes. In the normal baboon heart γ is about 0.46, in the human heart about 0.47. (From [22] with permission)

Recently fractal analysis was applied to myocardial perfusion measurements with $^{13}NH_3$ as a tracer measured with PET [2]. Healthy volunteers were compared with patients suffering from the cardiac syndrome X, who experience angina pectoris and show exercise induced electroencephalograph (EEG) abnormalities without coronary blood vessel deviations visible with coronary angiography. Healthy volunteers have values of γ which decrease gradually from 0.485 to 0.47 for the first eight bifurcations of the bifurcating blood vessel network model (Fig. 4a). However, the blood flow distribution is significantly more asymmetrical in the third to seventh bifurcation for the model analysis of syndrome X patients, with values of γ going down to 0.46, leading to greater perfusion heterogeneity. This suggests that syndrome X is an ischemic disease due to microvascular blood flow distribution disorders in small coronary vessels after three to seven vascular bifurcations. Thus fractal heterogeneity of blood flow distribution is found in the normal human heart, and deviations from the normal blood flow heterogeneity may indicate myocardial disease states.

Before the fractal analysis of the myocardial perfusion heterogeneity was performed, it was already known that syndrome X patients under baseline conditions had higher myocardial perfusion and coefficients of variation of myocardial perfusion [27–29]. The fractal analysis of perfusion heterogeneity confirmed the higher coefficient of variation found previously, but added to this the suggestion that the heterogeneity was due to asymmetry of the perfusion distribution at the third to seventh bifurcation level.

Under some conditions of reduced DO_2 or ischemia, the relative heterogeneity of blood flow or the fractal dimension of blood flow heterogeneity are not increased. The blood flow in small regions in rabbit hearts of size 0.1–1 mm, assessed by determining the deposition of the flow marker ^{3}H-desmethylimipramine, showed a smaller coefficient of variation (= SD/mean) when the arterial O_2 tension was lowered from 97 to 26 mm Hg by breathing a hypoxic gas mixture, which presumably increased average myocardial blood flow [30]. The spatial correlation between adjacent regional flows was higher in the hypoxic state than during normoxia, leading to the conclusion that the fractal dimension was lower during hypoxia (see above). Kleen et al. [31] assessed the fractal heterogeneity of blood flow to the pig heart during critical coronary stenosis which abolished reactive hyperemia without causing significant reduction of myocardial perfusion at rest. The stenosis did not lead to a reduction in the fractal dimension D of 1.39, nor in relative dispersion (SD/mean) of the flow. Then, hemorrhagic shock was induced in the presence of the stenosis and arterial blood pressure was reduced to about 50 mm Hg. Myocardial blood flow at rest was now substantially reduced. The relative dispersion of myocardial perfusion increased, but the fractal dimension decreased significantly to 1.26 and spatial correlation between adjacent regional flow values accordingly increased. Resuscitation with small volumes of normal saline or of a mixture of hypertonic saline and dextran did increase the average myocardial blood flow and the relative dispersion of flow, but did not increase the fractal dimension of myocardial perfusion. These findings indicate that fractal heterogeneity of perfusion does not always increase with hypoxia or ischemia.

It has been expected for a long time that despite the heterogeneous perfusion, blood flow and metabolism are matched to each other in the normal heart. Methods to measure local VO_2 to prove this point have only been developed very recently [32–37]. However, first we will look at earlier measurements of enzyme content and local metabolite levels which already suggested that metabolism and perfusion were matched in normal myocardium.

Metabolic Indicators of Metabolism-Perfusion Matching

The tissue contents of active enzymes can be determined using *in vitro* assays where formation of the product of the enzyme is assessed under optimal conditions. Succinate dehydrogenase (SDH) is an enzyme of oxidative metabolism via the tricarboxylic acid (TCA) cycle and is distributed very heterogeneously (Fig. 1B). Local blood flow in the resting porcine heart is significantly correlated with SDH activity in samples of about 0.9 gram [11], although a major part of the variability of flow is still not explained by the oxidative capacity as indicated by SDH (Fig. 5). This may not be surprising, because enzyme activity measurement under optimal conditions *in vitro* does not necessarily reflect the actual flux through the TCA cycle at the time of the blood flow measurement. In the dog heart, beating under resting conditions, no correlation was found between mitochondrial enzymes (citrate synthase and cytochrome c-oxidase) on the one hand and local blood flow on the other [38]. Correlations with creatine kinase and lactate dehydrogenase were low [39] and correlations with other glycolytic enzymes were absent [38]. There was a rather high correlation between local resting blood flow and contents of local adenosine triphosphate (ATP) or total creatine (creatine plus creatine phosphate) [40, 41]. These measurements of enzyme activity and metabolite content suggested indeed that blood flow and metabolism show some relation.

More direct tests of the existence of ischemia in low flow regions were measurement of inosine, a breakdown product of ATP and measurement of lactate, the end-product of anaerobic glycolysis, both of which are generated when aero-

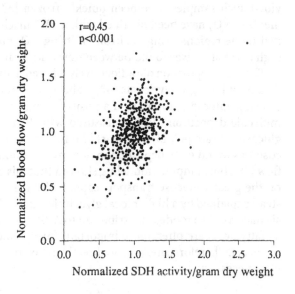

Fig. 5. The relation between local blood flow under resting conditions and activity of the mitochondrial enzyme succinate dehydrogenase (SDH) in pig left ventricle. Blood flow and enzyme activity were first expressed per gram dry weight and then normalized to the mean value in the left ventricle. Samples obtained from seven pigs. Correlation coefficient and level of significance are given in the figure. (From [11] with permission)

bic ATP synthesis cannot keep up with ATP demand. In normal myocardium, inosine and lactate were not increased in the regions with low blood flow, suggesting that there was no lack of blood flow to these regions. This suggested that metabolic demand was low in low-flow regions and that blood flow was matched to the metabolic demand [41]. This point was demonstrated elegantly by measuring the accumulation of S-adenosylhomocysteine in 83 mg myocardial tissue samples during homocysteine thiolactone infusion in anesthetized dogs under resting conditions [38]. Samples with blood flow below 0.2 ml g^{-1} min^{-1} in the resting state in the normal heart did not show increased intracellular adenosine levels, demonstrating that in these small regions with very low flow ATP was not broken down to purine products. Thus the net turnover of ATP was sustained in this region despite the fact that flow was one fourth the average myocardial flow or lower. As adenosine production is normally increased during ischemia or hypoxia, it was concluded that metabolic demand is adapted to the low DO$_2$. These measurements of inosine, adenosine and lactate therefore suggested that in the normal heart in the resting state there are no metabolic signs of ischemia in the low flow areas and that in the normal heart perfusion is matched to metabolism. To obtain more direct proof, measurement methods for local VO$_2$ had to be developed.

Measurement of Local Oxygen Consumption

Until recently the measurement of local VO$_2$ as a measure of aerobic energy metabolism has been problematic. Often the deposition of labeled deoxyglucose, a tracer indicator of glucose uptake in tissue was used to indicate local metabolic rate [38, 42, 43]. Two new measurement techniques now make the study of heterogeneity of aerobic metabolism possible. Local VO$_2$ can be measured by measuring the high-resolution ^{13}C-nuclear magnetic resonance (NMR) spectrum from an extract of a tissue sample of 50 mg dry mass taken from the organ *in situ*, provided such samples have been quickly frozen [32–36]. Non-invasive measurements of VO$_2$ have been obtained with a PET machine in slightly larger myocardial tissue regions using positron-emitting ^{15}O$_2$ molecules [37]. In both cases a high correlation was found between flow and local aerobic metabolic flux.

The local deposition of radioactively labeled deoxyglucose is considered an indicator of local glycolytic rate [42]. Label deposition can be imaged in tissue slices using autoradiography, or if a positron-emitting fluor label is attached to the molecule deposition can be measured with PET. Profiles of regional uptake of glucose in brain [42, 43] and heart [38] have thus been measured. [^{3}H]-deoxyglucose was found to be deposited in dog myocardium in proportion to local blood flow [38], but computer modeling showed that this deposition was not dependent on the greater glucose transport capacity by the higher blood flow, and was instead explained by a higher local glycolytic rate [44]. However, anaerobic glycolysis makes only a modest contribution to ATP synthesis, and other substrates such as fatty acids are often more important for aerobic metabolism, for instance in the heart. Therefore, methods to directly measure aerobic metabolic rate in tissue were necessary.

Our goal was to develop a method to study the heterogeneity of VO_2 in myocardium in animal experiments in the laboratory, to complement the labeled microsphere method to measure local blood flow. To this end we infuse ^{13}C-labelled substrate for the TCA cycle during a short, well-defined period. We then measure the enrichment of metabolites labeled via the TCA cycle in quick-frozen samples taken from the myocardium [32–36]. This method builds on existing methods to determine the TCA cycle flux by following the development of ^{13}C-NMR-peaks of glutamate sequentially over time [45–49]. However, what is new is that the flux is estimated from a frozen tissue sample, i.e., from ^{13}C-enrichment at one point in time.

Because glutamate is enriched with ^{13}C via the TCA cycle, by carbon-skeleton exchange with α-ketoglutarate, the extent of enrichment is dependent on the rate of turnover in the TCA cycle. The ^{13}C isotope from [2-^{13}C]-acetate, [3-^{13}C]-lactate or [3-^{13}C]-pyruvate enters first the 4-carbon position of glutamate in the first turn of the TCA cycle. During the next turn of the TCA cycle the ^{13}C-isotope enters the 2- or 3-carbon position of glutamate. Consequently, the ratio of 2- or 3-carbon to 4-carbon at a certain time after starting the infusion of the labeled substrate indicates the speed of the TCA cycle [36]. However, for accurate evaluation one must also know the flux of anaplerotic substrates into the TCA cycle. This anaplerotic flux normally consists of unenriched substrates which enter the TCA cycle via other pathways than acetyl CoA, for instance coming from carboxylation of pyruvate and breakdown of amino acids and fatty acids of uneven carbon-chain length. The anaplerotic flux can enlarge the pools of TCA cycle intermediates. Fortunately, splitting of the ^{13}C-NMR-peaks via so-called J-coupling between adjacent ^{13}C isotopes in glutamate gives a measurable fine structure in the spectrum (Fig. 6) from which the anaplerotic flux can be reliably estimated [50, 51].

We have adapted the model analysis [45, 48] so that the flux in the TCA cycle is determined from the high-resolution MR spectrum in extracts of tissue samples taken at one point in time [32, 36]. We do not only take the total amount of ^{13}C-isotope into account in the 4-, 3- and 2-carbon position of glutamate, which would be enough if the anaplerotic flux were known, but analyze the full fine-structure of the spectrum to estimate the anaplerotic flux and the fractional enrichment of acetyl CoA with ^{13}C simultaneously with the TCA cycle flux. With our computer models the distribution of ^{13}C in the TCA cycle during infusion of ^{13}C-enriched acetate is calculated.

In our simplest model the NMR-multiplet areas of ^{13}C-enriched glutamate, labeled by quick exchange with the TCA cycle, can be calculated using 32 differential equations for the 32 $^{12}C/^{13}C$-isotopomers of glutamate. Because glutamate usually contains > 80% of the total carbon pool labeled by ^{13}C, we modeled only one lumped metabolite pool. The mean transit time for transport of label from coronary artery to the acetyl CoA pool, which is about 0.5 min, is included in the model and can be estimated from the ^{13}C spectrum. With this simple model we analyzed ^{13}C-NMR data obtained after infusing [2-^{13}C]-acetate for 5 min [32, 35, 36] and found a high correlation with VO_2 and contractile performance in the heart. VO_2 in subendocardial and subepicardial samples were strongly correlated with local perfusate flow (Fig. 7). In this case we infused 5 mM acetate, but meas-

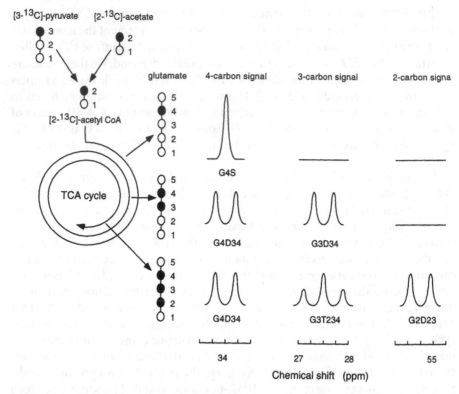

Fig. 6. Measurement of oxygen consumption with ^{13}C NMR spectroscopy. Schematic picture of ^{13}C incorporation in glutamate. The flux in the tricarboxylic acid (TCA) cycle is proportional to oxygen consumption. ^{13}C-enriched acetate or pyruvate is infused into the heart. The filled circles indicate ^{13}C isotope, the open circles indicate [12]C. The ^{13}C reaches glutamate via the TCA cycle. In the first turn of the cycle ^{13}C is only incorporated in the 4-position of glutamate. In the following turn of the cycle ^{13}C also reaches the 3- and 2- position of glutamate. The signals of the different carbon atoms are at different positions in the spectrum, given by frequency shift in parts per million (ppm) relative to a reference compound. If two ^{13}C isotopes are adjacent the peaks are split into a doublet (D) or if there are two ^{13}C neighbors, a triplet (T) may be found. G stands for glutamate. Analysis of the peak heights and multiplet fine structure gives the rate of turnover of the TCA cycle. (From [36] with permission)

urements were feasible with acetate concentrations as low as 0.5 mM, and the principle also applies to labeled pyruvate and lactate.

More accurate estimates of aerobic metabolism were obtained with a model consisting of 6 metabolite pools (acetyl CoA, citrate and other 6-carbon TCA cycle intermediates, the 5-carbon intermediate α-ketoglutarate, oxaloacetate and other 4-carbon intermediates, the amino acids glutamate and aspartate). The exchange rates between the TCA cycle and the associated amino acids pools (glutamate and aspartate) are taken into account. The six pool model consists of 132 differential equations [33, 34]. Computer simulations show that the TCA cycle flux can be estimated using parameter optimization, if 7 or more distinguishable ^{13}C-NMR-multiplets of glutamate are measured from extracts of samples frozen

Fig. 7. The relation between local perfusate flow and local oxygen consumption (VO₂) in samples from isolated rabbit heart. In this series [2-^{13}C]-acetate has been infused for 5 min. All samples from left ventricular free wall of seven rabbit hearts, obtained in pairs. Filled symbols: subendocardial samples. Open symbols: subepicardial samples. Symbol shapes indicate individual rabbits. Flow of Tyrode solution was measured with radioactively labeled microspheres. (From [36] with permission)

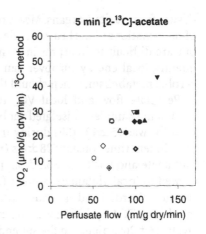

quickly at one point in time, after a short infusion (about 5 min) of ^{13}C-enriched acetate.

Experiments were done on isolated rabbit hearts under various conditions, including ischemia, hypoxia and cardioplegia. Four minutes of infusion of [2-^{13}C]-acetate were followed by 90 seconds of infusion of [1,2-^{13}C]-acetate. Computer analysis had shown that addition of the second, double label improved the accuracy of the estimation considerably. Samples of 50–150 mg dry mass were taken from the left ventricular free wall. The transmural resolution was 2 mm, so that subendocardium and subepicardium could be separately measured, even in the small rabbit heart. Eight distinct multiplet areas from high-resolution NMR spectra of an extract of the tissue sample were fitted, yielding four parameters (TCA cycle flux, mean transit time from the coronary ostium to the acetyl CoA pool in the mitochondria, fraction of labeling of acetyl CoA from the infused acetate, glutamate content). These parameters were estimated by non-linear least squares optimization. The anaplerotic flux was found to be about 6% of the TCA cycle flux, also estimated using the model. The VO₂ is equal to the estimated flux in the TCA cycle, multiplied by a stoichiometry factor which is known because it depends on the fraction of acetyl CoA that is derived from the ^{13}C-enriched acetate which we also estimate. There was excellent correspondence between the absolute values of VO₂ measured with a conventional coronary venous O₂ electrode and microsphere flow determination, and VO₂ measured independently with our new ^{13}C method in the same region (correlation coefficient = 0.9). This was also true for low perfusion pressures (20–40 mm Hg) and when O₂ concentration was lowered by about 80%.

With our new ^{13}C-method local VO₂ can be measured simultaneously in many small myocardial regions, provided quick-frozen tissue samples can be obtained. This technique yields absolute values of local VO₂, which can be related to local blood flow, independently measured with labeled microspheres. This measurement of the aerobic metabolic rate has a similar spatial resolution as the microsphere measurements of local blood flow. Given the generality of the biochemical principles underlying the method, this measurement is likely to be applicable to tissues from various organs. Measurements of local contractile function in terms of deformations of the heart muscle are feasible with NMR tagging methods [52], but are difficult to interpret in terms of cardiac mechanical work [53]. Consequently, local energy turnover can perhaps best be determined by measuring aerobic metabolism, which should then be related to local blood flow.

Perfusate flow and local VO_2 turned out to be highly interdependent in 50–150 mg samples in isolated rabbit heart [54]. The enrichment of acetyl CoA with ^{13}C was $95 \pm 1\%$ (SE) during infusion of 1.5 mM ^{13}C-enriched acetate, with enrichment time constant 28 ± 4 s (n = 32). The exchange flux from TCA cycle to glutamate and back was 36.5 ± 5.3 µmol g^{-1} min^{-1}. Local myocardial VO_2 was related to local glutamate content (r = 0.44, n = 44, $p < 0.01$). Myocardial VO_2 in the subepicardial and subendocardial halves of the left ventricle free wall calculated from TCA cycle flux was 14.2 ± 1.4 and 18.0 ± 1.7 µmol g^{-1} min^{-1}, respectively, $43 \pm 20\%$ higher in the subendocardial layer ($p < 0.05$, n = 16). So far only a few pilot experiments on hearts *in situ* have been carried out [54]. In a rabbit heart *in situ*, left ventricular subendocardial and subepicardial VO_2 were 26.0 ± 3.8 and 15.6 ± 1.4 µmol g^{-1} min^{-1} respectively, at 115 mm Hg systolic arterial pressure. At systolic pressure 60 mm Hg, the subendocardial and subepicardial VO_2 were 8.2 ± 3.0 and 5.2 ± 1.4 µmol g^{-1} min^{-1} respectively. Rabbit left ventricular VO_2 is slightly higher in subendocardium than in subepicardium, explaining greater subendocardial vulnerability to infarction.

Although measurements of VO_2 with PET have been applied to the brain, it turned out to be difficult in the heart because of the continuous movement of this organ. The time course of disappearance of ^{11}C-acetate was measured which is metabolized by the TCA cycle. It turned out that the time constant of the disappearance of the ^{11}C-signal was inversely related to VO_2. This approach has been applied often, but shows limited spatial resolution and is hard to quantify in absolute terms. Very recently the first measurements of local VO_2 using $^{15}O_2$ and PET measurements of the time course of disappearance of the ^{15}O label have been published. $^{15}O_2$ is metabolized to $H_2^{15}O$. The signal of the labeled water is slowly washed out of tissue and its PET signal is not distinguishable from $^{15}O_2$, but is separated by computer analysis of the time course using large distributed models [55]. A preliminary report [37] indicated that a close correlation is found between local VO_2 and blood flow, the latter measured by injection of $H_2^{15}O$ in closed-chest dogs. Pilot studies have been made on humans with $^{15}O_2$ inhaled via the lungs. The big advantage of PET is that it allows non-invasive measurements, but the ^{13}C method has potentially larger spatial resolution and has already allowed the measurement of transmural differences in VO_2 in the small rabbit heart, which has not yet been feasible with PET.

In conclusion, it was impossible to study the heterogeneity of myocardial aerobic metabolism until very recently, but now methods have been developed and validated which allow the measurement of absolute values of VO_2 either invasively by measuring high-resolution ^{13}C-NMR spectra or non-invasively with PET at slightly lower resolution. These methods must now be applied to study the heterogeneity of aerobic metabolism and its relation to local perfusion and function in health and disease.

Local Tissue Oxygenation

If local VO_2 and blood flow are known, the local venous O_2 concentration can be calculated. However, several measurements of local tissue oxygenation have been available for a considerable time: tissue O_2 electrodes, spectrophotometry of hemoglobin (Hb) in frozen tissue samples [56, 57], and an indirect method by measuring nicotinamide adenine dinucleotide (NADH) fluorescence to indicate hypoxic tissue [58]. Near infrared methods to image Hb oxygenation in tissue are under development, and O_2 concentration dependent NMR imaging of tissue, functional magnetic resonance imaging (MRI), has made a lot of progress. These measurements are covered in other chapters, so we will concentrate here on the Hb O_2 saturation and NADH measurements which throw direct light on whether perfusion and metabolism are locally matched.

If perfusion and aerobic metabolism are perfectly matched, the O_2 concentration in small veins should be the same everywhere. The arteriolar blood has the same O_2 content everywhere in the heart. Weiss and colleagues [56, 57] have shown that cardiac tissue in experimental animals can be frozen quickly, and that Hb oxygenation in arterioles and venules of 20–500 μm diameter can then be measured microspectrophotometrically in the frozen tissue samples. In this way it was found that there was a substantial spread in venular blood Hb oxygenation values [56], suggesting that in the heart under resting conditions perfusion and metabolism were not perfectly matched. It should be noted that even venules with almost zero blood O_2 content were found [56], which suggests that matching of blood flow and aerobic metabolism was not very good. However, a relatively weak point in these cryospectrophotometric measurements is that it took at least half a minute to freeze the center of the tissue samples, so that differences in venular O_2 content may have developed in irregularly beating tissue where metabolism continued and blood in the venous network might redistribute. Despite the potential elegance of this method, the results are therefore of somewhat uncertain accuracy. From the venular O_2 concentration measurements together with blood flow measurements with microspheres in adjacent samples, a value for local VO_2 can be calculated [57]. Pilot experiments with the ^{13}C-method (see above) showed similar values in the rabbit under comparable hemodynamic conditions [54]. Both methods show higher subendocardial than subepicardial VO_2. From the spread of venular Hb saturation, it can be concluded that imperfect matching between local perfusion and aerobic metabolism probably leads to some spread in O_2 extraction reflected in a range of values for venular Hb O_2 saturation.

It is of considerable interest that methods have been developed to measure Hb O_2 saturation in blood vessels of about 100 μm diameter in the eye *in situ* in humans using spectrophotometry [59]. Thus, at least in the eye, the microcirculation is accessible for O_2 measurements in small vessels in patients.

Low O_2 tension at the mitochondria leads to insufficient oxidation of NADH. NADH fluoresces in the blue when excited by ultraviolet radiation and this can be measured in the intact heart [58]. The NADH fluorescence can be visualized very well in the isolated heart perfused with Hb-free perfusate, and with somewhat less contrast in the blood-perfused heart. It was found that upon reduction of flow or O_2 tension in the perfusate a patchy pattern appears on the surface of the saline-perfused heart [58, 60], indicating that tissue hypoxia is not distributed homogeneously. The NADH fluorescent regions have a linear dimension of several hundred micrometer. Indeed, calculations of O_2 diffusion in perfused tissue [61] show that further flow heterogeneity within small regions of the order of 100–200 µm diameter has little effect on the tissue O_2 tension profile [23, 26]. Two explanations were put forward for the patchy NADH fluorescence pattern: local mismatch of perfusion to aerobic metabolism; and the arterial-to-venous intracapillary O_2 concentration gradient leads to hypoxia at the venous end of the capillary bed. Ince and colleagues [60] studied the patchy pattern of NADH fluorescence in saline-perfused rat hearts and proposed that these fluorescent patches reflected microcirculatory weak units which were prone to mismatch between perfusion and metabolism. However, Vetterlein et al. [20] studied the patchy patterns of NADH fluorescence in the blood perfused rat heart *in situ* at reduced perfusion pressure and concluded that NADH fluorescence was mainly found surrounding the venous end of the capillary bed. Thus, the arterial-to-venous O_2 gradient appears to be an important cause of the patchy nature of NADH fluorescence, which is found during reduced DO_2 in regions of several hundred micrometer diameter in rat heart. The patchy NADH fluorescence in small regions shows heterogeneity of local DO_2 to VO_2 ratios at a small scale. This emphasizes that heterogeneous DO_2 is demonstrated at various spatial scales, from large myocardial regions of about 1 cm linear dimension, to the smallest regions where flow can be measured with X-ray fluorescent microspheres which are a few mm across, to regions of a few hundred micrometer diameter. The finding of large, patchy infarction areas by the pathologist indicates that not only microcirculatory disturbances, but also blood flow distribution problems at macroscopic scales play important roles in pathophysiology.

Does Heterogeneity of Perfusion Exacerbate Tissue Ischemia?

It has been known for a long time that when coronary perfusion pressure is decreased, blood flow in the subendocardial muscle layer is decreased more than in the subepicardial muscle layer. The greater subendocardial vulnerability to infarction during ischemia was thought to be related to this factor. Even without reduction of coronary perfusion pressure the blood flow distribution within each of these transmural myocardial layers is very heterogeneous (see above). It is tempting to connect this perfusion heterogeneity to the patchy pattern of infarction often found after severe ischemia.

Do the infarcted regions for instance correspond to the regions which receive low flow before coronary stenosis or reduction of perfusion pressure? We measured local myocardial blood flow before and after acutely inducing partial coronary stenosis of the left anterior descending coronary artery, so that coronary pressure distal to the stenosis dropped from 107 to 39 mm Hg. In the ischemic region, dependent on the stenosed artery, blood flow in ~0.9 gram samples fell very heterogeneously [41]. On average, blood flow was reduced from 1.06 to 0.47

ml g^{-1} min^{-1}. As expected, perfusion was reduced more drastically in the suben-docardial region (by $57 \pm 13\%$, SE) than in the subepicardial region (by $34 \pm 19\%$). However, flow reduction within each transmural layer was quite variable (Fig. 9). Although there was a gradient of increasing flow reduction from subepicardium to subendocardium, within each of these layers there was no relation between control blood flow levels, measured before stenosis, and the flow reduction caused by the stenosis (Fig. 8). Consequently, some small regions are hit relatively hard by ischemia while others are to some extent spared. Consequently flow reduction during ischemia is very heterogeneous [62, 63] and independent of the level of perfusion before stenosis [41].

The metabolic effects of the flow reduction due to stenosis were investigated by measuring inosine, a breakdown product of ATP, and lactate after 20 min of flow reduction. Because local ATP content varies markedly itself, the inosine content was normalized to ATP content. In many samples in the ischemic region with flows in the range 0.5–0.8 ml g^{-1} min^{-1} the inosine/ATP ratio was higher than 0.05, but at similar low flow in the non-ischemic region this was never the case. At the lowest flows in the ischemic region lactate content was increased above that found in the non-ischemic region. There was a significant correlation between the flow reduction in the ischemic region during coronary stenosis and lactate. The inosine/ATP ratio was increased in a substantial fraction of the samples with 50–70% flow reduction. The accumulation of lactate or inosine was the same for samples which had low or high flow before stenosis (Fig. 9). Deussen et al. [64] recently published very similar findings for 125 mg wet weight samples in dog heart: for a similar partial coronary stenosis the S-adenosyl-homocysteine concentration after 30 min homocysteine infusion increased with the relative de-

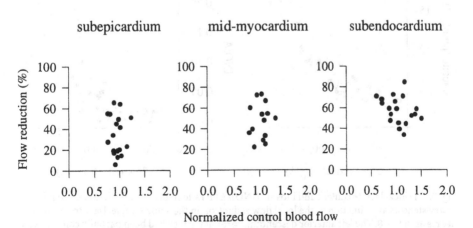

Fig. 8. Relation between the local blood flow reduction in the ischemic region caused by coronary stenosis in pig heart and myocardial blood flow before ischemia. The left anterior descending coronary artery was partially constricted to reduce distal coronary pressure to about 39 mm Hg and the flow reduction was assessed in the ischemic regions of about 0.9 g wet weight at 15 min after bringing about the stenosis. Pre-ischemic control blood flows were normalized to the median blood flow to compare data from four animals. (From [41] with permission)

crease in blood flow, and this increase was similar in areas with low flow or high flow under control conditions. Consequently, not the absolute blood flow level, but the relative extent of flow reduction during stenosis appears to determine the metabolic consequences of ischemia. Because the relative extent of flow reduction is not dictated by the blood flow level before stenosis, but is very heterogeneous, one should expect that tissue ischemia develops very heterogeneously during partial coronary stenosis. On the other hand, the aerobic metabolic rate is probably very heterogeneous (see above), so that one expects that regions with high metabolism and flow under control conditions are the most vulnerable to tissue damage during complete flow cessation. Indeed, a preliminary report [65] shows that infarcted regions in the area at risk had significantly higher perfusion before coronary occlusion than the non-infarcted areas in the same area at risk.

The myocardial blood flow distribution after endotoxin shock is heterogeneous, to a similar extent as in controls, but the blood flow is completely redistributed during shock [7]. These measurements were performed in dogs injected with endotoxin, and in controls. In the endotoxin group cardiac output (CO) and mean arterial pressure (MAP) were decreased by 44 and 48% respectively. De-

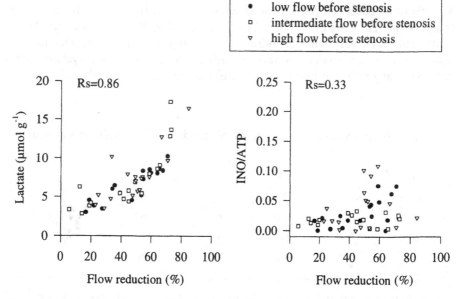

Fig. 9. The local lactate content and inosine (INO)/ATP ratio in pig left ventricle after 20 min coronary stenosis as a function of the local flow reduction in the same sample. Data from the same hearts as in Fig. 8. The left anterior descending coronary artery had been partially constricted to reduced distal coronary pressure to about 39 mm Hg. The flow reduction was calculated from local blood flows measured with radioactively labeled microspheres 5 min before and 15 min after partially constricting the coronary artery. Low flow before stenosis: 61–90% of median blood flow. Intermediate flow before stenosis: 90–107% of median flow. High flow before stenosis: 107–152% of median flow. Spearman rank correlation coefficients, (R_s), given in panels. (From [41] with permission)

spite the redistribution of myocardial blood flow, VO_2 by the heart was undiminished, and lactate uptake was not decreased although a lower percentage of lactate was extracted from a higher arterial lactate concentration in the endotoxin group. The redistribution of blood flow was termed a maldistribution by the authors [7], although the relation between local perfusion and VO_2 could not be determined at that time and global VO_2 was not significantly decreased. Aerobic metabolic energy was less efficiently used for the heart as a whole, because cardiac contractile performance indices were decreased while VO_2 was undiminished after endotoxin injection.

The question remains whether the heterogeneous response to tissue ischemia exacerbates tissue ischemia relative to a hypothetical homogeneous response. It might be beneficial that some parts of the tissue are still relatively well-perfused, at the expense of others which suffer more than average. Little data is available to decide on this question. However, it is remarkable that ischemic myocardium can often still take up lactate as fuel for aerobic metabolism while radioactive tracer measurements show that there is at the same time lactate production at some sites in the myocardium which is hidden by the net lactate extraction [66]. In healthy volunteers there is no myocardial lactate production hidden under the net lactate extraction of the heart, not even during strenuous exercise [67], and only during exercise while breathing air with reduced O_2 content is myocardial lactate production found in healthy persons [68].

The regions where flow is reduced most severely might reduce their function and lower their metabolism, a condition which is called hibernation, but this is not corroborated by the finding that lactate levels are high in all regions with severe flow reduction. The occurrence of coronary steal has been reported, where pharmacological vasodilation leads to luxury perfusion of relatively well-perfused areas, but leading to reduced blood flow in critically underperfused regions. The regional flow reserve is lost non-uniformly during reduction of coronary perfusion pressure [62]. It may be that pharmacological vasodilation increases blood flow to regions which do not need extra perfusion, but steals away blood from regions that need the blood more badly, and coronary vasodilation may often be of little or no benefit to alleviate ischemia. Inhibition of the production of the endogenous vasodilator nitric oxide (NO) causes ischemic areas to appear in isolated hearts of endotoxemic rats [60], although such areas do not appear in hearts isolated from non-endotoxemic control rats where overall perfusate flow has been reduced to a similar level after blocking NO synthase.

In an organ with 50% O_2 extraction, blood flow is decreased by one half, the tissue would become partially hypoxic. If flow is redistributed, however, some regions may still be relatively well oxygenated and local function may be well maintained, at the expense of other regions where even less O_2 is supplied than would be the case for homogeneous reduction of flow. If VO_2 is distributed evenly through the heart, heterogeneity of blood flow does decrease the average O_2 tension in the heart. Because of the inverse relation between blood flow and the arterial-to-venous O_2 concentration difference, a decrease in blood flow in one place leads to a larger decrease in end-capillary O_2 concentration than the corresponding increase during redistribution causes in another place. If these changes take place below the inflection point of the Hb-O_2 dissociation curve, the decrease of the local end-capillary O_2 tension is amplified by the sigmoidal shape of the Hb-O_2 dissociation curve.

At the present state of knowledge, it is uncertain whether the heterogeneous response of tissue to ischemia or shock leads to exacerbation of the condition relative to a hypothetical homogeneous flow reduction. The existence of lactate uptake in the ischemic heart for aerobic metabolism, while at the same time lactate is produced in other places [66], leads us to the hypothesis that some regions in the heart are kept relatively well perfused in order to maintain cardiac function as much as possible in a last ditch effort to survive. Making perfusion more homogeneous in the ischemic heart by giving vasodilators may not be beneficial.

Conclusion

In the healthy state, the perfusion of the left ventricle of the heart is quite heterogeneous, despite the fact that the contractile function of the heart is thought to be homogeneous. It is very likely that the heterogeneity of blood flow is paralleled by heterogeneity of VO_2, so that normally the metabolism/perfusion ratio is relatively homogeneous. Heterogeneity of perfusion is found at all scales, from centimeters to millimeters. Heterogeneity of DO_2 is shown by NADH fluorescence in regions of several hundred micrometer diameter. During coronary stenosis, blood flow is reduced very heterogeneously, and the relative reduction of flow determines to what extent metabolic indicators of tissue ischemia accumulate. Consequently, the metabolism/perfusion ratio becomes very heterogeneous during cardiac ischemia. Measurement of VO_2 in small regions was problematic until recently, but now an invasive ^{13}C-NMR method and a non-invasive PET method allow measurement of VO_2 in small myocardial regions, and one can begin to study the relationships between local blood flow, aerobic metabolism and function.

Acknowledgements. This work was supported by grants no. 89.100, 96.127 and D94.016 of the Netherlands Heart Foundation.

References

1. King RB, Bassingthwaighte JB, Hales JRS, Rowell LB (1985) Stability of heterogeneity of myocardial blood flow in normal awake baboons. Circ Res 57:285–295
2. Visser KR, Meeder JG, Van Beek JHGM, Van der Wall EE, Willemsen ATM, Blanksma PK (1998) A mathematical model for the heterogeneity of myocardial perfusion form ^{13}NH$_3$ PET data evaluated in patients with syndrome X compared with healthy volunteers. J Nucl Med (in press)
3. Piiper J, Marconi C, Heisler N, et al (1989) Spatial and temporal variability of blood flow in stimulated dog gastrocnemius muscle. Adv Exp Med Biol 248:719–728
4. Vicini P, Bonadonna RC, Utriainen T, et al (1997) Estimation of blood flow heterogeneity distribution in human skeletal muscle from positron emission tomography data. Ann Biomed Eng 25:906–910

5. Glenny RW, Robertson HT (1990) Fractal properties of pulmonary blood flow: characterization of spatial heterogeneity. J Appl Physiol 69:532–545.
6. Glenny RW, McKinney S, Robertson KT (1997) Spatial pattern of pulmonary blood flow distribution is stable over days. J Appl Physiol 82:902–907
7. Groeneveld ABJ, van Lambalgen AA, van den Bos GC, Bronsveld W, Nauta JP, Thijs LG (1991) Maldistribution of heterogeneous coronary blood flow during canine endotoxin shock. Cardiovasc Res 25:80–88
8. Arts T, Bovendeerd PH, Prinzen FW, Reneman RS (1991) Relation between left ventricular cavity pressure and volume and systolic fiber stress and strain in the wall. Biophys J 59:93–102
9. Bassingthwaighte JB, King RB, Roger SA (1989) Fractal nature of regional myocardial flow heterogeneity. Circ Res 65:578–590
10. King RB, Bassingthwaighte JB (1989) Temporal fluctuations in regional myocardial flows. Pflügers Arch 413:336–342
11. Bussemaker J, van Beek JHGM, Groeneveld ABJ, et al (1994) Local mitochondrial enzyme activity correlates with myocardial blood flow at basal workloads. J Mol Cell Cardiol 26:1017–1028
12. Mori H, Chujo M, Haruyama S, et al (1995) Local continuity of myocardial blood flow studied by monochromatic synchrotron radiation-excited X-ray fluorescence spectrometry. Circ Res 76:1088–1100
13. Wu X, Ewert DL, Liu YH, Ritman EL (1992) In vivo relation of intramyocardial blood volume to myocardial perfusion. Evidence supporting microvascular site for autoregulation. Circulation 85:730–737
14. Groeneveld ABJ, van Lambalgen AA, van den Bos GC, Nauta JP, Thijs LG (1992) Metabolic vasodilation with glucose-insulin-potassium does not change the heterogeneous distribution of coronary blood flow in the dog. Cardiovasc Res 26:757–764
15. Austin RE, Aldea GS, Coggins DL, Flynn AE, Hoffman JIE (1990) Profound spatial heterogeneity of coronary reserve. Discordance between patterns of resting and maximal myocardial blood flow. Circ Res 67:319–331
16. Sokoloff L (1981) Relationships among local functional activity, energy metabolism, and blood flow in the central nervous system. Fed Proc 40:2311–2316
17. Stapleton DD, Van Beek JHGM, Roger S, Baskin DG, Bassingthwaighte JB (1988) Regional myocardial flow heterogeneity assessed with 2-iododesmethylimipramine. Circulation 78 (Suppl II):405 (Abst)
18. Ellis CG, Wrigley SM, Groom AC (1994) Heterogeneity of red blood cell perfusion in capillary networks supplied by a single arteriole in resting skeletal muscle. Circ Res 75:357–368
19. Mandelbrot BB (1983) The fractal geometry of nature. Freeman, New York
20. Vetterlein F, Prange M, Lubrich D, Pedina J, Neckel M, Schmidt G (1995) Capillary perfusion pattern and microvascular geometry in heterogeneous hypoxic areas of hypoperfused rat myocardium. Am J Physiol 268:H2183–H2194
21. Van Beek JHGM, Roger SA, Bassingthwaighte JB (1989) Regional myocardial flow heterogeneity explained with fractal networks. Am J Physiol 257:H1670–H1680
22. Bassingthwaighte JB, Van Beek JHGM (1988) Lightning and the heart: fractal behavior in cardiac function. Proc IEEE 76:693–699
23. Van Beek JHGM (1992) Fractal models of heterogeneity in organ blood flow. In: Egginton S, Ross HF (eds) Oxygen transport in biological systems. Cambridge University Press, Cambridge, pp 135–163
24. Van Beek JHGM, Bassingthwaighte JB, Roger SA (1989) Fractal networks explain regional myocardial flow heterogeneity. In: Rakusan K, Biro G, Goldstick TK, Turek Z (eds) Oxygen transport to tissue XI. Plenum Press, New York, pp 249–257
25. Bassingthwaighte JB, Van Beek JHGM, King RB (1990) Fractal branchings: the basis of myocardial flow heterogeneities? Ann NY Acad Sci 591:392–401.
26. Van Beek JHGM, Barends JPF, Westerhof N (1994) The microvascular unit size for fractal flow heterogeneity relevant for oxygen transport. In: Vaupel P, Zander R, Bruley DF (eds) Oxygen transport to tissue XV. Plenum, New York, pp 901–908
27. Galassi AR, Crea F, Araujo LI, et al (1993) Comparison of regional myocardial blood flow in syndrome X and one-vessel coronary artery disease. Am J Cardiol 72:134–139

28. Meeder JG, Blanksma PK, Crijns HJGM, et al (1995) Mechanisms of angina pectoris in syndrome X assessed by myocardial perfusion dynamics and heart rate variability. Eur Heart J 16:1571-1577
29. Meeder JG, Blanksma PK, Van der Wall EE, et al (1997) Coronary vasomotion in patients with syndrome X: evaluation with positron emission tomography and parametric myocardial perfusion imaging. Eur J Nucl Med 24:530-537
30. Matsumoto T, Goto M, Tachibana H, Ogasawara Y, Tsujioka K, Kajiya F (1996) Microheterogeneity of myocardial blood flow in rabbit hearts during normoxic and hypoxic states. Am J Physiol 270:H435-H441
31. Kleen M, Welte M, Lackermeier P, Habler O, Kemming G, Messmer K (1997) Myocardial blood flow heterogeneity in shock and small-volume resuscitation in pigs with coronary stenosis. J Appl Physiol 83:1832-1841
32. Van Beek JHGM, Bussemaker J, Westerhof N (1996) Measurement of local oxygen consumption in small frozen tissue samples with a new method shows a higher metabolic rate in subendocardium than in subepicardium in isolated rabbit heart. J Physiol 491:158P (Abst)
33. Van Beek JHGM, Bussemaker J, Barends JPF, Westerhof N (1996) A ^{13}C-NMR technique to determine absolute oxygen consumption in quickly frozen small myocardial samples. FASEB J 10:A325 (Abst)
34. Van Beek JHGM, Csont T, Bussemaker J, Barends JPF (1996) Measuring local myocardial O_2 consumption in many samples. Ann Biomed Eng 24:S-19 (Abst)
35. Van Beek JHGM (1997) Is local metabolism the basis of the fractal vascular structure in the heart? Int J Microcirc 17:337-345
36. Van Beek JHGM, Csont T, De Kanter FJJ, Bussemaker J (1998) Simple model analysis of ^{13}C NMR spectra to measure oxygen consumption using frozen tissue samples. Adv Exp Med Biol (in press)
37. Li Z, Yipintsoi T, Caldwell JH, et al (1996) In vivo measurement of regional myocardial oxygen utilization with inhaled ^{15}O-oxygen and positron emission tomography. Ann Biomed Eng 42:S-32 (Abst)
38. Sonntag M, Deussen A, Schultz J, Loncar R, Hort W, Schrader J (1996) Spatial heterogeneity of blood flow in the dog heart. I. Glucose uptake, free adenosine and oxidative/glycolytic enzyme activity. Pflügers Arch 432:439-450
39. Franzen D, Conway RS, Zhang H, Sonnenblick EH, Eng C (1988) Spatial heterogeneity of local blood flow and metabolite content in dog hearts. Am J Physiol 257:H1670-H1680
40. Bussemaker J, van Beek JHGM, Groeneveld ABJ, et al (1994) Oxygen supply is not limiting in low-flow regions of normal pig left ventricle. In: Bussemaker J (thesis) The coupling of heterogeneous myocardial blood flow and energy metabolism. Vrije Universiteit, Amsterdam, pp 49-65
41. Bussemaker J, Groeneveld ABJ, Teerlink T, Hennekes M, Westerhof N, Van Beek JHGM (1997) Low- and high blood flow regions in the normal pig heart are equally vulnerable to ischaemia during partial coronary stenosis. Pflügers Arch 434:785-794
42. Sokoloff L, Reivich M, Kennedy C, et al (1977) The [^{14}C]deoxyglucose method for the measurement of local cerebral glucose utilization: theory, procedure, and normal values in the conscious and anesthetized albino rat. J Neurochem 28:897-916
43. Hibbard LS, McGlone JS, Davis DW, Hawkins RA (1987) Three-dimensional representation and analysis of brain energy metabolism. Science 236:1641-1646
44. Deussen A (1997) Local myocardial glucose uptake is proportional to, but not dependent on blood flow. Pflügers Arch 433:488-496
45. Chance EM, Seeholzer SH, Kobayashi K, Williamson JR (1983) Mathematical analysis of isotope labeling in the citric acid cycle with applications to ^{13}C NMR studies in perfused rat hearts. J Biol Chem 258:13785-13794
46. Chatham JC, Forder JR, Glickson JD, Chance EM (1995) Calculation of absolute metabolic flux and the elucidation of pathways of glutamate labeling in perfused rat heart by ^{13}C NMR spectroscopy and nonlinear least squares analysis. J Biol Chem 270:7999-8008
47. Lewandowski ED (1992) Nuclear magnetic resonance evaluation of metabolic and respiratory support of work load in intact rabbit hearts. Circ Res 70:576-582

48. Weiss RG, Gloth ST, Kalil-Filho R, Chacko VP, Stern MD, Gerstenblith G (1992) Indexing tricarboxylic acid cycle flux in intact hearts by carbon-13 nuclear magnetic resonance. Circ Res 70:392–408
49. Yu X, White LT, Doumen C, et al (1995) Kinetic analysis of dynamic ^{13}C NMR spectra: metabolic flux, regulation, and compartmentation in hearts. Biophys J 69:2090–2102
50. Malloy CR, Sherry AD, Jeffrey FMH (1990) Analysis of tricarboxylic acid cycle of the heart using ^{13}C isotope isomers. Am J Physiol 259:H987–H995
51. Malloy CR, Thompson JR, Jeffrey FMH, Sherry AD (1990) Contribution of exogenous substrates to acetyl coenzyme A: measurement by ^{13}C NMR under non-steady-state conditions. Biochemistry 29:6756–6761
52. Rademakers FE, Rogers WJ, Guier, et al (1994) Relation of regional cross-fiber shortening to wall thickening in the intact heart. Three-dimensional strain analysis by NMR tagging. Circulation 89:1174–1182
53. Hexeberg E, Homans DC, Bache RJ (1995) Interpretation of systolic wall thickening. Can thickening of a discrete layer reflect fibre performance? Cardiovasc Res 29:16–21
54. Van Beek JHGM, de Kanter FJ, Bussemaker J (1998) Measuring subendocardial versus subepicardial O$_2$ consumption in rabbit left ventricle using ^{13}C-NMR spectroscopy. J Mol Cell Cardiol (Abst)
55. Deussen A, Bassingthwaighte JB (1996) Modeling [^{15}O]oxygen tracer data for estimating oxygen consumption. Am J Physiol 270:H1115–H1130
56. Weiss HR, Sinha AK (1978) Regional oxygen saturation of small arteries and veins in the canine myocardium. Circ Res 42:119–126
57. Weiss HR (1979) Regional oxygen consumption and supply in the rabbit heart – effect of nitroglycerin and propanolol. J Pharmacol Exp Therap 211:68–73
58. Steenbergen C, Deleeuw G, Barlow C, Chance B, Williamson JR (1977) Heterogeneity of the hypoxic state in perfused rat heart. Circ Res 41:606–615
59. Delori FC (1988) Noninvasive technique for oximetry of blood in retinal vessels. Appl Optics 27:1113–1125
60. Avontuur JAM, Bruining HA, Ince C (1995) Inhibition of nitric oxide synthesis causes myocardial ischemia in endotoxemic rats. Circ Res 76:418–425
61. Van Beek JHGM, Loiselle DS, Westerhof N (1992) Calculation of oxygen diffusion across the surface of isolated perfused hearts. Am J Physiol 263:H1003–H1010
62. Coggins DL, Flynn AE, Austin RE, et al (1990) Nonuniform loss of regional flow reserve during myocardial ischemia in dogs. Circ Res 67:253–264
63. Flynn AE, Coggins DL, Austin RE, et al (1990) Nonuniform blood flow in the canine left ventricle. J Surg Res 49:379–384
64. Deussen A, Loncar R, Flesche CW (1996) The risk of ischemia is similar for low and high flow areas of the left ventricle. Int J Microcirc 16:229 (Abst)
65. Huang C-H, Kim S-J, Kudej RK, et al (1998) An adenosine A1 agonist protects myocardium by altering the spatial distribution of myocardial blood flow. FASEB J 12:A76 (Abst)
66. Gertz EW, Wisneski JA, Neese R, Bristow JD, Searle GL, Hanlon JT (1981) Myocardial lactate metabolism: evidence of lactate release during net chemical extraction in man. Circulation 63:1273–1279
67. Kaijser L, Berglund B (1992) Myocardial lactate extraction and release at rest and during heavy exercise in healthy men. Acta Physiol Scand 144:39–45
68. Grubbström J, Berglund B, Kaijser L (1993) Myocardial oxygen supply and lactate metabolism during marked arterial hypoxaemia. Acta Physiol Scand 149:303–310

The Microcirculation and Tissue Oxygenation

R. N. Pittman

Introduction

The microcirculation plays a central role in tissue oxygenation, because it is across the walls of the microvessels (arterioles, capillaries and venules) that oxygen (O_2) passes between the blood and the cells of each tissue. Each tissue possesses a microvasculature whose architecture is characteristic of that tissue, and presumably the arrangement of microvessels has been adapted to that tissue's specific requirements. A cursory examination of the global features of microvascular networks from different organs bears out this observation. Because of the wide range of microvascular network structures, it is not practical for one laboratory to investigate O_2 transport in many different tissues. However, an approach that has been useful is to study in detail the fundamental biophysical and physiological principles of O_2 transport that are common to all tissues, and apply those principles to tissues with different microvascular network geometries. In this chapter we will review the major aspects of what is currently known about O_2 transport at the level of the microcirculation.

Convective and Diffusive Transport of Oxygen

O_2 is transported within the microcirculation by convection (i.e., bulk flow of blood) and diffusion (i.e., random movement of free or bound O_2 molecules). Convection is a process by which substantial amounts of O_2 can be moved rapidly over large, macroscopic distances. The large vessels of the circulatory system are responsible for efficiently distributing blood, and the O_2 it carries, among the various organs. Convection continues to be an important means of distributing O_2 within the microvascular networks, since diffusion is an efficient mechanism of transport only over distances in the order of tens of microns.

Almost all of the O_2 carried by the blood is reversibly bound to the hemoglobin (Hb) contained within the erythrocytes or red blood cells (RBCs). At normal hematocrit (Hct), about 98% of the O_2 content of blood is due to the bound form. Thus, moving RBCs represent a substantial and mobile source of O_2. The low solubility of O_2 in plasma results in a negligible amount being carried in the dissolved form, except at very high oxygen tensions (PO_2). Later in this chapter, the effects of enhancing the effective O_2 solubility of the plasma by Hb-based O_2 carriers (HBOCs) or perfluorocarbon emulsions (PFCs) will be discussed.

The diffusive transport of free O_2 molecules between two locations is described by Fick's first law of diffusion, according to which the driving force for the net movement of O_2 is the difference in PO_2 between the two sites. Based in part on his histologic studies of fixed tissues, August Krogh [1] concluded that the most likely vascular site for O_2 transport from blood to tissue was the capillary network. The primary reasons for this conclusion were that the capillaries appear to be ideal gas exchangers due to their thin walls (single layer of endothelial cells), large surface area-to-volume ratio, low RBC velocity (due to their large collective cross-sectional area), and the short diffusion distances between capillaries and neighboring parenchymal cells (most cells are in contact with at least one capillary). Krogh, with the help of Erlang, formulated a simple mathematical model in which a capillary was surrounded by a concentric cylinder of tissue. The model was used to predict the magnitude of the PO_2 difference needed to adequately supply the tissue cylinder with O_2 (i.e., no hypoxic regions). This model (Fig. 1) formed the basis of our quantitative understanding of tissue oxygenation for many years, and is still used by some investigators to interpret their data.

For many years after Krogh's ideas [1] appeared in the literature, most investigators assumed that all O_2 exchange occurred in the capillaries. Based on this concept, one would predict that the O_2 content of blood would change (decrease) only in the capillaries, and that the arterial and venous vessels would behave as relatively O_2-impermeable conduits for the blood (Fig. 2A). In 1970, fifty years after Krogh introduced his model of O_2 exchange, Duling and Berne [2] reported that there were losses of O_2 from the pre-capillary vessels. Direct measurements of PO_2 within and on the outside walls of arterioles, using O_2-sensitive microcathodes, demonstrated that there was a progressive fall in PO_2 from the largest arterioles entering a tissue down to the terminal arterioles. These first systematic microcirculatory measurements of blood PO_2 were carried out in thin tissues, the

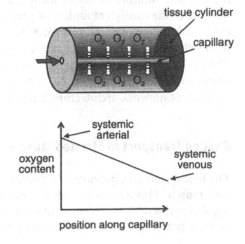

Fig. 1. Krogh cylinder model of oxygen transport, showing a single capillary surrounded by a cylinder of tissue with uniform properties in regard to oxygen (uniform Krogh diffusion coefficient and consumption). Under these conditions, oxygen content should fall linearly with distance along the capillary from the systemic arterial value to the systemic venous value. (From [34] with permission)

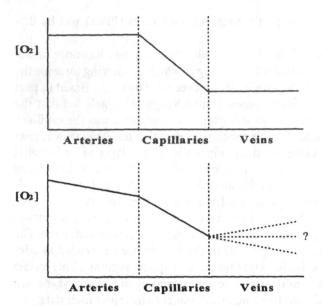

Fig. 2. Variation of oxygen content, [O$_2$], within the circulatory system. Panel A: This schematic diagram represents the consequences of the Krogh cylinder model, where all oxygen exchange is assumed to take place only across the walls of the capillaries, with both arterial and venous vessels negligibly permeable to oxygen. Panel B: Revised picture of oxygen exchange, according to the results of Duling and Berne [2] and others, showing the loss of oxygen from the pre-capillary network. As indicated by the diagram, there remains some uncertainty regarding the variation of [O$_2$] in the venous network

hamster cheek pouch and hamster and rat cremaster muscles, with relatively low metabolic rates, but subsequent investigations have found similar results for cat cerebral cortex [3], rabbit cerebral cortex [4], hamster retractor muscle [5–7], and rat spinotrapezius muscle [8]. More recently, these results have been confirmed in the hamster skinfold chamber, using a different technique to measure PO$_2$ [9]. Because of the consistent finding of precapillary O$_2$ losses in many tissues covering a wide range of metabolic rates, the current view of the distribution of O$_2$ within the circulatory system has been revised, as shown schematically in Fig. 2B. The existence of a pre-capillary O$_2$ loss is qualitatively similar among all tissues examined so far; the magnitude of the loss for a given tissue depends upon the specifics of network architecture, blood flow, Hct and metabolic rate.

Oxygen Transport in Striated Muscle

The first systematic, quantitative studies of O$_2$ transport were carried out in striated muscle. Muscle was chosen as a model tissue because most muscles have a regular, predictable vascular architecture, and the behavior of muscle in regard to O$_2$ transport is governed by the same physical principles that apply to other tissues. Much is also known about how muscles respond to alterations in O_2 supply (DO_2) and demand at a macroscopic, as well as a microscopic, level. Striated muscle is an important tissue in its own right, because of the unique ability of this tissue to increase its rate of oxygen consumption (VO_2) more than 10-fold from rest to contraction, and because it comprises about 40% of body mass. The majority of the data reviewed below was obtained from studies of the retractor muscle of the Syrian hamster [10].

Experimental Approach

The approach to studying O_2 transport in microvascular networks is based upon considerations of mass balance, and is illustrated schematically in Fig. 3. Namely, the rate at which O_2 diffuses across the wall of an unbranched vascular segment is equal to the difference between the rates at which O_2 enters and leaves the segment by convection. In symbolic terms, this statement can be represented by the following expression:

$$QO_2^D = QO_2^C(in) - QO_2^C(out) \tag{1}$$

where QO_2^D is the rate at which O_2 diffuses across the wall of the vascular segment and QO_2^C (in or out) is the rate at which O_2 flows into or out of the segment by convection. The QO_2^C (in or out) can be estimated by the following expression:

$$QO_2^C = \pi R^2 v \, [Hb] \, SO_2 \, C_B \tag{2}$$

where R is the radius of the segment, v is the average velocity of blood, [Hb] is the average concentration of Hb, SO_2 is the average O_2 saturation of the Hb, and C_B is the O_2 binding capacity of Hb. The amount of O_2 dissolved in the blood is considered to be negligible compared with that bound to Hb. Thus, it is necessary to measure the quantities in eqn. 2 at two sites along a vascular segment in order to compute QO_2^C at the two sites, and then substitute these values into eqn. 1 to obtain the diffusive flow of O_2 from the segment.

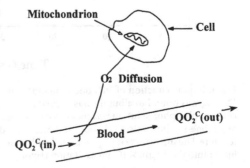

Fig. 3. Illustration of approach to quantify diffusion of oxygen from a single microvessel. The diffusive flow of oxygen is given by application of the Fick principle (i.e., conservation of mass) as the difference between the convective oxygen inflow and outflow, respectively. Refer to eqns. 1–2 and the accompanying text

Experimental Methods

In order to measure the quantities used in eqn. 2, intravital video microscopy and microphotometry are employed. After a suitable microscopic field is chosen for study, the temporal and spatial features of the light intensity in the microscopic image are processed to obtain RBC velocity [11], Hb concentration [12] and SO_2 [13]. For arterioles and venules, the light intensity is sampled above the centerline of the vessel in a region that is small compared with the diameter of the vessel, and the photometric signals are processed to yield v, [Hb] and SO_2. For capillaries, video recordings are made and analyzed off-line to obtain RBC velocity [14], number of RBCs per unit length (lineal density) [15] and SO_2 [16]. For all the microvessels, video recordings are used to obtain geometric data, including luminal diameter, segment length and distances from other microvessels.

In some cases tissue PO_2 has been measured using O_2 microcathodes [17]. More recently, the technique of phosphorescence quenching microscopy has been used to measure PO_2 [18]. In this approach, a phosphorescent metallo-porphyrin compound is bound to albumin and introduced into the circulation. The albumin-bound phosphor thus reports PO_2 of the plasma, although in tissues

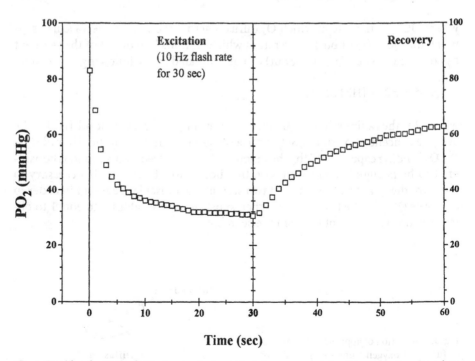

Fig. 4. Rapid reduction of PO_2 due to photo-activated oxygen uptake. Pd-porphyrin phosphor (2.5 mg/ml) bound to albumin was excited at a flash rate of 10 Hz for 30 sec. PO_2 of the Saran-covered phosphor solution was measured continuously with a PO_2 microcathode [17] and plotted at one-sec intervals. Excitation flash was turned off during the 30-sec recovery period plotted here. During recovery, PO_2 increased with time as oxygen diffused from the surrounding solution into the 10 μm × 10 μm excitation region

with leaky microvessels, some of the phosphor can appear in the interstitial fluid. After the phosphor is excited by a brief (μsec to 10's of μsec) flash of light of the appropriate excitation wavelength, it decays by emitting light at a characteristic wavelength with a lifetime that depends on the PO_2 of the local environment of the phosphor. For a medium with uniform PO_2, the time course of the decay is monoexponential and the relationship between lifetime and PO_2 can be calibrated using the Stern-Volmer equation. One must exercise caution when interpreting the phosphorescence decay curve, however, because, in the microvessels and tissue, PO_2 is generally not uniform, thereby violating the assumption leading to the monoexponential time course. These PO_2 gradients are due to O_2 diffusion from microvessels (producing local intravascular radial gradients in PO_2) and VO_2 in the tissue. By using fitting models for heterogeneous spatial distributions of PO_2, one can account for the intrinsic non-uniformities [19]. In the tissue, an additional concern arises, due to the artifactual lowering of PO_2 by photo-activated VO_2 by the phosphor [18]. Each time the phosphor is excited, a small amount of molecular O_2 is converted to the highly reactive species singlet oxygen, resulting in an apparent VO_2. At the high flash rates commonly used, this can result in a substantial reduction in PO_2 for stationary samples such as interstitial fluid. Figure 4 shows an example in which the PO_2 falls by over 40 mm Hg in 5 seconds at a flash rate of 10 Hz. Although this effect (i.e., photo-activated O_2 uptake) also occurs in microvessels, the resulting fall in PO_2 is negligible at normal blood flow, since the excited volume is replaced by a fresh volume with high PO_2 between flashes and the cumulative effect that occurs in a stationary fluid does not take place [20]. PO_2 measurements in microvessels can also be used to estimate $HbSO_2$ through the O_2 dissociation curve for Hb.

Oxygen Transport in Arterioles and Venules

Using the techniques described above, Swain and Pittman [5] reported that in the resting retractor muscle of the hamster, about two-thirds of the O_2 utilized by the muscle diffused across the walls of the arterioles and about one-third diffused across the walls of the capillaries. This conclusion was based upon changes in SO_2 in the arteriolar and venular networks. Thus, in resting muscle, the arterioles appear to be the major source of O_2 for the tissue, a conclusion supported by the measurements of Duling and Berne [2], but contrary to the expectations of Krogh [1].

A more detailed examination of the convective and diffusive movement of O_2 in the four largest branching generations of the arteriolar network revealed a progressive fall in SO_2 along the arteriolar tree, again consistent with the finding of a longitudinal fall in PO_2 by Duling and Berne [2] in another tissue. After normalizing the segmental differences in SO_2 (ΔSO_2) to the lengths (ΔL) of the serial branching generations, yielding the longitudinal gradient in SO_2, one observes in Fig. 5 a large increase in $\Delta SO_2/\Delta L$ on progressing from the largest arterioles (1A, average diameter = 60 μm) to the smallest ones measured in this study (4A, average diameter = 20 μm). Most of this 20-fold increase in longitudinal gradient

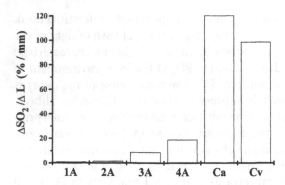

Fig. 5. Variation of longitudinal gradient in oxygen saturation, $\Delta SO_2/\Delta L$, across arteriolar and capillary networks. Bars represent average value of $\Delta SO_2/\Delta L$ in four consecutive branching generations of arterioles (1A–4A), arteriolar end of capillaries (C_a) and venular end of capillaries (C_v) in retractor muscle of Syrian hamster. (Data from [5, 31])

can be explained by the accompanying 10-fold decrease in RBC velocity, yielding a progressively longer residence time for RBCs in the successive branches of the arteriolar network, thereby allowing them more time to release O_2. Kuo and Pittman subsequently investigated the effects of varying the DO_2 by decreasing [6] and increasing [7] the systemic Hct (hemodilution and hemoconcentration, respectively). The control situations (normal Hct) were consistent with the results of Swain and Pittman [5]. Compared with the control situation (52% Hct), moderate hemodilution (to 33% Hct) produced higher RBC velocity and reduced the pre-capillary O_2 loss, whereas hemoconcentration (control of 50% to 65% Hct) produced lower RBC velocity and increased pre-capillary O_2 loss.

The question naturally arises, "What is the destination of the O_2 that diffuses from the arterioles?" Three obvious sites to receive the O_2 are: (1) the parenchymal cells near an arteriole; (2) a nearby venule; and (3) a nearby capillary. Certainly the tissue surrounding an arteriole could utilize any diffused O_2, since the source of the O_2 for cellular metabolism is immaterial to a cell consuming it. In striated muscle and some other tissues, the arterioles and venules with the largest diameters are often in close proximity for the first few branching generations. This proximity provides a necessary geometric condition that promotes diffusion between the two neighboring vessels, provided the likely circumstance that there is a PO_2 difference between them. Although theoretical calculations have suggested that the magnitude of such diffusive shunting of O_2 should be relatively small [21], several studies have provided evidence for its existence [5, 22, 23]. Further work is required to provide a definitive answer as to whether, and under what conditions, this phenomenon is an important determinant of O_2 distribution within the microcirculation and tissue. The third possibility is similar to the second, involving arteriolar-capillary diffusive exchange, rather than arteriolar-venular exchange, and it will be discussed below when O_2 transport in capillaries is considered.

A careful analysis of O_2 diffusion from arterioles revealed that the rate of O_2 diffusion as determined from eqns. 1 and 2, was an order of magnitude higher than predicted by standard models of diffusive biotransport [24]. This surprising result was consistent among the three studies described above [5–7]. Since the experimental methods used to determine the variables of eqn. 2 were found to be reliable, it was concluded that the assumed permeability of the tissue to O_2 could be in error. The permeability in question is Krogh's diffusion coefficient, the product of the solubility and diffusion coefficient of O_2 in the muscle. Since the diffusion coefficient had been determined only under *in vitro* conditions at room temperature [25], experiments were carried out to measure it under conditions that more closely resembled the *in vivo* conditions of the intravital microscopic measurements [26–28]. Although it was not possible to measure the diffusion coefficient under *in vivo* conditions, the results of these studies indicated that Krogh's diffusion coefficient was larger than had been assumed, by at least a factor of 2.5, thereby reducing the discrepancy between observed and predicted O_2 diffusion from arterioles. Part of the increase in the Krogh coefficient was due to an upward revision in the value of O_2 solubility [29] and the rest was due to a higher than expected temperature dependence of the diffusion coefficient [27–28]. Although the source of the remaining discrepancy is not completely resolved, it appears to be related to the approximate nature of the calculation of the convective O_2 flow in eqn. 2 [30]. A more accurate determination of the variables in eqn. 2, particularly their spatial variation across the arteriolar lumen, should lead to a resolution of this remaining puzzle.

In a later chapter, Intaglietta presents an alternative explanation of the observed pre-capillary O_2 loss. The explanation is based on the conclusion that the microvessel wall consumes O_2 at a rate more than two orders of magnitude greater than that of resting skeletal muscle. The principal factor leading to this conclusion is the observation of a large transmural difference in PO_2, based on paired measurements of PO_2 in the luminal and perivascular regions near the microvessel wall, using the phosphorescence quenching technique. Since the measurements in both regions have potential sources of error leading to inaccurate determination (generally, underestimation) of PO_2, the results need to be interpreted with caution. In regard to the near-wall luminal measurement, one would expect a large intravascular radial gradient in PO_2 to accompany the proposed high VO_2 of the wall. This gives rise to two problems: (1) a monoexponential analysis of the phosphorescence emission curve will result in an underestimation of PO_2 due to the non-uniformity of PO_2 (and, hence, range of phosphorescence lifetimes) in the measured volume [19]; and (2) the PO_2 dependence of the initial phosphorescence intensity (higher for lower PO_2) will result in a greater contribution to the measured signal from microregions with lower PO_2 [20]. An additional problem associated with the perivascular measurement is the photo-activated conversion of O_2 to the highly reactive singlet state, and its subsequent reaction with nearby organic molecules, resulting in a net consumption of O_2 as described earlier in this chapter. Furthermore, although the smooth muscle and endothelial cells of the microvessel wall require energy to maintain normal function, there does not appear to be any independent evidence in the literature to support a large O_2 requirement of either cell type. In particular, mitochondrial content, the generally accepted index of capacity for VO_2, is quite small in both vascular smooth muscle and endothelial cells. Thus, additional studies, that take into account these potential sources of error, are needed before one can determine with more certainty whether a much larger than expected VO_2 by the microvessel wall is the major determinant of the pre-capillary O_2 loss.

Oxygen Transport in Capillaries

The most striking observation regarding the DO_2 in capillaries is the high degree of heterogeneity of perfusion, a circumstance made more obvious by the single-file flow of RBCs through capillaries [31]. The heterogeneity expresses itself in the wide range of RBC velocity, RBC spacing and RBC supply rate (i.e., the number of RBCs passing through a capillary segment per unit time). Measurements of SO_2 in 100 μm segments at the arteriolar (A, entrance) and venular (V, exit) ends of capillary networks yielded the results for $\Delta SO_2/\Delta L$ shown in the two rightmost bars of Fig. 5. Examination of the change of SO_2 along neighboring capillaries indicated that there was substantial diffusion of O_2 between adjacent capillaries, with some capillaries losing O_2 and their neighbors gaining some of it. Thus, in resting muscle, there is considerable diffusive exchange of O_2 among neighboring capillaries, especially near their arteriolar ends. The measurements of RBC SO_2 in resting muscle [22, 31] also show a significant degree of heterogeneity in tissue oxygenation manifested by a wide distribution of end-capillary SO_2. This appears to be due to a large heterogeneity of RBC-perfused capillary path lengths. Although no experiments were carried out on contracting muscle, computer simulations indicated that the degree of diffusive interactions among capillaries in a network would be greatly attenuated during the hyperemia accompanying exercise [31], and predicted that the heterogeneities of end-capillary SO_2 would be enhanced in contracting muscle [31–32]. A more detailed examination of the issue of heterogeneity is taken up in the chapter by van Beek, and additional data on O_2 transport in capillary networks is discussed by Ellis in another chapter.

An important finding, that bears on the question of the destination of O_2 that diffuses from arterioles, was that considerable diffusion of O_2 occurred from arterioles to capillaries that passed nearby. The solid lines in Figure 6B represent the average longitudinal decline in SO_2 at the arteriolar and venular ends of a typical capillary (400 μm total length) in the retractor muscle of the hamster. The longitudinal gradient in SO_2 is about 0.1%/μm and is the same at both ends of the capillary. Note that, if the decline in SO_2 from the input value of 60% continued until the end of the capillary, the end-capillary SO_2 would be 20%, corresponding to a PO_2 of 14 mm Hg. However, the observed value of end-capillary SO_2 was 40%, corresponding to a PO_2 of 24 mm Hg. This puzzling result was resolved when it was realized that small arterioles (often out of focus in the microscopic field) commonly cross the paths of capillaries, as shown schematically in Figure 6A [33]. Thus, this common architectural feature of arteriolar and capillary networks in striated muscle operates in such a way that the arteriole is a diffusive source of O_2 that replenishes the O_2 released from an RBC as it traverses the capillary. An important consequence of this phenomenon is that the end-capillary, and hence tissue, PO_2 is elevated considerably (10 mm Hg in this example) above what it would be with the usual textbook arrangement of parallel capillaries supplied with O_2 only by convection from the arterioles.

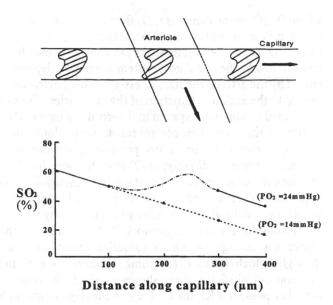

Distance along capillary (μm)

Fig. 6. Diffusive exchange of oxygen between arteriole and capillary. Panel A: Schematic diagram of capillary crossing the path of an arteriole. Panel B: Variation of SO_2 along a typical capillary in retractor muscle of hamster [31,33]. Solid lines represent observed variation of SO_2 along capillary at arteriolar and venular ends. Dashed lines extended from arteriolar end of capillary shows extrapolated variation of SO_2 along the capillary. Curved dashed/dotted line shows actual variation of SO_2 along the capillary due to diffusive uptake of oxygen from arteriole by RBCs traversing the capillary. Mid-course uptake of oxygen results in an increased end-capillary SO_2 and PO_2

Local Regulation of the Oxygen Supply

One of the most important functions of the circulatory system is to provide an adequate DO_2 to all the tissues of the body. A range of mechanisms exists for regulating the DO_2 in response to varying needs, such as occurs during exercise. It is generally thought that the arterioles and the capillaries are the most important vascular elements of the system [30, 34]. The microcirculation of striated muscle is a particularly good example of the interplay of different parts of the O_2 transport system, since the demand for O_2 can be changed by an order of magnitude during intense muscle contraction and the normally functioning circulation responds by providing the appropriate DO_2 to the tissue [35–37].

One approach to examining regulation of the DO_2 is to consider the Fick principle applied to O_2 mass balance. It can be represented by the following expression:

$$VO_2 = Q[CaO_2 - CvO_2] \tag{3}$$

where Q is blood flow, and $Ca_{or}vO_2$ is arterial or venous O_2 content, respectively. By factoring out the term C_aO_2, this equation can be rewritten in the equivalent form:

$$VO_2 = Q\,CaO_2 \cdot \{[CaO_2 - CvO_2]/CaO_2\} \tag{4}$$

where $Q C_a O_2$ is the convective O_2 flow in the arterial blood (DO_2) and the ratio in parentheses is the fractional extraction of O_2 from the arterial blood. By separating DO_2 from O_2 extraction, one can gain some insight into how the DO_2 might be regulated by the circulatory system, since DO_2 depends upon blood flow (controlled by the arterial resistance vessels) and O_2 extraction depends upon factors related to the exchange function of the capillaries. Pinsky has discussed the role of the cardiopulmonary system in determining overall DO_2 in an earlier chapter.

How do the vessels that control resistance to blood flow know when the DO_2 is lower than a desirable level? Two popular hypotheses are: (1) that the resistance vessels can sense O_2 directly; or (2) that they are signaled indirectly through alterations in parenchymal cell metabolism (metabolic hypothesis of blood flow regulation). There is conflicting evidence on whether one or more elements of the resistance vessel wall has the ability to sense changes in PO_2 over the range normally found in the arterial network [38]. It is unlikely that mural PO_2 ever becomes low enough to inhibit oxidative metabolism of the microvessel wall through mitochondrial cytochrome oxidase. However, there are other oxygenases, some of which have been shown to exist in the vessel wall (e.g., cyclooxygenase) that possess a K_m for O_2 (10's of mm Hg) much higher than that of cytochrome oxidase. Thus, it is possible that one or more of these molecules could link O_2 to the excitation-contraction coupling cascade of vascular smooth muscle. The cell type(s) involved in O_2 sensing and the location of such sites within the microvascular network remain the subject of much speculation. There is considerable evidence in support of O_2-linked vasodilator metabolites (e.g., adenosine) that are released from active parenchymal cells in response to a reduction in the ratio of DO_2 to VO_2.

A more recent proposal by Ellsworth et al. [39] is that the RBC is a regulator of vascular tone. This idea is particularly appealing because it allows the principal carrier of O_2 to act as a mobile messenger, continuously reporting the oxygenation state of the circulation. The mechanism works like this: Adenosine triphosphate (ATP) is released from the RBC in response to low PO_2 and low pH and binds to P_{2y} receptors on the vascular endothelium, inducing the formation of nitric oxide (NO) or prostacyclin (PGI_2). These, in turn, would initiate a vasodilation that is propagated along the vasculature to upstream sites. This proposal allows the entire vasculature to act as the sensor; what is needed is for the PO_2 and pH of the RBC to fall to sufficiently low levels to trigger the release of ATP. Other aspects of O_2 signaling are discussed by Gorlach in a later chapter.

Tissue Oxygenation

So far, this chapter has dealt almost exclusively with the DO_2 in the microcirculation, with the implicit assumption that if the supply is adequate, then tissue oxygenation will allow normal cellular function. Tissue oxygenation is determined by a balance between the microcirculatory DO_2 and the parenchymal cell O_2 demand. The primary characteristics of the tissue are: (1) the permeability of the tissue to O_2 (dependent on the effective solubility and diffusion coefficient for

O_2); and (2) the spatial distribution and activity of the sinks for O_2, the mitochondria, relative to the sources of O_2, primarily the capillaries.

O_2 is unique among the nutrients supplied by the microcirculation in that the permeability of most tissue structures, including the microvessels, to O_2 is quite high. In situations of high demand for O_2, however, the heterogeneities associated with RBC perfusion might place an overall limitation on the DO_2. Weibel [40] has put forward the concept of symmorphosis in which there is an appropriate matching of structure and function, in regard to the body's O_2 transport system. It is appealing to hypothesize that the vasculature of each tissue whose function might be severely limited by a reduction in the DO_2, relative to demand, has been adapted to compensate in some unknown way for the intrinsic heterogeneities of perfusion and DO_2.

Muscle function can be critically affected if the DO_2 is limited. Limitations of DO_2 can be attributed primarily to two factors: (1) convective delivery of oxygenated RBCs to the exchange vessels, i.e., capillaries and small arterioles and venules; and (2) diffusive transport of O_2 from the Hb inside the RBC to the muscle fiber mitochondria. This diffusive transport is dependent on the rates of free and facilitated diffusion along the pathway for O_2 and on the characteristics of O_2 binding to, and release from Hb, and myoglobin. The role and determinants of the RBC-to-mitochondrion diffusive pathway are poorly understood. Such understanding is of fundamental and practical importance because some of the determinants of this pathway may be controlled, thus opening the possibility of improving DO_2 to parenchymal cells under conditions of critical DO_2. In all tissues, spatial heterogeneities of the factors that determine DO_2, including, but not limited to, blood flow, may significantly affect the convective and diffusive pathways and result in undersupplied and oversupplied tissue regions, even when the organ, on average, receives an adequate DO_2 (i.e., mismatch of DO_2 and O_2 demand).

Implicit in the Krogh model of O_2 transport is the concept that all of the resistance to O_2 transport is located in the tissue (i.e., simple diffusion of O_2 through the tissue). A number of recent theoretical studies, using different geometrical models of RBCs and different boundary conditions, point to the significant role of extracellular, primarily intracapillary, resistance [41–48]. The principal determinant for the high fraction of the resistance attributable to the capillary is the low solubility of O_2 in plasma, which results in only a small fraction of the available O_2 being transferred to the capillary wall through the plasma gaps between the RBCs. Roy and Popel [48] have recently reported theoretical calculations that predict oxygenation variables in 24 muscles (skeletal muscles, diaphragm, myocardium) in groups of athletic and non-athletic animals, working under maximal aerobic conditions, and they concluded that the extracellular (outside the muscle fiber) resistance accounts for over 50% of the total transport resistance in these muscles. Cryomicrospectrophotometric measurements in dog gracilis muscle [49] and hearts in different species [50] at a resolution of ~ 120 microns [51] are consistent with these theoretical conclusions. Whole organ experiments of Wagner and his co-workers on isolated dog gastrocnemius muscle [52, 53] and human quadriceps [54] appear to support the theoretical predictions that a significant fraction of the resistance to O_2 transport is intracapillary, but a contribution of heterogeneity of DO_2 to limitation of the DO_2 also remains a possibility. Therefore, at the present time the theoretical prediction that about one-half of the PO_2 drop from an RBC to distant mitochondria occurs outside the muscle fiber, has not been validated by direct microcirculatory measurements.

Enhancing the Oxygen Supply with Therapeutic Interventions

As stated previously, Krogh's original model was formulated on the premise that all the resistance to O_2 transport was associated with diffusion through the tissue (i.e., located external to the capillary). More recent theoretical studies [48, 55] have pointed out that, due to the particulate nature of blood and the binding of O_2 to Hb in the erythrocytes, about half of the resistance to O_2 transport is located inside the capillary. This realization opens a window for therapeutic interventions to enhance the diffusive DO_2 under a variety of conditions associated with a reduced DO_2 relative to O_2 demand (e.g., hypoxic, circulatory and anemic hypoxia). Thus, achievable goals are the reduction of the intracapillary component of resistance to O_2 transport or the increase in the partial pressure difference that drives O_2 diffusion.

Several key intravascular factors limit the movement of O_2 from the RBC to the mitochondria in parenchymal cells: (1) RBC spacing; (2) the solubility of O_2 in plasma; and (3) the affinity of RBC Hb for O_2. The action of interventions that alter one or more of these factors can be observed only crudely at the level of the whole organism or a whole organ. Thus, it is generally not possible to clearly delineate the mechanism by which the global response is elicited. An understanding of the basic mechanisms of action of specific interventions require detailed measurements of O_2 transport at the level of the microvessels where the O_2 exchange actually takes place, particularly the capillaries. This quantitative understanding of how O_2 transport is affected should allow one to design better therapeutic measures to compensate for a decreased DO_2.

Based on the large increase in effective O_2 solubility caused by HBOCs following their intravascular administration, one would expect a decrease in the intracapillary resistance to O_2 transport, with a concomitant increase in the diffusive supply of O_2 between capillary blood and the mitochondria of parenchymal cells. If the cells are hypoxic prior to the introduction of the HBOC, then cellular oxygenation would be expected to increase up to a maximum provided by the new PO_2 difference. If the improved DO_2 exceeds the cellular demand, then there will be a generalized increase in tissue PO_2. Theoretical predictions by Roy and Popel [48] also indicate that the presence of Hb between and around the RBCs should further reduce the intracapillary resistance to O_2 transport (i.e., Hb facilitated diffusion of O_2), enhancing the supply of O_2 to the mitochondria even more (Fig. 7). The positive, but usually negligible, convective transport of O_2 in the plasma gap between RBCs should also become more important with the higher effective O_2 solubility produced by the HBOC. *In vitro* studies and theoretical calculations by Page et al. [56] indicate that these effects can be substantial. Further discussion of blood substitutes and HBOCs are taken up by other authors in subsequent chapters.

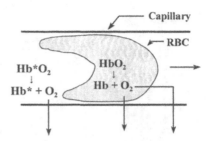

Fig. 7. Schematic diagram of RBC and plasma in a capillary. Introduction of a hemoglobin-based oxygen carrier (Hb* in plasma space) provides higher effective solubility of oxygen and also potential for facilitated diffusion of oxygen in medium surrounding RBC. Perfluorocarbon emulsion would also provide increased solubility of oxygen and potential rheological effect due to near-wall excess of submicron emulsion particles. Allosteric effectors of hemoglobin would act within the RBC to facilitate release of oxygen from hemoglobin at higher than normal PO_2

One would also expect a decrease in the intracapillary resistance to O_2 transport with PFCs, based on the high solubility of O_2 in this medium. In addition to the increased solubility of O_2 afforded by the PFC, there could be an improvement in DO_2 due to altered capillary blood rheology and a near-wall excess of submicron emulsion particles that will further decrease the intracapillary resistance to O_2 transport. The positive, but usually negligible, convective transport of O_2 in the plasma gap between RBCs should also become more important with the higher O_2 solubility produced by the PFC.

Another class of agents that can improve the DO_2 are drugs that shift the O_2 dissociation curve. A rightward shift of the O_2 dissociation curve caused by these compounds should produce an initial increase in the PO_2 difference between blood and the mitochondria, and increase the DO_2 to parenchymal cells by increasing the driving force for diffusion [57]. Theoretical predictions by Roy and Popel [48] also indicate that an increased P_{50} of the Hb and altered Hill coefficient, n, will decrease the intracapillary resistance to O_2 transport, further enhancing the supply of O_2 to the mitochondria.

Application of Mathematical Models of Oxygen Transport

It can be anticipated that future experimental and theoretical studies will also be important for tissues and organs other than striated muscle. It is likely that mathematical models will be developed that will supplant the classical Krogh model of O_2 transport and would serve as a basis and prototype for formulating new quantitative models of O_2 transport in different organs and tissues (e.g., myocardium, tissues engineered *in vitro*). Such models could be combined with modern imaging methods (e.g., high resolution magnetic resonance imaging (MRI)) and could be used for designing physiologically-based pharmacologic treatments and surgical procedures. For example, a model of left ventricular coronary hemodynamics and oxygenation based on methods of cardiac MRI currently being devel-

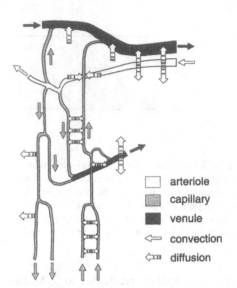

Fig. 8. Schematic diagram showing possible diffusive interactions among arterioles, capillaries and venules. Diffusion of oxygen is shown by interrupted arrows and convection of oxygen in the different vessels is indicated by the solid arrows, shaded according to the inset key. (From [34] with permission)

☐ arteriole

▨ capillary

■ venule

⇐ convection

⇚⫿ diffusion

oped, including assessment of regional blood flow and SO_2, could be used to predict the effectiveness of coronary vascular surgery aimed at providing adequate DO_2 to the myocardium. As another example, recent progress in angiogenesis and tissue engineering will make it possible, in the near future, to grow vascular networks and tissues with desired properties under controlled *in vitro* conditions. Mathematical models will then be most useful in determining desirable characteristics of these artificial vascular networks from the standpoint of adequate tissue oxygenation.

Conclusion

In the early years of this century, Krogh [1] laid the foundation for future work on O_2 transport. As we come to the end of the twentieth century, many of Krogh's ideas have been revised, as a result of new technology that has made possible direct measurements of O_2 transport in the microcirculation. One of the most important findings is the realization that O_2 can diffuse across the walls of all the vessels of the microcirculation (Fig. 8). Although this result necessarily complicates our interpretation of experimental data, the incorporation of this finding into mathematical models should lead to a better understanding of O_2 transport. The reasons for the current gap in our quantitative understanding of O_2 transport and its limitations at the microcirculatory level are two-fold: (1) there is a lack of direct measurements of microvascular O_2 distribution; and (2) there is a lack of a theoretical model for O_2 exchange in a realistic microvascular network with heterogeneous blood flow distribution that would facilitate a quantitative interpretation of these data. Whole organ and microcirculatory studies have focussed on heterogeneity of RBC flow in resting and contracting muscle [58–64] and heart [65–67] with the goal of assessing exchange of O_2, but the relationship between the heterogeneity of hemodynamic variables and O_2 transport remains poorly understood in muscle and other tissues. Knowledge of the magnitude of the resistances to O_2 transport and of the heterogeneity of DO_2 are of crucial importance for understanding the limitations of O_2 transport in skeletal muscle and other organs under normal conditions and in disease; lack of such detailed knowledge is a major concern of clinical scientists [68–71]. Improved understanding of these important issues should also allow us to make more enlightened decisions regarding the use of therapeutic interventions (such as HBOCs, PFCs and allosteric effectors of Hb) aimed at improving the DO_2 to tissues.

Acknowledgements. I gratefully acknowledge the contributions of the following colleagues to our collaborative studies and to our numerous discussions that have clarified the ideas presented here: Dr. Christopher G. Ellis, Dr. Mary L. Ellsworth, and Dr. Aleksander S. Popel. I also thank Li Wang and Lei Zheng for producing Figs. 2–7. The work of the author and his colleagues reported here was supported in part by research grant HL18292 from the National Heart, Lung and Blood Institute.

References

1. Krogh A (1959) The anatomy and physiology of capillaries. Hafner Pub, New York
2. Duling BR, Berne RM (1970) Longitudinal gradients in periarteriolar oxygen tension: A possible mechanism for the participation of oxygen in local regulation of blood flow. Circ Res 27:669–678
3. Duling BR, Kuschinsky W, Wahl M (1979) Measurements of the perivascular PO_2 in the vicinity of the pial vessels in the cat. Pflügers Arch 383:29–34
4. Ivanov KP, Derii AN, Samoilov MO, Semenov DG (1982) Diffusion of oxygen from the smallest arteries of the brain. Pflügers Arch 393:118–120
5. Swain DP, Pittman RN (1989) Oxygen exchange in the microcirculation of hamster retractor muscle. Am J Physiol 256:H247–H255
6. Kuo L, Pittman RN (1988) Effect of systemic hemodilution on microvascular oxygen transport in hamster striated muscle. Am J Physiol 254:H331–H339
7. Kuo L, Pittman RN (1990) Influence of hemoconcentration on arteriolar oxygen transport in hamster striated muscle. Am J Physiol 259:H1694–H1702
8. Lash JM, Bohlen HG (1987) Perivascular and tissue PO_2 in contracting rat spinotrapezius muscle. Am J Physiol 252:H1192–H1202
9. Torres-Filho IP, Kerger H, Intaglietta M (1996) PO_2 measurements in arteriolar networks. Microvasc Res 51:202–212
10. Sullivan SM, Pittman RN (1982) Hamster retractor muscle: A new preparation for intravital microscopy. Microvasc Res 23:329–335
11. Wayland H, Johnson PC (1967) Erythrocyte velocity measurements in microvessels by a two-slit photometric method. J Appl Physiol 22:333–337
12. Lipowsky HH, Usami S, Chien S, Pittman RN (1982) Hematocrit determination in small bore tubes by differential spectrophotometry. Microvasc Res 24:42–55
13. Pittman RN, Duling BR (1975) Measurement of percent oxyhemoglobin in the microvasculature. J Appl Physiol 38:321–327
14. Tyml K, Sherebrin MH (1980) A method for on-line measurements of red cell velocity in microvessels using computerized frame-by-frame analysis of television images. Microvasc Res 20:1–8

15. Ellis CG, Fraser S, Hamilton G, Groom AC (1984) Measurement of the lineal density of red blood cells in capillaries in vivo, using a computerized frame-by-frame analysis of video images. Microvasc Res 27:1–13
16. Ellis CG, Ellsworth ML, Pittman RN (1990) Determination of red blood cell oxygenation in vivo by dual video densitometric image analysis. Am J Physiol 258:H1216–H1223
17. Whalen WJ, Riley J, Nair P (1967) A microelectrode for measuring intracellular PO_2. J Appl Physiol 23:798–801
18. Vanderkooi JM, Maniara G, Green TJ, Wilson DF (1987) An optical method for measurement of dioxygen concentration based on quenching of phosphorescence. J Biol Chem 262:5476–5482
19. Zheng L, Golub AS, Pittman RN (1996) Determination of PO_2 and its heterogeneity in single capillaries. Am J Physiol 271:H365–H372
20. Pittman RN, Golub AS, Popel AS, Zheng L (1998) Interpretation of phosphorescence quenching measurements made in the presence of oxygen gradients. In: Hudetz A, Bruley D (eds) Oxygen transport to tissue XX. Plenum Press, New York (in press)
21. Sharan M, Popel AS (1988) A mathematical model of countercurrent exchange of oxygen between paired arterioles and venules. Math Biosci 90:17–34
22. Stein JC, Ellis CG, Ellsworth ML (1993) Relationship between capillary and systemic venous PO_2 during nonhypoxic and hypoxic ventilation. Am J Physiol 265:H537–H542
23. Shonat RD, Johnson PC (1997) Oxygen tension gradients and heterogeneity in venous microcirculation: a phosphorescence quenching study. Am J Physiol 272:H2233–H2240
24. Popel AS, Pittman RN, Ellsworth ML (1989) The rate of oxygen loss from arterioles is an order of magnitude higher than expected. Am J Physiol 256:H921–H924
25. Ellsworth ML, Pittman RN (1984) Heterogeneity of oxygen diffusion through hamster striated muscles. Am J Physiol 246:H161–H167
26. Meng H, Bentley TB, Pittman RN (1992) Oxygen diffusion in hamster striated muscle: comparison of in vitro and near in vivo conditions. Am J Physiol 263:H35–H39
27. Bentley TB, Meng H, Pittman RN (1993) Temperature dependence of oxygen diffusion and consumption in mammalian striated muscle. Am J Physiol 264:H1825–H1830
28. Bentley TB, Pittman RN (1997) Influence of temperature on oxygen diffusion in hamster retractor muscle. Am J Physiol 272:H1106–H1112
29. Mahler M, Louy C, Homsher E, Peskoff A (1985) Reappraisal of diffusion, solubility, and consumption of oxygen in frog skeletal muscle, with applications to muscle energy balance. J Gen Physiol 86:105–134
30. Pittman RN (1995) Microvascular architecture and oxygen exchange in skeletal muscle. Microcirculation 2:1–18
31. Ellsworth ML, Popel AS, Pittman RN (1988) Assessment and impact of heterogeneities of convective oxygen transport parameters in capillaries of striated muscle: Experimental and theoretical. Microvasc Res 35:341–362
32. Popel AS, Charny CB, Dvinsky AS (1986) Effect of heterogeneous oxygen delivery on oxygen distribution in skeletal muscle. Math Biosci 81:91–113
33. Ellsworth ML, Pittman RN (1990) Arterioles supply oxygen to capillaries by diffusion as well as by convection. Am J Physiol 258:H1240–H1243
34. Ellsworth ML, Ellis CG, Popel AS, Pittman RN (1994) Role of microvessels in oxygen supply to tissue. News Physiol Sci 9:119–123
35. Granger HJ, Meininger GA, Borders JL, Morff RJ, Goodman AH (1984) Microcirculation of skeletal muscle. In: Mortillaro NA (ed) The physiology and pharmacology of the microcirculation, Vol 2. Academic Press, New York, pp 181–265
36. Segal SS (1992) Convection, diffusion, and mitochondrial utilization of oxygen during exercise. In: Lamb DR, Gisolfi CG (eds) Energy metabolism in exercise and sport. Brown and Benchmark, New York, pp 269–344
37. Wagner PD (1996) Determinants of maximal oxygen transport and utilization. Annu Rev Physiol 58:21–50
38. Pittman RN (1986) Interaction between oxygen and the blood vessel wall. Can J Cardiol 2:124–131
39. Ellsworth ML, Forrester T, Ellis CG, Dietrich HH (1995) The erythrocyte as a regulator of vascular tone. Am J Physiol 269:H2155–H2161

40. Weibel ER (1984) The pathway for oxygen. Harvard Univ Press, Cambridge
41. Hellums JD (1977) The resistance of oxygen transport in the capillaries relative to that in the surrounding tissue. Microvasc Res 13:131–136
42. Federspiel WJ, Sarelius IH (1984) An examination of the contribution of red cell spacing to the uniformity of oxygen flux at the capillary wall. Microvasc Res 27:273–285
43. Federspiel WJ, Popel AS (1986) A theoretical analysis of the effect of the particulate nature of blood on oxygen release in capillaries. Microvasc Res 32:164–189
44. Groebe K, Thews G (1989) Effect of red cell spacing and red cell movement upon oxygen release under conditions of maximally working skeletal muscle. Adv Exp Med Biol 248:175–185
45. Groebe K, Thews G (1990) Calculated intra- and extracellular PO_2 gradients in heavily working red muscle. Am J Physiol 259:H84–H92
46. Wang C-H, Popel AS (1993) Effect of red blood cell shape on oxygen transport in capillaries. Math Biosci 116:89–110
47. Groebe K (1995) An easy-to-use model for O_2 supply to red muscle. Validity of assumptions, sensitivity to errors in data. Biophys J 68:1246–1269
48. Roy TK, Popel AS (1996) Theoretical predictions of end-capillary PO_2 in muscles of athletic and non-athletic animals at VO_{2max}. Am J Physiol 271:H721–H737
49. Honig CR, Gayeski TEJ (1993) Resistance to O_2 diffusion in anemic red muscle: Roles of flux density and cell PO_2. Am J Physiol 265:H868–H875
50. Gayeski TEJ, Honig CR (1991) Intracellular PO_2 in individual cardiac myocytes in dogs, cats, rabbits, ferrets, and rats. Am J Physiol 260:H522–H531
51. Voter WA, Gayeski TEJ (1995) Determination of myoglobin saturation of frozen specimens using a reflecting cryospectrophotometer. Am J Physiol 269:H1328–H1341
52. Hogan MC, Bebout DE, Wagner PD (1991) Effect of hemoglobin concentration on maximal O_2 uptake in canine gastrocnemius muscle. J Appl Physiol 70:1105–1112
53. Wagner PD (1995) Muscle O_2 transport and O_2 dependent control of metabolism. Med Sci Sports Exerc 27:47–53
54. Richardson RS, Noyazewski EA, Kendrick KF, Leigh JS, Wagner PD (1995) Myoglobin O_2 desaturation during exercise. Evidence of limited O_2 transport. J Clin Invest 96:1916–1926
55. Popel AS (1989) Theory of oxygen transport to tissue. Crit Rev Biomed Eng 17:257–321
56. Page TC, Light WR, McKay CB, Hellums JD (1998) Oxygen transport by erythrocyte/hemoglobin solution mixtures in an in vitro capillary as a model of hemoglobin-based oxygen carrier performance. Microvasc Res 55:54–64
57. Khandelwal SR, Randad RS, Lin P-S, et al (1993) Enhanced oxygenation in vivo by allosteric inhibitors of hemoglobin saturation. Am J Physiol 265:H1450–H1453
58. Sarelius IH (1986) Cell flow path influences transit time through striated muscle capillaries. Am J Physiol 250:H899–H907
59. Sarelius IH (1990) An analysis of microcirculatory flow heterogeneity using measurements of transit time. Microvasc Res 40:88–98
60. Sarelius IH (1993) Cell and oxygen flow in arterioles controlling capillary perfusion. Am J Physiol 265:H1682–H1687
61. Duling BR, Damon DH (1987) An examination of the measurement of flow heterogeneity in striated muscle. Circ Res 60:1–13
62. Laughlin MH (1991) Heterogeneity of blood flow in striated muscle. In: Crystal RG, West JB (eds) The Lung: Scientific foundations. Raven Press, New York, pp 1507–1516
63. Kurdak SS, Grassi B, Wagner PD, Hogan MC (1995) Effect of [Hb] on blood flow distribution and O_2 transport in maximally working skeletal muscle. J Appl Physiol 79:1729–1735
64. Tyml K, Cheng L (1995) Heterogeneity of red blood cell velocity in skeletal muscle decreses with increased flow. Microcirculation 2:181–194
65. Wieringa PA, Stassen HG, Van Kan JJI, Spaan JAE (1993) Oxygen diffusion in a network model of the myocardium. Int J Microcirc Clin Exp 13:137–169
66. Bassingthwaighte JB, Beard DA (1995) Fractal ^{15}O-labelled water washout from the heart. Circ Res 77:1212–1221
67. King RB, Raymind GM, Bassingthwaighte JB (1996) Modeling blood flow heterogeneity. Ann Biomed Eng 24:352–272

68. Yu M, Levy MM, Smith P, Takaguchi SA, Miyasaki A, Myers SA (1993) Effect of maximizing oxygen delivery on morbidity and mortality rates in critically ill patients: a prospective, randomized, controlled study. Crit Care Med 21:830–838
69. Leach RM, Treacher DF (1994) The relationship between oxygen delivery and consumption. Disease-a-Month 60:303–368
70. Hayes MA, Timmins AC, Yau EHS, Palazzo M, Hinds CJ, Watson D (1994) Elevation of systemic oxygen delivery in the treatment of critically ill patients. N Engl J Med 330: 1717–1722
71. Bishop MH, Shoemaker WC, Appel PL, et al (1995) Prospective, randomized trial of survivor values of cardiac index, oxygen delivery, and oxygen consumption as resuscitation endpoints in severe trauma. J Trauma 38:780–787

Oxygen Distribution and Consumption by the Microcirculation and the Determinants of Tissue Survival

A. G. Tsai, H. Kerger, and M. Intaglietta

Introduction

In most organisms oxygen (O_2) requirements cannot be supplied directly from the environment and circulatory systems have evolved to meet these needs. Provision and extraction of the necessary gases to/from the tissue cell mass, follows a scheme embedded into the origins of physiological thinking that starts with the observation that lung capillaries are the interface between the atmosphere and the circulation. The subsequent observation that capillaries permeate all tissues of upper forms of life led to the "mirror image" conclusion that these conduits, where red blood cells transit in single file, reverse their function, yielding the O_2 acquired in the lung to the tissues and *vice versa* for carbon dioxide.

Experimental evaluation of the role of capillaries in tissues is elusive due to the lack of experimental techniques that allow the direct examination of capillaries within the tissue. Lung capillaries are equally intractable from an experimental viewpoint, although the lung presents defined gas and blood inputs and outputs that give a firm basis for modeling lung capillary transport events. This situation is not present in tissues, and gas exchange to and from tissue capillaries has relied on theoretical analysis that began with Krogh [1] and Erlangen, who assumed that capillaries are the primary sites of O_2 delivery (DO_2). They described analytically how gases are exchanged between blood flowing in a cylindrical conduit, the single capillary, and a surrounding tissue cylinder, and tissue oxygenation was extrapolated as the summation of the contribution of each of the unitary components. This idealization implies that most O_2 is exchanged by the capillaries which therefore must have large blood/tissue O_2 gradients. Since most capillaries have O_2 tensions (PO_2) in the range of 30–20 mm Hg a substantial fraction of the arterial O_2 has left the blood vessels prior to arriving at the capillaries. Furthermore, venous blood PO_2, presumed to be representative of tissue PO_2, is in the range of 30 to 40 mm Hg in most organs with the exception of the heart where it is 20 mm Hg [2]. Given that tissue PO_2 is about 25 mm Hg, capillaries should be in virtual O_2 equilibrium with the tissue, and therefore void of the steep gradients needed for supplying O_2 to the tissue.

Considerations of DO_2 on the basis of the blood O_2 content must include the O_2 carrying capacity of hemoglobin (Hb), which shows that O_2 saturation at 25 mm Hg is 50%. Most studies of O_2 distribution in the microcirculation show that capillary PO_2 is seldom below 20 mm Hg, while values above 30 mm Hg correspond to the PO_2 in arterioles. Therefore in most tissues, capillaries deliver at most 20% of the O_2 gathered by the lungs, if the PO_2 in capillaries becomes as low as 20 mm Hg, which is difficult to reconcile with a mixed venous PO_2 of 40 mm Hg.

The Role of Capillaries in Tissue Oxygenation

The concept that capillaries constitute the primary site of gas exchange within the tissue probably originates from the observation that as a consequence of their large number they provide a large surface area for material and gas exchange. Gas exchange however, is determined by additional parameters such as the permeability/diffusion/metabolism characteristics of the exchange barrier, and the concentration gradient that drives the exchange. For gases such as O_2, carbon dioxide (CO_2) and nitric oxide (NO), the fact that tissue is mostly water (more than 80% composition) and the physical similarity of these molecules determine that their diffusion constant is nearly the same and similar to the diffusion constant for these gases in water, throughout the organism.

Concentration gradients that drive the material transfer are different. Capillary/tissue O_2 gradients are maximal in the lung (50 mm Hg/μ) and minimal in the tissues (0.5 mm Hg/μ). This large disparity is in part compensated by the large tissue versus lung capillary surface area; however, as tissue and lung respiration are quantitatively different they may also be qualitatively different.

Experimental findings indicate that capillaries may not have a predominant role in supplying O_2 in some tissues. There is much to be learned in this respect. It is generally accepted that in all tissues capillary PO_2 is about 25 mm Hg, and is actively regulated to that value. When this finding is related to the properties of the dissociation of O_2 from Hb, it indicates that at least half of the O_2 in blood exits the blood vessels prior to arrival to the tissue. It should be noted that in a few instances tissue PO_2 has been reported to be below 20 mm Hg under normal conditions.

Microvascular Evidence for PO_2 Distribution

The nature of O_2 distribution in the tissue at the microscopic level has been known since the 70s when data was obtained with polarographic microelectrode measurements [3]. These results have been repeatedly tested with the development of the spectrophotometric technique for the measurement of O_2 saturation in blood [4], showing that a substantial portion of arterial O_2 is delivered prior its arrival in the capillaries. In fact, O_2 maps of the arteriolar network revealed that arterioles deliver O_2 to the tissue at such a rate that it could not be accounted for by the O_2 gradients measured by electrode techniques in the surrounding tissue [5]. Pittman [6] recently reviewed the existing data and confirmed again that arterioles play a significant role in delivering O_2 to the tissue.

Examination of the PO_2 distribution in the microcirculation has been considerably simplified through the introduction of technology based on phosphorescence quenching of metallo-organic compounds for measuring PO_2 optically in the microvessels and surrounding tissue [7–11]. This technology was used by us to map PO_2 in the hamster window preparation which allows the *in vivo* analysis of PO_2, in the absence of anesthesia, in blood and in tissue. The tissue of this preparation includes subcutaneous connective tissue and a skin muscle layer perfused by a capillary network. The distribution of tissue is approximately two thirds connective tissue and one third skin muscle.

The technology has been validated *in vitro* and *in vivo* by comparison with microelectrode measurements and found to satisfactorily portray microscopic PO_2, providing results that are equivalent in all aspects with those of all other methods for measuring PO_2 where the microanatomy is evident. Therefore this methodology does not necessarily agree with the multiwire method of Kessler et al. [12], or surface electrodes, techniques that are not sufficiently spatially selective for detailed tissue versus blood vessel discrimination.

The principal findings on PO_2 distribution are given in Figure 1 which shows that arteriolar blood enters the microcirculation of the hamster skin fold model at about 58 mm Hg (65% saturated), capillary PO_2 is about 30 mm Hg (52% saturation), venular capillary PO_2 is the same as capillary PO_2 [13]. Therefore virtually no or little O_2 is delivered as blood transits from the capillaries to the collecting

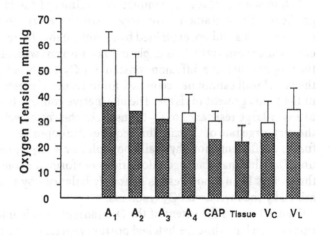

Fig. 1. Distribution of PO_2 in the microcirculation of the awake hamster skin fold. A_1: Major arterioles in this model with diameter in the range 50–60 micrometers (μ). A_{2-3}: Descending order of arterioles. A_4: Terminal arterioles, 5–8 μ diameter. CAP: Capillaries. V_c: Collecting venules. V_L: Large venules. The full length of the bar represents intravascular blood PO_2. The white portion of the bar is the gap in PO_2 between the blood-tissue interface and the measurement in the tissue at a distance about 3 μ from the interface. This difference in PO_2 divided by the distance over which it is measured is the wall PO_2 gradient that determines the rate of exit of oxygen by diffusion from the arterioles, which is confirmed by mass balance calculations. This rate of diffusional exit is responsible for the decline in PO_2 from the A_1 arterioles to the capillaries. The increase in PO_2 in the large venules is due to shunting. The hatched portion of the bar represents the oxygen in the tissue outside of the blood vessel wall, showing that virtually no oxygen is given by the capillaries to tissue. (From [25] with permission)

venules. Large venule PO_2 is 34 mm Hg, indicating that O_2 has been acquired by either convective or diffusive shunting.

This data shows that even though this tissue uses comparatively little O_2, most of the O_2 is delivered by the arterioles, and virtually no O_2 is delivered by the capillaries.

Detailed Analysis of Blood Vessel Oxygen Microenvironment

The phosphorescence decay technology allows us to measure PO_2 in the tissue and therefore explore PO_2 in the immediate vicinity of the microvessels. This methodology has been criticized in the past under the assumption that oxygen consumption (VO_2) by phosphorescence emission yields abnormally low values for tissue PO_2. Calibration of the technique with fluid samples has demonstrated that the VO_2 by the probe is between 100 to 1000 times smaller than the rate of DO_2 from the neighboring vessels. Furthermore measurements with the polarographic and phosphorescence techniques in tissue give identical results for tissue PO_2, and values obtained are essentially identical to those produced by all other methods. Therefore we conclude that PO_2 measurements in tissue are accurate and not subject to artifacts.

PO_2 measurements in the immediate vicinity of the blood vessels reveal large gradients. These gradients are larger than those expected solely from diffusion considerations and are explained by assuming that there is a large VO_2 in the microvascular vessel wall. This explanation conforms with physical principles, while the proposal that the diffusion constant for O_2 may be a factor of 10 greater [5] in the vessel wall cannot be accounted for in terms of mechanisms for O_2 transport in the fluids present in tissue. The alternative concept that the gradients are due to a very large resistance to O_2 diffusion in the vessel wall is not compatible with the very large rate of O_2 exit. This requires the opposite, namely, either a large diffusion coefficient (not physically possible) or a large gradient (which we measure). Detailed mass balance calculations performed in our laboratories show that the O_2 loss from blood vessels is exactly balanced by the diffusional exit determined by the measured PO_2 gradients.

Figure 1 shows the extent of the O_2 gradient, which amounts to the white portion of each bar, while the hatched portion represents the tissue PO_2 in the immediate vicinity of the blood vessels. It is important to consider that measurements are made in a region that is about 3 micrometers from the blood tissue interface. It is therefore apparent that a large amount of the O_2 delivered by the blood vessel does not reach the tissue. In fact virtually none of the O_2 delivered by capillaries reaches the tissue, since there is no PO_2 gradient outside a capillary tissue cylinder that is about 3 micrometers thicker than the inner capillary radius.

These findings have the following implications:
1) Capillaries deliver most of their O_2 to a thin tissue layer that surrounds them. This layer is about 3 micrometers thick and includes the endothelium.
2) Arterio/venous capillary PO_2 differences are virtually non–existent.

3) The only tissue region with large PO_2 inhomogeneity is the immediate vicinity of the microvessels, namely the microvascular wall.
4) Blood O_2 is delivered to the tissue by the arterioles.
5) The vessel wall serves as a metabolic barrier that protects the tissue from the high O_2 content of blood.
6) Capillary O_2 mostly serves to supply O_2 to the endothelium.
7) Arterio/venous shunts ensure that venular endothelium is oxygenated at the same level as capillary endothelium.

Cellular and Systemic Evidence for Arteriolar Endothelial Oxygen Consumption

The biological activity of the cellular components of the microvascular vessel wall suggests the need for large VO_2. The endothelium performs many biochemical functions that require O_2 [14, 15]. These include synthesis and secretion of renin, prostaglandins, collagen, endothelin, prostacyclin, NO, interleukins, factors V and VIII, degradation of bradykinin and prostaglandins, clearance of proteins, lipids and lipoproteins, conversion of angiotensin I to II, expression of antigens, synthesis of thrombomodulin, heparan sulfate proteoglycans, plasminogen activator, cell adhesion factor (CAM) and antiplatelet factors, to cite a few [16]. From purely mechanical considerations the endothelium in conjunction with smooth muscle undergoes a continuous expenditure of energy in performing mechanical work in contracting against blood pressure due to vasomotion in arterioles [17] and capillaries [18].

Experimental findings in whole organs further support the concept that endothelium is metabolically very active. Curtis et al. [19], denuded the vasculature of isolated dog hindlimbs and perfused the tissue with 40 mg/kg deoxycholate (DOC), a detergent extensively used in *in vitro* studies to remove endothelium. They found that removal of the endothelium caused O_2 extraction to decrease from 3.8 ± 1.1 to 2.5 ± 0.9 ml O_2/min kg, a decrease in VO_2 of about 35%.

When the vasculature of organs as diverse as the rat hindlimb, the kidney, intestine and the mesentery are caused to constrict and develop tone from a relaxed state, their VO_2 virtually doubles if blood flow is maintained constant. This finding is evidence of the high metabolic cost of vascular tone, and an indication of the partition of O_2 distribution and VO_2 between tissue and vascular compartments. In a study of the perfusion of rat hind limbs, Ye et al. [20] found that VO_2 increased from 5.4 ± 0.2 to a maximum value of 8.6 ml O_2/min kg, an increase of 59% in VO_2 that was directly attributable to the metabolic requirement of the development of tone by the vasculature. In the same study [20], it is reported that the mesenteric macro and microvasculature consumes O_2 at the rate of 42.8 ml O_2/min kg.

Tissue Oxygenation Versus Functional Capillary Density in Tissue Survival

A model that illustrates some of the concepts discussed is that of survival in long term hemorrhagic shock [21] and the analysis of microvascular conditions that lead to microvascular failure. These studies were conducted in the awake hamster skin fold chamber without anesthesia. In this study, animals were subjected to a period of 4 hours of hypotension at 40 mm Hg caused by blood withdrawal. Such a prolonged period has little clinical significance, but is crucial for observing the mechanisms that are operational. Analysis was made by differentiating between surviving (S) and non surviving animals (NS), where 30% of the animals subjected to the protocol did not survive.

A specific finding was that there is no difference between survivors and non-survivors in mixed venous PO_2 and Hb, while arterial PO_2 is significantly higher in non-survivors (120 mm Hg vs. 100 mm Hg for survivors). A preliminary conclusion that can be obtained from this result is that the intrinsic O_2 carrying capacity of blood as well as O_2 extraction are not determinant factors for outcome, a result that is also important for the design of blood volume restoration fluids [22]. In both survivors and non-survivors arterial PCO_2, standard bicarbonate and pH decreased during shock for both groups, and were significantly lower in non-survivors. Since this difference was not associated with O_2 availability we may assume that outcome is determined by functional differences that hinder the O_2 metabolic pathway.

Hemorrhage causes a global decrease of blood flow, which has been reported to be as much as 90% in skeletal muscle [23]. Although the decrease in blood flow was evident in all groups, non-survivors had significantly lower blood flow in the microcirculation by at least a factor of 2 relative to survivors. Surviving animals maintained some level of oxygenation in the arterioles and the tissue after 4 hours of shock, while the non-survivors presented lower values. However tissue PO_2 was near zero for both NS and S animals after 4 hours of shock. Severe shock conditions reduce DO_2 to the microcirculation of the skin fold chamber to less than 10% of the systemic control, with the result that tissue PO_2 was in the range of 1.0–0.5 mm Hg regardless of outcome.

There were neither qualitative nor quantitative differences in systemic DO_2 which, although depressed, was similar for both survivors and non-survivors after 4 hours of shock in the tissue investigated. Thus tissue oxygenation does not appear to be the sole determinant in determining outcome. Conversely, functional capillary density (FCD) is significantly affected by shock, with important differences between survivors and non-survivors since survivors present about 40% FCD after 4 hours of shock, while non-survivors have no functional capillaries at the end of the shock period. It should be noted that since tissue PO_2 is essentially zero for either group, the capillary density failure appears to be unrelated to the capacity of the capillaries to deliver the little available O_2, suggesting that in these conditions the critical role of capillaries may be linked to the extraction of metabolites rather than the supply of O_2.

Conclusion

The development of a new technique for the measurement of intravascular and tissue PO_2 has produced new findings on the distribution of PO_2 in the microcirculation. These findings corroborate previous intravascular measurements by other methods, but taken as a whole show that there is a very large O_2 sink at the microvascular vessel wall. Our results show that capillaries do not appear to play a mayor role in oxygenating the tissue, a fact that was intrinsic to older data on PO_2 distribution in the microcirculation. The discovery of the arteriolar vessel wall O_2 gradient is in accordance with available systemic data on VO_2 by the endothelium *in situ* and the vasculature. The existence of this gradient determined by the high metabolism of this microvascular tissue is also in conformity with the physical phenomenon needed for extracting comparatively large amounts of O_2 from the arterioles, an effect that cannot be explained by increased diffusivity. The large consumption of O_2 by the microvasculature could not be inferred from systemic measurement in the past because the metabolism of microvessels cannot be separated from the tissue on a systemic basis.

Capillary failure in shock appears to be one of the causes that leads to the demise of the organism. This phenomenon, although documented only in skeletal muscle and connective tissue, appears to be independent of O_2 availability. Although it is undeniable that tissue oxygenation is necessary for tissue survival, these studies indicate that functional capillaries are equally important in ensuring tissue viability, a fact explored in some detail in the clinical analysis of ischemia [24]. Therefore, attention should be given to the factors that contribute to capillary viability, since low O_2 states appear to be survivable when capillaries are open and functioning, but not otherwise.

These findings have critical consequences for the understanding of ischemic disease, because microvessel wall metabolism appears to be a regulator of O_2 transfer to the tissue. In this context an increase in metabolism caused by inflammation or other pathologies may deprive the tissue of O_2, a fact noted in many diseases where blood perfusion is adequate, but the tissue does not survive. These findings taken as a whole suggest that metabolism of the arteriolar endothelium may be a target for the treatment of ischemia.

Acknowledgement. The research described was supported by grants from the Heart and Lung Institute of the NIH and the Program Project NHLBI HL-48818.

References

1. Krogh A (1918) The number and distribution of capillaries in muscle with the calculation of the oxygen pressure necessary for supplying the tissue. J Physiol 52:409–515
2. Rothe CF, Friedman JJ (1984) Control in the cardiovascular system. In: Selkurt EE (ed) Physiology, 5th Edn. Little, Brown and Co, Boston, ch 17
3. Duling BR, Berne RM (1970) Longitudinal gradients in periarteriolar oxygen tension. A possible mechanism for the participation of oxygen in the local regular of blood flow. Circ Res 27:669–678

4. Pittman RN, Duling BR (1975) Measurement of percent hemoglobin in the microvasculature. J Appl Physiol 38:321–327
5. Popel AS, Pittman RN, Ellsworth ML (1989) Rate of oxygen loss from arterioles is an order of magnitude higher than expected. Am J Physiol 256:H921–H924
6. Pittman RN (1995) Influence of microvascular architecture on oxygen diffusion from arteriolar networks. Microcirculation 2:1–18
7. Vanderkooi JM, Maniara G, Green TJ, Wilson DF (1987) An optical method for measurement of dioxygen concentration based on quenching of phosphorescence. J Biol Chem 262: 5476–5482
8. Torres Filho IP, Intaglietta M (1993) Micro vessel PO_2 measurements by phosphorescence decay method. Am J Physiol 265:H1434–H1438
9. Torres Filho IP, Fan Y, Intaglietta M, Jain RK (1994) Non-invasive measurement of microvascular and interstitial oxygen profiles in a human tumor in SCID mice. Proc Natl Acad Sci USA 91:2081–2085
10. Shonat RD, Wilson DF, Riva CE, Pawlowski M (1992) Oxygen distribution in the retinal and choroidal vessels of the cat as measured by a new phosphorescence imaging method. Applied Optics 31:3711–3718
11. Wilson DF (1993) Measuring oxygen using oxygen dependent quenching of phosphorescence: A status report. Adv Exp Med Biol 333:225–232
12. Kessler M, Hoeper J, Krumme BA (1976) Monitoring of tissue perfusion and cellular function. Anesthesiology 45:184–197
13. Kerger H, Torres Filho IP, Rivas M, Winslow RM, Intaglietta M (1995) Systemic and subcutaneous microvascular oxygen tension in conscious Syrian golden hamsters. Am J Physiol 267:H802–H810
14. Bruttig SP, Joyner WL (1983) Metabolic characteristics of cells cultured from umbilical blood vessels: Comparison with 3T3 fibroblasts. J Cell Physiol 116:173–180
15. Kjellstrom BT, Ortenwall P, Risberg R (1987) Comparison of oxidative metabolism in vitro in endothelial cells from different species and vessels. J Cell Physiol 132:578–580
16. Kirkpatrick CJ, Wagner M, Hermanns I, et al (1997) Physiology and cell biology of the endothelium: A dynamic interface for cell communication. Int J Microcirc Clin Ex 17:231–240
17. Colantuoni A, Bertuglia S, Intaglietta M (1984) Quantitation of rhythmic diameter changes in arterial microcirculation. Am J Physiol 246:H508–H517
18. Tsai AG, Friesenecker B, Intaglietta M (1995) Capillary flow impairment and functional capillary density. Int J Microcirc 15 (Suppl 5):238–243
19. Curtis SE, Vallet B, Winn MJ, Caufield JB, King CE, Chapler CK, Cain SM (1995) Role of vascular endothelium in O_2 extraction during progressive ischemia in canine skeletal muscle. J Appl Physiol 79:1351–1360
20. Ye J-M, Colquhoun EQ, Clark MG (1990) A comparison of vasopressin and noradrenaline on oxygen uptake by perfused rat hind limb, kidney, intestine and mesenteric arcade suggests that it is in part due to contractile work by blood vessels. Gen Pharmac 21:805–810
21. Kerger H, Saltzman DJ, Menger MD, Messmer K, Intaglietta M (1996) Systemic and subcutaneous microvascular PO_2 dissociation during 4-h hemorrhagic shock in conscious hamsters. Am J Physiol 270:H827–H836
22. Intaglietta M (1997) Whitaker Lecture 1996: Microcirculation, biomedical engineering and artificial blood. Ann Biomed Eng 25:593–603
23. Zhao K-S, Junker D, Delano FA, Zweifach BW (1985) Microvascular adjustments during irreversible hemorrhagic shock in rat skeletal muscle. Microvasc Res 30:143–153
24. Fabrell B (1977) The skin microcirculation and the pathogenesis of ischemic necrosis and gangrene. Scand J Clin Lab Invest 37:473–476
25. Intaglietta M, Johnson PC, Winslow RM (1996) Microvascular and tissue oxygen distribution. Cardiovasc Res 32:632–643

Oxygen Signaling Cascades in Mammalian Cells

A. Görlach

Introduction

With the evolution from single prokaryotic cells to more complex multicellular organisms, oxygen (O_2) became essential for the survival of all higher life forms due to its role in mitochondrial respiration permitting adenosine triphosphate (ATP) synthesis by oxidative phosphorylation. Thus, the supply of O_2 to respiring tissues provides a fundamental physiological challenge for the organism. Inadequate O_2 supply will impair metabolic efficiency whereas overprovision of O_2 is not only wasteful but can, through excessive generation of reactive O_2 species (ROS), be potentially harmful. Thus the maintenance of an adequate supply of O_2 to the organs is mandatory, a process which requires the coordination of pulmonary, cardiac, vascular and central nervous function with cellular growth and metabolism. Therefore specialized O_2 sensing cells localized in chemoreceptive organs, vascular smooth muscle cells, in central neurons as well as in the kidney and liver, exist, which can be activated to induce adaptive responses at the systemic, local and cellular level by modulating O_2-sensitive ion channel activity and regulating O_2 dependent gene expression in order to restore appropriate O_2 availability to the cells. For example, a fall in O_2 tension (PO_2) is sensed by the carotid body which increases, by stimulating nerve discharge, the respiratory motoneuronal output. O_2 sensing cells in the lung smooth muscle cells mediate the constriction of pulmonary arteries in response to hypoxia, thereby allowing the shunt of blood from hypoxic to less hypoxic alveolar zones. The decrease in the ventilation/perfusion mismatch helps to sustain O_2 availability. However, the increase in cardio-respiratory output might not be sufficient in certain cases to compensate the decreased O_2 availability and eventually may not be able to adjust and protect other organs from the lack of O_2. Therefore, in addition to these classical O_2 sensors most, if not all, nucleated cells are able to sense and to respond to hypoxia by modulating O_2 dependent gene expression or ion channel activity [1]. For example, genes encoding important enzymes of carbohydrate metabolism are expressed zonally in the liver matching the heterogeneous O_2 distribution in this organ [2].

On the other hand, limited O_2 supply (DO_2) is found in various pathophysiological conditions including atherosclerosis, resulting in clinical syndromes such as angina pectoris, claudication, gangrene and infarctions of the myocardial and nervous system. Angiogenesis, organ fibrosis and wound repair are other conditions where limited DO_2 is crucial for the outcome and prognosis of disease. Hypoxic areas are frequently found in growing solid tumors and have been responsible for tumor resistance to radio- and chemotherapy as well as for progressive tumor growth and metastasis due to neoangiogenesis. Depending on the severity and duration of hypoxia, a cascade of events can be triggered which can lead to permanent injury or death or to adaptation and survival. Crucial in this cascade is how the cascade is initiated, how lack of O_2 is detected by the cells, and how these initial steps can activate further processes.

Oxygen Sensing and the Response to Hypoxia

Chemoreceptors such as the carotid body, as well as the cells producing erythropoietin under hypoxia are regarded as the classical O_2 sensors. In the carotid body, type I cells are able to respond to hypoxia twofold [3]. First, O_2-sensitive potassium (K^+) channels are inhibited thus allowing calcium (Ca^{2+}) influx and a fast release of neurotransmitters which excite sensory afferent terminals thereby stimulating the brain stem respiratory centers to increase respiration. Second, hypoxia induces the expression of tyrosine hydroxylase starting at 1 h and peaking after 6 h. This enzyme is responsible for the production of neurotransmitters enabling the type I cells to exert enhanced nervous activity to improve the ventilatory drive and blood circulation in acute and chronic hypoxia. In addition to this classical O_2 sensor there is increasing evidence that O_2-sensitive ion channels, for example K^+ and Ca^{2+} channels, are more broadly distributed in different cell types than previously thought, including neurons, myocytes and endothelial cells. Such O_2 sensitive channels might be involved in the regulation of vasomotor tone under hypoxia [4].

One of the best examples of O_2 regulated gene expression is the regulation of erythropoiesis by erythropoietin [5]. The major signal appears to arise from reduced tissue DO_2 resulting in mainly transcriptional activation of gene expression in the liver and kidney. Hypoxic erythropoietin production cannot be induced by 'chemical hypoxia' such as inhibition of the respiratory chain or by other cell stresses such as heat shock, but can be stimulated by certain transition metals including cobalt (Co^{2+}), manganese (Mn^{2+}), and nickel (Ni^{2+}) as well as by the iron chelator desferrioxamine. O_2 can influence the expression of many different genes responsible for various important cellular functions. In the vascular system O_2 dependent gene expression is involved in the proliferation of fibroblasts, smooth muscle cells and endothelial cells [6], in angiogenesis and neovascularization in tumors and ischemic tissues [7], endothelial specific functions such as coagulation, cell adhesion and permeability [8], as well as in the regulation of vasomotor activity [9]. O_2 dependent gene regulation plays a role in glucose metabolism and transport [10, 11], as well as in catecholamine metabolism [12]. Cellular proliferation on one side, but also apoptosis and cell death on the other side, are influenced by genes regulated by hypoxia. These genes might contribute to the uncontrolled growth behavior of tumors, enabling cells within the tumor to survive and to proliferate in areas with limited DO_2 due to insufficient vessel architecture [13–15].

Evidence for a widely operative regulatory mechanism mediating the response to O_2 availability arose from two observations. First, striking similarities were found in these genes in their response not only to hypoxia, but also to stimuli initially described to induce the erythropoietin gene such as Co^{2+}, or desferrioxamine. Second, analysis of cis-acting elements of these different genes has revealed the critical importance of common regulatory elements and transcription factors. However, it is far from understood how cells are able to sense O_2 availability. Classically, the paradigm for gene regulation in response to an external stimulus would involve a ligand-receptor interaction followed by a series of chemical steps that transduce the signal leading to the expression of appropriate genes, for example by induction or repression of transcription or changes in messenger ribonucleic acid (mRNA) stability or through translational control. Thus a working model to study O_2 signaling cascades would include a cellular sensor protein as a receptor to interact with O_2 thereby inducing or inhibiting signal transduction cascades which then either modulate ion channel activities or lead to the induction or repression of desoxyribonucleic acid-(DNA-) and/or RNA-binding proteins which eventually modulate gene expression or transmitter release in order to adapt to the initial stimulus (Fig. 1).

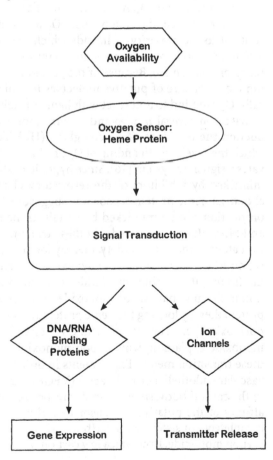

Fig. 1. A working model to study oxygen signaling cascades includes a cellular oxygen sensor protein as a receptor to interact with oxygen thereby inducing or inhibiting signal transduction cascades. The modulation of ion channel activities or the induction or repression of DNA- and/or RNA-binding proteins leads to adaptive responses to oxygen availability by altered gene expression or transmitter release

Identification of the Oxygen Sensor

Any process which is affected by O_2 in a concentration dependent manner could in theory form the basis of O_2 sensing. Under hypoxic conditions a variety of events are caused by the compromise of energy metabolism. Thus, gene expression by hypoxia could be triggered by one or several of these processes. However, inhibition of the respiratory chain does not affect the expression of a number of O_2 dependent genes including erythropoietin, indicating that the signaling mechanisms are not directly related to energy metabolism.

In principle, O_2 sensing could be based on two different forms of molecular interaction with O_2. First, O_2 could act as an electron acceptor in a redox based sensing system. O_2 dependent signals could be generated through the rate of production of ROS, or by diversion of electrons from an alternate acceptor by O_2, or by changing the redox state of one component of a reducing system. Alternatively, a chain of redox reactions, with O_2 as the terminal electron acceptor, could take place where signals could be generated by the redox state of components quite distant from the reaction with O_2 itself, as long as such a system would be close enough to equilibrium in order to preserve the dependence of the redox state on the concentration of O_2. A second form of O_2 sensing would involve the classical ligand-receptor configuration where O_2 would represent the ligand. However, in contrast to the majority of ligands which act solely as messengers, O_2s central role in metabolic respiration is dominant over its role in signaling via a sensor-receptor mechanism. Because of the peculiar chemical properties of O_2 there is a limited repertoire of putative molecules to which it can combine. Characteristically, O_2 can bind to and react with heme proteins.

Based on several *in vivo* and *in vitro* models of hypoxic erythropoietin production the existence of a hemoglobin(Hb)-like sensor has been proposed in which the reversible liganding of O_2 produces a conformational change and activates a signaling system [16]. Since hypoxic erythropoietin production cannot be mimicked by inhibitors of the respiratory chain such as cyanide, a non-mitochondrial heme protein sensor was suggested. However, hypoxic erythropoietin production can be mimicked by certain transition metals such as Co^{2+}, Ni^{2+}, and Mn^{2+}. It was suggested that these transition metals could substitute for the iron atom in the heme moiety, thereby locking the protein in the deoxy configuration which then mimics the hypoxic state. Further evidence was provided by the finding that carbon monoxide could inhibit hypoxic erythropoietin induction indicating that carbon monoxide would ligand the ferrous iron of the heme protein thereby locking the heme protein in the oxy configuration and simulating normoxia. Heme substituted with Co^{2+} or Ni^{2+}, in contrast, fails to bind carbon monoxide explaining why carbon monoxide did not abrogate the response to these transition metals. Experiments in other cell types producing, for example, vascular endothelial growth factor (VEGF) in an O_2 dependent manner, as well as in the carotid body, showed similar responses to hypoxia and an apparently low affinity of the putative O_2 sensor to carbon monoxide. These findings are not completely consistent with a Hb-like O_2 sensor since Hb has a high affinity to carbon monoxide. However, a low carbon monoxide affinity O_2 sensor would still be responsive in carbon monoxide-mediated hypoxic stress. Furthermore, inhibitors of heme synthesis as well as iron chelators such as desferrioxamine are able to abrogate the hypoxic response of erythropoietin. Thus, four experimental criteria for O_2 sensing via a heme based sensor protein have been developed:

1) normoxia should negate the response even in the presence of metabolic inhibitors such as cyanide
2) Co^{2+}, and Ni^{2+}, as well as desferrioxamine should mimic the hypoxic effects
3) Carbon monoxide should reverse hypoxic responses
4) inhibitors of heme synthesis should abrogate the effects of hypoxia, Co^{2+}, Ni^{2+}, and desferrioxamine.

Whereas the nature of such a heme protein O_2 sensor remains rather obscure in mammalian cells, heme proteins that play a role in O_2 sensing have been detected in bacteria. The best studied example is found in nitrogen fixing bacteria such as *Rhizobium meliloti* where nitrogen fixing genes are regulated by O_2 via the FixLJ network [17]. A two-domain heme protein termed FixL defines a heme-based sensor protein. In the absence of O_2 it becomes autophosphorylated to FixL phosphate, and the phosphate is then transferred to FixJ. Since its phosphatase function is inhibited under hypoxia, FixL can respond to O_2 by regulation of both its autokinase as well as its phosphatase activities. Although this two-domain heme protein is ideally suited to sense O_2 and transduce its presence via kinase activity no evidence has been provided yet that a similar O_2 sensing system is also present in mammalian cells.

In addition, some further aspects of erythropoietin regulation by hypoxia do not fit with a Hb-like sensor protein; acute exposure of normoxic cells to desferrioxamine stimulates erythropoietin production whereas pre-incubation of cells with desferrioxamine reduces hypoxic erythropoietin production [18, 19]. It was suggested that desferrioxamine might interact with the heme-bound iron or act via interference with the synthesis of a rapid turn over heme protein. Since heme iron is, in contrast to the "free" cellular iron pool, not directly chelatable by desferrioxamine, these suggestions are not compatible with a simple Hb-like sensor system and are not sufficient to explain why desferrioxamine can mimic hypoxia. Alternatively, desferrioxamine might prevent O_2 dependent radical production which is sensitive to iron chelation such as described in the Fenton reaction. Indeed, evidence has been provided recently that desferrioxamine interferes with the iron mediated degradation of hydrogen peroxide (H_2O_2) as described in the Fenton reaction in hepatoma cells [20]. These findings would also be consistent with an O_2 sensing system involving chelatable non-heme iron moieties such as iron sulfur (Fe-S) clusters. O_2-responsive Fe-S clusters are known in *E. coli* for example, where the transcriptional regulator FNR (fumarate and nitrate reductase regulator) is required for the switch from aerobic to anaerobic metabolism. It is suggested that O_2 is supplied to the cytoplasmic FNR by diffusion and inactivates FNR by direct interaction. The reactivation under anoxic condition requires cellular reductants [21].

Furthermore, a heme protein as part of a multicomponent electron transport system, in which non-heme and/or heme iron moieties are involved, would also be a consistent candidate. Based on spectrophotometric studies in erythropoietin producing human hepatoma cells, a low potential b-type cytochrome was identified that was reoxidized by hypoxia but not by cyanide and that had a low affinity to carbon monoxide [22]. Treatment with cobalt chloride could abolish the hypoxic reduction of this cytochrome, whereas the redox state of mitochondrial cytochromes remained unaffected [23]. A heme protein with similar characteristics is known as cytochrome b558 and is part of the nicotinamide adenine dinucleotide (phosphate) (NAD(P)H) oxidase of phagocytes [24]. This multicomponent enzyme is able to generate, on stimulation with bacteria and other toxins, large amounts of ROS in the respiratory burst by transferring electrons from NAD(P)H via flavin and heme moieties to molecular O_2. Immunohistochemistry and Western blot analysis provided evidence for the presence of components of the NAD(P)H oxidase termed p22, p47, p67 and gp91, in these erythropoietin producing cells [23]. Furthermore erythropoietin producing hepatoma cells were able to generate H_2O_2 in an O_2-dependent manner although with a much lower rate than the phagocyte enzyme, consistent with the idea that a "low output" NAD(P)H oxidase might generate ROS dependent on the O_2 availability. The change in the cellular redox state might then transfer the stimulus from the O_2 sensor to the effector. The redox state of the cell is determined by the amount of different species of ROS generated mainly by membrane bound oxido-reductases such as the NAD(P)H oxidase or the respiratory chain, as well as by the amount of scavenger systems such as catalase, thioredoxin, Ref1, glutathione peroxidase, vitamins C and E, cysteine and histidine residues, including the content of "free" iron [25]. ROS may serve as second messengers and induce the expression of the genes described above, regulate cell cycle and cell division and modulate ion channel activity. Signaling might either involve direct interactions of ROI with certain transcription factors or indirectly modulate activity of transcription factors by tyrosine kinases, Ras/Raf/MAP kinases, or scavenger systems [26, 27]. In human hepatoma cells, H_2O_2 production by a NAD(P)H oxidase decreased under hypoxic conditions. Inhibition of the NAD(P)H oxidase with concomitant reduction of the intracellular H_2O_2 concentration on the other hand induced erythropoietin production [28].

Similar studies were performed in chemoreceptive organs such as the carotid body or neuroepithelial bodies of the lung known to be crucially involved in O_2 sensing in the body. The addition of H_2O_2 inhibited the hypoxic nerve discharge in the carotid body [29]. The spectrophotometric detection of cytochrome b558 together with the identification of four NAD(P)H oxidase components by immunofluorescence in hypoxia-responsive type I cells in the carotid body suggested the presence of NAD(P)H oxidase in this organ [30]. In pulmonary neuroepithelial bodies representing airway chemoreceptive organs in the lung, all NAD(P)H oxidase components were identified in close vicinity to O_2 sensitive K^+ channels in the membrane. Since the activity of these channels could be modulated by H_2O_2 it was suggested that an NAD(P)H oxidase might be involved in O_2-dependent regulation of channel activity in neuroepithelial bodies [31]. Moreover, the expression of the small subunit of cytochrome b558, p22, as well as H_2O_2 production have also been demonstrated in small intensely fluorescent cells (SIF), hypoxia-sensitive paraganglionic structures found throughout the body [32], indicating that NAD(P)H oxidase might play a specific role in O_2 sensitive cells. The molecular identity of these components remains, however, to be clarified. In patients with defective NAD(P)H oxidase function due to mutations in the genes encoding any of four subunits, O_2 sensing does not appear to be impaired, indicating that either multiple overlapping O_2 sensing systems are present, or that NAD(P)H oxidase isoforms exist in O_2 sensing cells. Furthermore, other b-type cytochromes including cytochrome P450 forms [33, 34] cannot be excluded as O_2 sensors. Interestingly, diphylene iodonium (DPI), initially known as an inhibitor of the NAD(P)H oxidase, decreased hypoxic gene expression but could not impair gene expression induced by Co^{2+} or desferrioxamine. Although DPI has been shown to be a rather unspecific inhibitor of flavoprotein oxidoreductases, these findings suggest that such an oxidoreductase might be involved in O_2 sensing, and that the site of action of Co^{2+} and desferrioxamine differs from O_2 signaling [35].

Oxygen Regulated Transcription Factors

In the search for the molecular basis of O_2 dependent regulation of erythropoietin, a hypoxia responsive enhancer element was identified in the 3′ flanking region [16]. This enhancer has been shown to operate in an inducible manner also in a variety of non erythropoietin producing cells in response to hypoxia [36]. The response was critically dependent on the binding of a nucleoprotein termed hypoxia inducible factor-1 (HIF-1) and could be blocked by cycloheximide indicating the involvement of *de novo* protein synthesis [37]. Affinity purification revealed the existence of at least two DNA binding proteins, HIF-1α and HIF-1β, which bind as heterodimers to DNA and belong to the basic helix-loop-helix/PAS family of transcription factors. Members of this subgroup of transcription factors are characterized by NH2 terminal bHLH domains which mediate DNA binding and protein dimerization, as well as a homology region termed PAS domain after the first transcription factors detected in this family (Per, ARNT, Sim). This domain might be involved in protein dimerization, DNA binding and transactivation [38]. Recently, highly conserved regions termed S boxes have been identified in PAS domains in a large family of sensor proteins present in all kingdoms [39]. The sensory signals for these activator proteins are O_2 (redox) or light. Interestingly, not only HIF-1α and HIF-1β contained this sensory signal, but also the only true O_2 sensor identified so far, namely the oxygen-dependent kinase FixL from *Rhizobium meliloti* (see above).

Whereas HIF-1α is a new member of this family, HIF-1β is identical to the previously identified transcription factor aryl hydrocarbon receptor nuclear translocator (ARNT), known as a heterodimerization partner of arylhydrocarbon receptor (AhR) [27]. AhR/ARNT play a key role in genes involved in the xenobiotic metabolism. Under physiological conditions AhR is held in a latent complex with the chaperone hsp90 which is released on ligand binding to dioxin and related aromatic hydrocarbons allowing the AhR/ARNT complex to translocate to the nucleus and bind to xenobiotic response elements in detoxifying genes such as cytochrome P450A1. Thus the HIF-1β/ARNT transcription factor apparently provides a surprising link between the xenobiotic and hypoxic signaling pathways. However, HIF-1α and AhR-mediated signal transduction mechanisms were not mutually exclusive, since hypoxic induction of HIF-1α dependent genes was not impaired by activation of the AhR pathway. Although HIF-1α was found to be associated with hsp90 it is not clear if translocation similar to AhR occurs upon hypoxic stimulation [40].

Both HIF-1α and ARNT are expressed in a wide variety of tissues [41]. Moreover, an increasing number of genes have been identified as targets for HIF-1α (Table 1). These genes are involved in wound repair, iron metabolism, angiogenesis such as VEGF, vascular tone, glycolytic metabolism and glucose transport. All of them are also induced by hypoxia, transition metals and the iron chelator desferrioxamine. A tentative HIF-1 consensus motif, with CGTG as a conserved core motif, was identified in these genes, suggesting again that closely related mechanisms of O_2 sensing and transcriptional activation are involved in a variety of physiological and pathophysiological relevant processes [38].

Recently the essential role of HIF-1α in the hypoxic response was demonstrated in HIF-1α knock out embryonic stem cells and mouse embryos [42]. Absence of HIF-1α resulted in malformation, developmental arrest, and lethality of HIF-1α $-/-$ embryos by day 11. Mice heterozygous for the HIF-1α deficient allele developed to adulthood normally, but when exposed to chronic hypoxia their he-

Table 1. Induction characteristics of mammalian oxygen regulated genes

Expression of mRNA	Hypoxia	Cobalt chloride	Desferri- oxamine	Hypoxia + carbon monoxide	Functional HIF-1 site
Erythropoietin	+	+	+	−	yes
Vascular endothelial growth factor	+	+	+	−	yes
Glucose transporter-1	+	+	+		yes
Phosphoglycerate kinase 1	+	+	+		yes
Lactate dehydrogenase A	+	+	+		yes
Phosphofructokinase-L	+	+	+		yes
Aldolase A	+	+	+		yes
Enolase 1	+	+	+		yes
Phosphoenolpyruvate carboxykinase	−	−		+	no
Inducible nitric oxide synthase	+		+		yes
Heme oxygenase-1	+				yes
Transferrin	+	+	+		yes
Tyrosine hydroxylase	+	+			yes

Induction characteristics of oxygen-regulated genes by hypoxia, cobalt chloride or the iron elator desferrioxamine. Many of these genes contain a functional HIF-1 binding site. + indicates upregulation of gene expression, − indicates downregulation of gene expression. Carbon monoxide abolished the hypoxic induction (−) or downregulation (+)

matological and cardiovascular responses were significantly impaired relative to wildtype litter-mates. HIF-1α −/− embryonic stem cells which did not express HIF-1α showed reduced expression of 13 glycolytic enzymes under hypoxia, and proliferation was also impaired under these conditions. Also, mouse embryonic stem cells containing a targeted disruption of the ARNT locus failed to respond to hypoxia by adequate modulation of gene expression [43]. ARNT −/− embryos were not viable past embryonic day 10.5 and showed defects of angiogenesis in the yolk sac and branchial arches, stunted development and often embryo wasting. Apparently, vasculogenesis remained intact whereas angiogenesis was abnormal resembling the phenotypes observed in VEGF +/− and tissue factor deprived (TF −/−) yolk sacs. Local hypoxic conditions during organogenesis might stimulate ARNT transcriptional activity causing VEGF and tissue factor production and blood vessel development.

Two transactivation domains have been identified in HIF-1α which repressed transcriptional activation under normoxia, and greatly enhanced hypoxic HIF-1α transcriptional activity [44, 45]. HIF-1α transactivation domains were also stimulated by exposure to $CoCl_2$ and desferrioxamine. Concomitantly, HIF-1α protein levels were increased by these treatments. Thus, the enhanced transcriptional activity in hypoxic cells by HIF-1α might result from a dual mechanism involving the increased activity of inducible HIF-1α transactivation domains and enhanced HIF-1α protein levels. Post-translational modifications that enhance transactivation might include phosphorylation, ligand-dependent conformation changes or co-factor recruitment. Such post-translational modifications might also explain differences in transcriptional activation observed among different cell lines. Protein phosphorylation events have been shown to regulate HIF-1 DNA binding activity but are also involved in multiple steps in the hypoxia signal-transduction pathway that lead to the synthesis of HIF-1α and ARNT [46]. Based on *in vitro* data of HIF-1 regulation it was proposed that HIF-1α acquires a new conformational state upon dimerization with ARNT, rendering HIF-1α more resistant to proteolytic attack [47]. Furthermore, the transcriptional coactivator p300/CBP has been shown to bind to HIF-1α [48] and ARNT [49]. Hypoxic gene activation was abolished by the viral oncoprotein E1A, an inhibitor of p300/CBP. Overexpression of p300 greatly enhanced hypoxia-induced transcription suggesting a critical role of p300/CBP in hypoxic activation of HIF-1. Since p300/CBP is probably involved in chromatin rearrangement it might be crucial for the accessibility of HIF-1 to its target DNA-binding site [50].

HIF-1α protein stability appears to be greatly enhanced under hypoxic conditions, and the ubiquitin-proteasome system can rapidly degrade HIF-1α under normoxic conditions [51]. Furthermore, the addition of H_2O_2 prevented hypoxia induced HIF-1α DNA binding by blocking HIF-1α protein accumulation whereas H_2O_2 had no effect on hypoxic cells indicating that an intact redox-dependent signaling pathway is required for destabilization of HIF-1α [52]. These findings were supported by experiments where overexpression of reducing proteins such as thioredoxin and Ref-1, both of them inducible themselves by hypoxia [53, 54], significantly potentiated induction of HIF-1α reporter gene constructs by hypoxia. Furthermore, HIF-1 DNA binding was abolished by sulfhydryl oxidation, whereas reducing thiol donors mimicked the hypoxic response of reporter genes under the control of a hypoxia responsive enhancer [51]. In addition, an important role for hydroxylradicals, generated by non-mitochondrial sources, for the survival rate of HIF-1α protein was suggested [55]. An O_2 dependent destabilization domain (ODD) localized between the two transactivation domains of HIF-1α was responsible for the control of (in)stability of HIF-1α under hypoxia. Complete deletion of this domain enabled HIF-1α to heterodimerize with HIF-1β/ARNT already under normoxic conditions. This dimer was functionally active and transactivated an erythropoietin 3' enhancer reporter gene [57].

In addition to HIF-1, the redox-mediated transcription factors activator protein-1 (AP1), nuclear factor-κB (NF-κB) and p53 as well as nuclear factor-interleukin 6 (NF-IL6) have been described to mediate O_2-dependent gene regulation [13, 53, 57, 58]. Whereas HIF-1 can specifically be activated by limited O_2 availability, the range of stimuli involved in activation of the other transcription factors is much broader. Furthermore, HIF-1 protein levels and HIF-1 DNA binding activity increased exponentially when decreasing the PO_2, with a half-maximal response around 10 mm Hg, and a peak induction at 3 mm Hg [59]. This range of O_2 values nicely matches the critical range of O_2 concentrations measured in tissues *in vivo*. In contrast, in the majority of studies induction of AP-1 was obtained at PO_2 levels around or even lower than 1 mm Hg [53, 57]. HIF-1 DNA binding activity and expression, however, rapidly declined at PO_2 levels below 3 mm Hg [59]. Although no PO_2 titration curve has been performed, Prabhakar et al. [60] demonstrated that among the immediate early genes such as c-fos, junB, jun D, and c-jun, c-fos mRNA can be stimulated 11-fold by PO_2 values of 40 mm Hg compared to two- to three-fold induction of the other immediate early genes. The hypoxic response was cell specific with higher induction rates in fibroblasts and hepatoma cells than in neuroblastoma cells and could be observed after 15 min with peak values after 1 h. However, it is not clear whether under these conditions AP-1 was actually functional. Hypoxic induction of p53 DNA-binding activity has been related to cell cycle control [13]. Although induction of NF-κB by hypoxia has also been reported [61], this transcription factor is normally induced by ROS and pro-oxidant states such as occur, for example, during reoxygenation [58]. Interestingly, AP-1 can be induced by reduced and oxidant states whereas NF-κB and p53 are activated by oxidant states [62]. Thus it might be speculated that O_2 dependent gene regulation involves an array of transcription factors which are maximally induced by different O_2 concentrations and redox states. HIF-1 might confer hypoxic stimuli in a physiologically relevant PO_2 range whereas other transcription factors are activated by anoxic or re-oxygenation stress.

Although the relevance of these processes is clear it is not immediately obvious how apparently closely related mechanisms of sensing and transcriptional activation could satisfy the requirements of regulated gene expression in diverse systems. It has become increasingly clear that a single HIF-1 site present in a hypoxia response element is not sufficient to induce hypoxic gene transcription. In the erythropoietin enhancer, for example, two additional DNA binding sites are necessary for the hypoxic response, one of these has been identified as the tissue specific transcription factor, hepatic nuclear factor 4 (HNF-4) [16]. In the LDH-A promoter a cAMP response element (CRE) potentiates hypoxic activation [16], whereas in the VEGF promoter an AP-1 site has been shown to be involved in the hypoxic response [63]. Tyrosine hydroxylase upregulation by hypoxia also requires binding of AP-1 and HIF-1 to their respective binding sites in the proximal promoter region [12]. None of these additional sites mediates the hypoxic response by themselves, but mutations within these sites abolish the hypoxic response. Furthermore, in many cell lines a complex consisting of activating transcription factor (ATF)-1 and CRE binding protein (CREB)-1 binds constitutively to the HIF-1 DNA binding site [64]. Thus it appears likely that co-operative factors influence the transcriptional activity of HIF-1 in order to modulate the overall characteristics of inducible and tissue-specific gene expression.

Finally, several other bHLH-PAS domain proteins with high homology to ARNT or HIF-1α have been identified very recently. ARNT2 whose expression is restricted to brain and kidney [65], can also heterodimerize with HIF-1α. EPAS1, homolog to HIF-1α, is preferentially expressed in the endothelium [66]. EPAS1 can heterodimerize with ARNT or ARNT2 under hypoxia and bind to the HIF-1 binding site. In addition to VEGF, it induces the endothelial specific receptor tyrosine kinase Tie2, which by binding of angiopoietin plays a role in vascular remodeling. Two other HIF-1α homologues, HIF-1 related factor (HRF) [67] and HIF-1 like factor (HLF) [68] were recently identified. The high sequence similarity to EPAS1 suggests that the three proteins are very closely related or even identical [39]. In contrast to the ubiquitous expression pattern of HIF-1α, EPAS1/HLF/HRF expression is restricted to endothelial cells in the embryo and to highly vascularized tissues and alveolar epithelial cells postnatally and in the adult. It has been suggested that EPAS1/HLF/HRF might be a candidate for a regulator of tubulogenesis in vertebrates similar to the master regulator trachealess (trh) in *Drosophila* [67]. Two other bHLH-PAS domain proteins were recently identified in mice, mSim1 and mSim2, which can also heterodimerize with ARNT but act as transcriptional repressors [69]. Sim regulates neuronal development in *Drosophila*, and a human homolog has been related to Down's syndrome [70]. Evidence for the presence of more bHLH-PAS domain proteins has already been provided and they now await identification and functional characterization [71]. The elucidation of the physiological importance of this complex pattern of heterodimerization partners, as well as the regulatory network involved, will be a challenging task and will hopefully provide new insights into the mechanisms of O_2-regulated gene expression.

Conclusion

Although evidence is overwhelming that cellular O_2 sensing is a general property of cells enabling them to stay functional during variations in O_2 availability, our knowledge concerning the specific mechanisms involved in O_2 sensing and O_2 signaling is still limited. Despite recent progress especially in the identification of O_2-regulated transcription factors and their target genes, large gaps remain in our understanding of how O_2 is sensed by cells, and which signaling cascades might mediate adequate responses to the current availability of O_2. Although the nature of the putative O_2 sensor remains obscure, evidence has accumulated that a heme protein might be involved, eventually exhibiting oxidase activity. This is supported by the increasing appreciation of redox-mediated mechanisms that regulate transcription factor and ion channel activities in O_2 signaling. Future challenges will face the identification of the O_2 sensor(s), the elucidation of the complex signaling network, the activation mechanisms of O_2-regulated transcription factors and ion channels and their possible interplay, as well as the complex interaction and crosstalk between energy metabolism and other major cellular functions in order to adequately respond to variations in O_2 availability.

References

1. Acker H (1994) Mechanisms and meaning of cellular oxygen sensing in the organism. Respir Physiol 95:1–10
2. Jungermann K, Kietzmann T (1997) Role of oxygen in the zonation of carbohydrate metabolism and gene expression in liver. Kidney Int 51:402–412
3. Acker H, Xue D (1995) Mechanisms of oxygen sensing in the carotid body in comparison with other O_2-sensing cells. News Physiol Sci 10:211–216
4. Lopez-Barneo J (1996) Oxygen-sensing by ion channels and the regulation of cellular functions. Trends Neurosci 19:435–444
5. Jelkmann W (1992) Erythropoietin: structure, control of production, and function. Physiol Rev 72:449–489
6. Scott PH, Belham CM, Peacock AJ, Plevin R (1997) Intracellular signaling pathways that regulate vascular cell proliferation: effect of hypoxia. Exp Physiol 82:317–326
7. Shweiki D, Itin A, Soffer D, Keshet E (1992) Vascular endothelial growth factor induced by hypoxia may mediate hypoxia-initiated angiogenesis. Nature 359:843–845
8. Ogawa S, Gerlach H, Esposito C, Pasagian-Macaulay A, Brett J, Stern D (1990) Hypoxia modulates the barrier and coagulation function of cultured bovine endothelium. J Clin Invest 85:1090–1098
9. Wadsworth RM (1994) Vasoconstrictor and vasodilator functions of hypoxia. Trends Pharm Sci 15:49–55
10. Semenza GL, Roth PH, Fang HM, Wang GL (1994) Transcriptional regulation of genes encoding glycolytic enzymes by hypoxia-inducible factor 1. J Biol Chem 269:23757–23763
11. Ebert BL, Firth JD, Ratcliffe PJ (1995) Hypoxia and mitochondrial inhibitors regulate expression of glucose transporter-1 via distinct cis-acting sequences. J Biol Chem 270:29083–29089
12. Millhorn DE, Raymond R, Conforti L, et al (1997) Regulation of gene expression for tyrosine hydroxylase in oxygen sensitive cells by hypoxia. Kidney Int 51:527–535
13. Graeber TG, Peterson JE, Tsai M, Monica K, Fornace AJ, Giaccia AJ (1994) Hypoxia induces accumulation of p53 protein, but activation of a G1-phase checkpoint by low-oxygen conditions is independent of p53 status. Mol Cell Biol 14:6264–6277
14. Shimizu S, Eguchi Y, Kamiike W, et al (1996) Induction of apoptosis as well as necrosis by hypoxia and predominant prevention of apoptosis by Bcl-2 and Bcl-XL. Cancer Res 56:2161–2166
15. Tucci M, Hammerman SI, Furfaro S, Saukonnen JJ, Conca TJ, Farber HW (1997) Distinct effects of hypoxia on endothelial cell proliferation and cycling. Am J Physiol 272:C1700–1708
16. Bunn HF, Poyton RO (1996) Oxygen sensing and molecular adaptation to hypoxia. Physiol Rev 76:839–885
17. Gilles-Gonzales MA, Ditta GS, Helinski DR (1991) A haemoprotein with kinase activity encoded by the oxygen sensor of *Rhizobium meliloti*. Nature 350:170–172

18. Wang GL, Semenza GL (1993) Desferrioxamine induces erythropoietin gene expression and hypoxia-inducible factor 1 DNA-binding activity: implications for models of hypoxic signal transduction. Blood 82:3610–3615
19. Gleadle JM, Ebert BL, Firth JD, Ratcliffe PJ (1995) Oxygen regulated expression of angiogenic growth factors: effects of hypoxia, transition metals and chelating agents. Am J Physiol 268:C1362–C1368
20. Unden G, Schirawski J (1997) The oxygen-responsive transcriptional regulator FNR of Escherichia coli – the search for signals and reactions. Mol Microbiol 25:205–210
21. Ehleben W, Porwol T, Fandrey J, Kummer W, Acker H (1997) Cobalt and desferrioxamine reveal crucial members of the oxygen sensing pathway in HepG2 cells. Kidney Int 51:483–491
22. Görlach A, Holtermann G, Jelkmann W, Hancock JT, Jones SA, Jones OTG, Acker H (1993) Photometric characteristics of haem proteins in erythropoietin-producing hepatoma (HepG2). Biochem J 290:771–776
23. Görlach A, Fandrey J, Holtermann G, Acker H (1994) Effects of cobalt on haem proteins on erythropoietin producing HepG2 cells in multicellular spheroid culture. FEBS Lett 348:216–218
24. DeLeo FR, Quinn M (1996) Assembly of the phagocyte NADPH oxidase: molecular interaction of oxidase proteins. J Leukoc Biol 60:677–691
25. Powis G, Briehl M, Oblong J (1995) Redox signalling and the control of cell growth and death. Pharmacol Therapeut 68:149–173
26. Lander HM (1997) An essential role for free radicals and derived species in signal transduction. FASEB J 11:118–124
27. Wang GL, Semenza GL (1996) Oxygen sensing and response to hypoxia by mammalian cells. Redox Report 2:89–96
28. Fandrey J, Frede S, Jelkmann W (1994) Role of hydrogen peroxide in hypoxia-induced erythropoietin production. Biochem J 303:507–510
29. Acker H, Bölling B, Delpiano MA, Dufau E, Görlach A, Holtermann G (1992) The meaning of H_2O_2 generation in carotid body cells for pO_2 chemoreception. J Auton Nerv Syst 41:41–52
30. Kummer W, Acker H (1995) Immunohistochemical detection of four subunits of neutrophil NAD(P)H oxidase in type I cells of carotid body. J Appl Physiol 78:1904–1909
31. Wang D, Youngson C, Wong V, et al (1996) NADPH-oxidase and a hydrogen peroxide-sensitive K+ channel may function as an oxygen sensor complex in airway chemoreceptors and small lung cell carcinoma cell lines. Proc Natl Acad Sci USA 93:13182–13187
32. Kummer W, Acker H (1997) Cytochrome b558 and hydrogen peroxide production in small intensely fluorescent cells of sympathetic ganglia. Histochem Cell Biol 197:151–158
33. Fandrey J, Seydel FP, Siegers CP, Jelkmann W (1990) Role of cytochrome p450 in the control of the production of erythropoietin. Life Sci 47:127–134
34. Harder DR, Narayanan J, Birks EK, et al (1996) Identification of a putative microvascular oxygen sensor. Circ Res 79:54–61
35. Gleadle JM, Ebert BL, Ratcliffe PJ (1995) Diphenylene iodonium inhibits the induction of erythropoietin and other mammalian genes by hypoxia. Implications for the mechanism of oxygen sensing. Eur J Biochem 234:92–99
36. Maxwell PH, Pugh CW, Ratcliffe PJ (1993) Inducible operation of the erythropoietin 3' enhancer in multiple cell lines: evidence for a widespread oxygen-sensing mechanism. Proc Natl Acad Sci USA 90:2423–2427
37. Wang GL, Semenza GL (1993) Purification and characterization of hypoxia-inducible factor-1. J Biol Chem 270:1230–1237
38. Wenger RH, Gassmann M (1997) Oxygen(es) and the hypoxia-inducible factor-1. Biol Chem 378:609–616
39. Zhulin IB, Taylor BL, Dixon R (1997) PAS domain S-boxes in archaea, bacteria and sensors for oxygen and redox. Trends Biochem Sci 22:331–333
40. Gradin K, McGuire J, Wenger RH, et al (1996) Functional interference between hypoxia and dioxin signal transduction pathways: competition for recruitment of the Arnt transcription factor. Mol Cell Biol 16:5221–5231
41. Wiener CM, Booth G, Semenza GL (1996) In vivo expression of mRNAs encoding hypoxia inducible factor 1. Biochem Biophys Res Commun 225:485–488

42. Iyer NV, Aimee YY, Agani F, et al (1998) Cellular and developmental control of O$_2$ homeostasis by hypoxia-inducible factor 1-alpha. Genes Dev 12:149–162
43. Maltepe E, Schmidt JV, Baunoch D, Bradfield CA, Simon MC (1997) Abnormal angiogenesis and responses to glucose and oxygen deprivation in mice lacking the protein ARNT. Nature 386:403–407
44. Pugh CW, O'Rourke JF, Nagao M, Gleadle JM, Ratcliffe PJ (1997) Activation of hypoxia-inducible factor-1; definition of regulatory domains within the α subunit. J Biol Chem 272: 11205–11214
45. Jiang BH, Zheng JZ, Leung SW, Roe R, Semenza GL (1997) Transactivation and inhibitory domains of hypoxia-inducible factor 1α. J Biol Chem 272:19253–19260
46. Wang GL, Jiang BH, Semenza GL (1995) Effect of protein kinase and phosphatase inhibitors on expression of hypoxia-inducible factor 1. Biochem Biophys Res Comm 216:669–675
47. Kallio PJ, Pongratz I, Gradin K, McGuire J, Poellinger L (1997) Activation of hypoxia-inducible factor 1α: posttranscriptional regulation and conformational change by recruitment of the ARNT transcription factor. Proc Natl Acad Sci USA 94:5667–5672
48. Arany Z, Huang E, Eckner R, et al (1996) An essential role for p300/CBP in the cellular reponse to hypoxia. Proc Natl Acad Sci USA 93:12969–12973
49. Kobayashi A, Numayama-Tsurata K, Sogawa K, Fujii-Kuriyama Y (1997) CBP/p300 functions as a possible trancriptional coactivator of Ah receptor nuclear translocator (Arnt). J Biochem 122:703–710
50. Shikama N, Lyon J, La Thangue NB (1997) The p300/CBP family: integrating signals with transcription factors and chromatin. Trends Cell Biol 7:230–236
51. Salceda S, Caro J (1997) Hypoxia-inducible factor 1α (HIF-1α) protein is rapidly degraded by the ubiquitin-proteasome system under normoxic conditions. J Biol Chem 272: 22642–22647
52. Huang LE, Arany Z, Livingston DM, Bunn DF (1996) Activation of hypoxia-inducible transcription factor depends on stabilization of its α subunit. J Biol Chem 271:32253–32259
53. Yao KS, Xanthoudakis S, Curran T, O'Dwyer PJ (1994) Activation of AP-1 and a nuclear redox factor Ref-1, in the response of HT29 colon cancer cells to hypoxia. Mol Cell Biol 14: 5997–6003
54. Berggren M, Gallegos A, Gasdaska JR, Gasdaska PY, Warneke J, Powis G (1996) Thioredoxin and thioredoxin reductase gene expression in human tumors and cell lines, and the effects of serum stimulation and hypoxia. Anticancer Res 16:3459–3466
55. Salceda S, Srinivas V, Caro J (1997) Hydroxyradical inhibition induces erythropoietin gene expression by affecting the proteasomal degradation of HIF-1α: implications for oxygen sensing. Blood 90:56a (Abst)
56. Huang LE, Gu J, Schau M, Bunn HF (1997) Erythropoietin gene is regulated by modulating HIF-1α stability through an oxygen dependent destabilization domain. Blood 90:303a (Abst)
57. Rupec RA, Baeuerle PA (1995) The genomic response of tumor cells to hypoxia and reoxygenation. Differential activation of transcription factors AP-1 and NF-kappa B. Eur J Biochem 234:632–640
58. Yan SF, Zou YS, Mendelsohn M, et al (1997) Nuclear factor interleukin 6 motifs mediate tissue-specific gene transcription in hypoxia. J Biol Chem 272:4287–4294
59. Jiang BH, Semenza GL, Bauer C, Marti HH (1996) Hypoxia-inducible factor 1 levels vary exponentially over a physiologically relevant range of O$_2$ tension. Am J Physiol 271: C1172–C1180
60. Prabhakar NR, Shenoy BC, Simonson MS, Cherniack NS (1995) Cell selective induction and transcriptional activation of immediate early genes by hypoxia. Brain Res 697:266–270
61. Koong AC, Chen EY, Giaccia AJ (1994) Hypoxia causes the activation of nuclear factor κB through the phosphorylation of IkBαα on tyrosine residues. Cancer Res 54:1425–1430
62. Sun Y, Oberley LW (1996) Redox regulation of transcriptional activators. Free Radic Biol Med 21:335–348
63. Damert A, Ikeda E, Risau W (1997) Activator-protein-1 binding potentiates the hypoxia-inducible factor-1 mediated hypoxia-induced transcriptional activation of vascular-endothelial growth factor expression in C6 glioma cells. Biochem J 327:419–423

64. Kvietikova I, Wenger RH, Marti HH, Gassmann M (1995) The transcription factors ATF-1 and CREB-1 bind constitutively to the hypoxia-inducible factor 1. Nucl Acid Res 23:4542–4550
65. Hirose K, Morita M, Ema M, et al (1996) cDNA cloning and tissue-specific expression of a novel basic helix-loop-helix/PAS factor (ARNT2) with close sequence similarities to the aryl hydrocarbon receptor nuclear translocator (Arnt). Mol Cell Biol 16:1706–1713
66. Tian M, McKnight SL, Russel DW (1997) Endothelial PAS domain protein 1 (EPAS1), a transcription factor selectively expressed in endothelial cells. Genes Dev 11:72–82
67. Flamme I, Fröhlich T, von Reuitern M, Kappel A, Damert A, Risau W (1997) HRF, a putative basic helix-loop-helix-PAS domain transcriptin factor is closely related to hypoxia-inducible factor-1α and developmentally expressed in blood vessels. Mech Dev 63:51–60
68. Ema M, Taya S, Yobotani N, Sogawa K, Matsuda Y, Fuji-Kuiryama Y (1997) A novel bHLH-PAS factor with close sequence similarity to hypoxia-inducible factor 1α regulates the VEGF expression and is potentially involved in lung and vascular development. Proc Natl Acad Sci USA 94:4273–4278
69. Probst MR, Fan CM, Tessier-Lavigne M, Hankinson O (1997) Two murine homologs of the Drosophila single-minded protein that interact with the mouse aryl hydrocarbon receptor nuclear transclocator protein. J Biol Chem 272:4451–4457
70. Dahmane N, Charron G, Lopes C, et al (1995) Down syndrome-critical region contains a gene homologous to Drosophila sim expressed during rat and human central nervous system development. Proc Natl Acad Sci USA 92:9191–9195
71. Hogenesch JB, Chan WK, Jackiv VH, Brown RC, Gu YZ, Perdew GH, Bradfield CA (1997) Characterization of a subset of the basic helip loop helix PAS superfamily that interacts with components of the dioxin signaling pathway. J Biol Chem 272:8581–8593

Hypoxia and Its Consequences

Hypoxic Hypoxia

K. R. Walley

Introduction

Adequate availability of oxygen (O_2) is essential for cellular respiration to produce sufficient adenosine triphosphate (ATP) to maintain normal organ function [1, 2]. Why is O_2 so important? O_2 is simply a garbage can, a metabolic dump, the lowest common metabolic denominator. In essence, obtaining energy from metabolic substrate (food) is the process of taking electrons in high energy states within covalent bonds and finding a low energy state to leave them in. The available energy is the difference between the starting high energy state and the final low energy state. The most readily available low energy acceptor for electrons is O_2. A two atom O_2 molecule can readily accept two electrons per atom, each of which can then combine with two protons (and protons are ubiquitous) to form two molecules of water. A number of organisms living near hydrothermal vents thousands of meters below the ocean surface use sulfur rather than O_2 as their electron garbage can, and some organisms and eukaryotic cells leave their unwanted electrons on other molecules to form lactate or ethanol. However, electrons left within the lactate molecule are at a much higher energy than those left with O_2 so that the metabolism of carbohydrates and other substrates to lactate generates relatively little ATP [3]. Subsequent aerobic metabolism of lactate, for example, by the heart, skeletal muscle, and liver, can still produce a great deal of ATP [4]. Thus lactate, as an electron garbage can, could be likened to the garbage outside a posh mansion the day after an elaborate feast; for the right scavenger, there is lots of good food left. In this analogy, O_2 as an electron acceptor is similar to a beat up trash can in the worst part of town; garbage in this can is truly garbage, there is nothing left to be had. Thus, O_2 is the aerobic garbage can for electrons. If the refuse of cellular metabolism is not taken out, the metabolic machinery shuts down. Hence, the central importance of O_2 to the maintenance of life.

To address the role of O_2, and specifically the effect of limited O_2 availability, this chapter first identifies hypoxic hypoxia with diffusion dependent steps in O_2 transport from the atmosphere to the mitochondria. It follows that low arterial O_2 partial pressure (PaO_2) is a key feature of hypoxic hypoxia. Therefore, the main physiologic causes of arterial hypoxemia are reviewed. Then the question of what limits O_2 transport is addressed, and it is pointed out that diffusion limitation is usually not the cause. In analogy to the lungs, "physiologic" arterial-venous shunt in tissues appears to limit O_2 extraction. Physiologic mechanisms that optimize O_2 extraction are discussed. Finally, the effects of hypoxic hypoxia on tissues are reviewed, finishing with a focus on the heart, a key organ in hypoxic hypoxia.

What is Hypoxic Hypoxia?

The meaning of hypoxic hypoxia can be understood by considering the pathway of O_2 transport from the air we breathe to the final step of the electron transport chain that occurs on the inner membrane surface of mitochondria. First, O_2 must be transported by bulk flow ventilation of the lungs to the alveolar capillary membrane. Next, O_2 must diffuse down a PO_2 gradient onto hemoglobin (Hb) molecules in the blood. Hb in the blood carries O_2 so that the next step in O_2 transport is bulk flow of blood from the lungs to tissue capillaries. When the oxygenated Hb is delivered to tissue capillaries, O_2 must again diffuse down a PO_2 gradient from the capillaries into the surrounding tissue. In the surrounding tissue, different carriers for O_2, such as myoglobin, are available to facilitate O_2 transport [5]. Over the small distances encountered within cells, diffusion plays an important role. However, it is essential to note that O_2 carriers within the cells increase cellular O_2 content tremendously so that diffusion limitation of O_2 transport is generally not encountered in life. Finally, O_2 in the mitochondria accept low energy electrons at the end of the ATP-producing electron transport chain.

Transport of O_2 from the air we breathe to the mitochondria can be limited at any of the above steps. Failure of bulk flow of O_2 from the air to the alveoli is called hypoventilation [6]. Failure to supply adequate Hb to bind O_2 is called anemic hypoxia [7]. Failure of bulk flow of blood from the lungs to the capillaries is called stagnant hypoxia or ischemia [7]. Poisoning of any of the carrier molecules along the way, so that they are no longer able to transport O_2 or carry out electron transport, is called histotoxic hypoxia [8]. Hypoxic hypoxia refers to the steps that depend on diffusion of O_2; namely, diffusion from the lungs into arterial blood and diffusion from oxygenated capillary blood into the tissues. Thus, the term hypoxic hypoxia is sometimes used when discussing low arterial PO_2 and sometimes used when discussing low tissue PO_2, both sites just downstream of a diffusion-dependent step in the transport of O_2 from the air to the mitochondria.

Low PO₂ is the Hallmark of Hypoxic Hypoxia

Hypoxic hypoxia refers to limited O_2 transport at steps that depend on diffusion, and diffusion is driven by PO_2 differences. Fick's law [5] states that the diffusion of a gas through a sheet of tissue (V_{gas}) depends on the gas partial pressure difference ($P_1 - P_2$) across the tissue, on the area of the tissue (A), on the diffusivity of the gas (D), and inversely on the tissue thickness (T). Thus, Fick's law is:

$$V_{gas} = (P_1 - P_2) \times A \times D/T \tag{1}$$

Diffusivity of a gas is a physical constant that is proportional to the solubility of the gas in the tissue sheet divided by the square root of the molecular weight of the gas. The area for diffusion and the thickness for diffusion depend on anatomy. Thus, PO_2 is crucial in limiting the diffusion-dependent steps in O_2 transport. PaO_2 is the downstream partial pressure for diffusion of O_2 across the pulmonary alveolar capillary membrane, and PaO_2 is closely related to the upstream pressure for diffusion from capillaries to tissues. Because of its key role in diffusion-dependent steps in O_2 transport, a low PaO_2 (hypoxemia) is a hallmark of hypoxic hypoxia.

Causes of Arterial Hypoxemia

Diffusion Limitation

A number of important pathophysiologic mechanisms underlie a low P_aO_2. Diffusion limitation of O_2 transport in the lungs is a potential theoretical cause of arterial hypoxemia. However, this mechanism of arterial hypoxemia is rarely clinically important. Transport of poorly diffusive gases such as carbon monoxide can be used to measure the diffusing capacity of the lungs, D_LCO [9]. A low D_LCO reflects decreased surface area for diffusion (A) and, to a much lesser extent, the thickness of the alveolar capillary membrane (T). While significant reductions in D_LCO can be found in various disease states, diffusion limitation of O_2 transport from alveoli to arterial blood in the lungs only becomes the limiting step to overall O_2 transport in exceptional circumstances. In athletes exercising maximally at high altitude, the transit time of blood through the pulmonary capillaries can become shorter than the loading time of O_2 onto Hb [10], resulting in diffusion limitation of gas transport. However, in almost all other circumstances, diffusion does not limit gas transport [11].

Hypoventilation

Fick's law also indicates that limitation of O_2 transport from the alveolus to pulmonary capillary blood can occur when the PO_2 difference from the alveolus to the blood is low. Alveolar PO_2 can be low due to a low PO_2 of inspired gas, for example, at high altitude. Breathing gas with a low inspired O_2 fraction, FiO_2, is a rare cause of hypoxemia. Most frequently, a low alveolar PO_2 is caused by hypoventilation. Since nitrogen is an inert gas it is pretty much in equilibrium everywhere. Since nitrogen uses up almost four-fifths of the atmosphere only one-fifth remains for O_2 and carbon dioxide (CO_2). The alveolar gas equation describes these ideas in a more rigorous form [5]. In simplified form, the alveolar gas equation is:

$$P_AO_2 = PiO_2 - (PaCO_2/R), \qquad (2)$$

where P_AO_2 is the partial pressure of oxygen in the alveolus, PiO_2 is the partial pressure of inspired oxygen, $PaCO_2$ is the partial pressure of arterial carbon dioxide, and R is the respiratory quotient, VCO_2/VO_2.

The alveolar gas equation indicates that P_AO_2 must decrease as $PaCO_2$ rises. A decrease in P_AO_2 then results in a decrease in PaO_2. $PaCO_2$ is proportional to CO_2 production and inversely proportional to alveolar ventilation. Thus, hypoventilation, specifically alveolar hypoventilation, results in an elevated alveolar $PaCO_2$ and, according to the alveolar gas equation, a decrease in alveolar PO_2. The alveolar gas equation (eqn. 2) shows that this effect can be overcome in a number of ways. Steps can be taken to increase alveolar ventilation, including using mechanically assisted ventilation to lower $PaCO_2$. In addition, high FiO_2 can prevent hypoxemia even in the setting of alveolar hypoventilation with high $PaCO_2$.

Shunt

Shunting of mixed venous blood past gas exchanging alveoli directly into the pulmonary veins can be an important contributor to arterial hypoxemia, for example, in some congenital heart diseases. Significant shunt can also occur within the lungs, for example, in acute respiratory distress syndrome (ARDS) where pulmonary arterial blood shunts past flooded alveoli [12]. Shunt has a particularly dramatic effect on arterial PO_2 due to the non-linear O_2-Hb dissociation curve (Fig. 1). Consider a 50 percent mixture of oxygenated blood, with a PO_2 of 100, and deoxygenated venous blood with an O_2 saturation (SO_2) of 60 percent. This half-and-half mixture will result in arterial blood with an SO_2 very close to 80 percent. Because of the curvilinearity of the O_2-Hb dissociation curve, a reduction in SO_2 by 20 percent results in far greater than a 20 percent reduction in

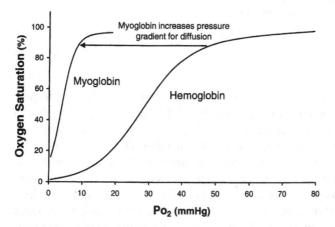

Fig. 1. Oxygen-hemoglobin and oxygen-myoglobin dissociation curves. The oxygen-hemoglobin curve is not linear so that, at high PO_2, substantial decreases in PO_2 do not decrease oxygen saturation much. The oxygen-myoglobin dissociation curve is greatly left-shifted providing a partial pressure gradient for diffusion of oxygen from the capillaries into the tissues

PaO_2. The arterial PO_2 of 80 percent saturated blood is approximately 45 mm Hg. Thus, shunt of deoxygenated venous blood into the arterial circulation can be a significant contributor to arterial hypoxemia in several disease states.

V/Q Mismatch

The most important cause of clinically significant arterial hypoxemia is ventilation/perfusion, V/Q, mismatch [13]. That is, O_2 ventilation of alveoli is not adequately matched to blood perfusing the alveolar capillaries. As a result, some regions have ventilation in excess of perfusion while other regions have perfusion in excess of ventilation. The regions with excess ventilation contribute to dead space, while the regions with excess perfusion contribute to a "physiologic shunt". Physiologic shunt contributes to arterial hypoxemia just as anatomic shunt does. An important difference between anatomic and physiologic shunt is that anatomic shunt does not respond to increasing FiO_2 because blood that does not come close to alveoli will not benefit by increasing alveolar PO_2. However, when FiO_2 is increased in the setting of V/Q mismatch, a doubling or tripling of FiO_2 doubles or triples alveolar ventilation of O_2. Many lung units with previously low V/Q ratios now normalize their O_2 V/Q ratios, ameliorating hypoxemia. Thus, while anatomic shunt is not responsive to changes in FiO_2, V/Q mismatch is very responsive.

Contribution of Low Mixed Venous Oxygen Saturation

Many discussions of the mechanism of arterial hypoxemia stop at this point. However, in critically ill patients with high physiologic or anatomic shunt fractions, mixed venous SO_2 (SvO_2) becomes exceedingly important. If SvO_2 is decreased in the setting of a high shunt fraction, then arterial saturation can decrease substantially (Fig. 2). The corollary is that increasing SvO_2 can be a very ef-

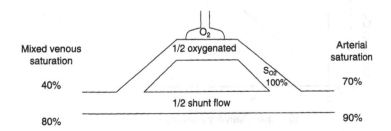

Fig. 2. The effect of mixed venous oxygen saturation on arterial oxygen saturation, in the presence of shunt, is illustrated. Oxygen in a stylized alveolus increases oxygen saturation (SO_2) to 100%. In this example a mixed venous oxygen saturation of 40% in the setting of a 50% shunt results in an arterial saturation of approximately 70% – severe hypoxemia. Without altering the lungs, increasing mixed venous oxygen saturation to 80% increases arterial oxygen saturation to 90%

fective approach to improving arterial SO_2 (SaO_2) in the setting of high shunt fraction. SvO_2 is set by the SaO_2 and the fraction of whole body O_2 delivery (DO_2) that is consumed (VO_2).

$$SvO_2 = SaO_2 \times (1 - VO_2/DO_2) \tag{3}$$

Increasing whole body DO_2 means that VO_2 is a smaller fraction of the total so that SvO_2 increases. An alternative approach to increasing SvO_2 is to minimize whole body VO_2. Clinical approaches to increase SvO_2 in order to improve arterial hypoxemia include increasing cardiac output (CO) and the O_2 carrying capacity of blood (to increase DO_2), and minimizing whole body VO_2 by the use of sedation and paralysis [14].

Limiting Steps in Tissue Oxygen Consumption

Important features of the O_2 extraction capacity of tissues can usefully be illustrated using the relationship between DO_2 and VO_2 (Fig. 3). In the whole body and in other organs, a biphasic relationship is found [15, 16]. At high DO_2 sufficient to maintain aerobic metabolism, VO_2 is relatively constant and independent of DO_2. If DO_2 is decreased then, at some low value, VO_2 must fall because it is not possible to extract more O_2 than is delivered. Decreasing VO_2, dependent upon decreasing DO_2, is associated with evidence of anerobic metabolism including mounting lactic acidosis and decreased organ function [1,17,18]. The critical O_2 extraction ratio (O_2ER, VO_2 divided by DO_2) at the transition from plateau (aerobic metabolism) to downslope (anaerobic, supply-dependent metabolism) is a

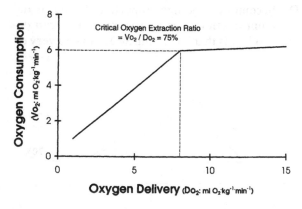

Fig. 3. A typical relationship between oxygen delivery (DO_2) and oxygen consumption (VO_2) is shown. At high oxygen deliveries VO_2 is independent of DO_2 and relatively constant; being set by oxygen demand. At low DO_2, VO_2 becomes dependent upon DO_2, associated with evidence of tissue hypoxia and anaerobic metabolism. The oxygen extraction ratio (O_2ER) (oxygen consumption divided by oxygen delivery) at the transition from plateau to downslope is the critical O_2ER and is a measure of the ability of tissues to extract oxygen

key measure of the O_2 extraction ability of a tissue or organ. The critical O_2ER in health is remarkably constant, at approximately 75% in many studies in various animal species and in various tissues [15–20].

At least two important mechanisms may account for a critical O_2ER. One possibility is that diffusion becomes limited at the critical O_2ER because a critical capillary PO_2 is reached at the critical DO_2/VO_2 point [21]. A second important potential mechanism is that, similar to the lungs, a physiologic arterial-venous shunt may be present. Because the O_2 in the shunt fraction of blood is not available for tissue uptake, the critical O_2ER is, at most, 1 minus the shunt fraction. Any form of arterial-venous O_2 shunt could conceivably contribute to apparent shunting including anatomic shunt [21], O_2 diffusional shunt [22, 23] from adjacent arterioles to venules, and mismatching of VO_2 and DO_2 [24].

In the whole body, the importance of diffusion limitation has been tested by left-shifting of the O_2-Hb dissociation curve [25]. When the dissociation curve is left-shifted, no substantial change in the whole body critical O_2ER is observed. At the same SO_2, left-shifting of the O_2-Hb dissociation curve greatly decreases capillary PO_2. If diffusion limitation were the explanation for the onset of anaerobic metabolism then the critical O_2ER should decrease. Since the critical O_2ER does not change, Schumacker and colleagues [25] conclude that "diffusion limitation does not initiate the early fall in oxygen consumption below the critical oxygen delivery". These results suggest that, in many organ systems, physiologic arterial-venous shunt may be the most important mechanism accounting for the critical O_2ER.

In contrast to the whole body and some organs, the heart [26] and working skeletal muscle [27, 28] appear to be characterized by a critical capillary PO_2 rather than by a critical O_2ER. Left-shifting the O_2-Hb dissociation curve significantly decreases the critical myocardial O_2ER but has no effect on the coronary venous PO_2 [26]. This finding suggests that maximal VO_2 by the myocardium is diffusion limited, rather than limited by a physiologic arterial-venous shunt fraction. Based on O_2 tracer studies Rose and Goresky [29] also conclude that a critical capillary PO_2 limits myocardial aerobic metabolism. They found that the limiting step to O_2 diffusion appears to occur in O_2 transfer across the red cell membrane-capillary wall. Interestingly, working skeletal muscle is also characterized by a critical venous PO_2, rather than by a critical O_2ER [27, 28]. During progressive hypoxemia using a rabbit hind limb preparation, Gutierrez and colleagues [27] found that venous PO_2, and not a critical O_2ER, accounted for limitation of aerobic metabolism. In contracting muscle, King et al. [28] concluded that capillary PO_2 limited VO_2. Thus, working heart and skeletal muscle with high VO_2 may not be encumbered with physiologic shunt to the same extent as other tissues.

In most organs, and on average in the whole body, diffusion is not the limiting step in the transport of O_2 from the atmosphere to the mitochondria as DO_2 becomes limited [25]. The heart and working muscle are therefore exceptions. Much more important to the limitation of O_2 transport is interruption of the other O_2 transport-optimizing mechanisms by hypoventilation, shunt, V/Q mismatch, anemia, low CO, or mismatch of VO_2 and DO_2 in peripheral tissues.

Mismatch of Oxygen Demand and Supply: Physiologic Arterial-Venous Shunt

Just as V/Q mismatch appears to be the most clinically important mechanism for limiting O_2 transport by the lungs, it has been postulated that mismatch between VO_2 and DO_2 is an important limiting factor for O_2 extraction by the tissues [19, 24, 30]. In a theoretical assessment of the effect of mismatching of VO_2 to DO_2 within tissue beds, it was found that biphasic $VO_2 - DO_2$ relationships, with many features of those measured in humans and in animal models, were predicted [24]. Small regions of tissue can be characterized by their VO_2 to DO_2 ratios. Regions with limited DO_2 in relation to VO_2 result in relatively hypoxic areas of tissue, while regions with excess DO_2 in relation to VO_2 contribute to physiologic shunting of arterial blood past the capillary bed into the venous drainage. When the distribution of microvascular VO_2/DO_2 is closely regulated with little variation, at a value near the average O_2ER, then O_2 extraction is efficient, with relatively few hypoxic regions and little shunt of oxygenated blood past the tissues. The critical O_2ER is high in this setting. Increasing the dispersion of the distribution of VO_2/DO_2 decreases the critical O_2ER (Fig. 4). That is, mismatching between VO_2 and DO_2 impairs O_2 transport much as it does in the lungs [24].

Theoretical analysis suggests that for relative dispersion less than 20%, the critical O_2ER is optimized (Fig. 4). However, when relative dispersion is increased beyond 30% the critical O_2ER decreases sharply [24]. Due to the difficulty of measuring variation in microregional VO_2, this hypothesis has not been tested directly. However, capillary transit time distributions may be reasonable surrogate measurements reflecting distributions of VO_2/DO_2 [19, 30]. Humer and colleagues [19] found that following endotoxin infusion, the relative dispersion of capillary transit times increased by approximately 15% compared to non-endotoxemic controls. The increase in heterogeneity of transit times was associated with a reduction in the critical O_2ER to approximately 60% from 74%. The theoretically predicted reduction in critical O_2ER due to increased DO_2/VO_2 mismatching, corresponded closely to the experimentally measured reduction in crit-

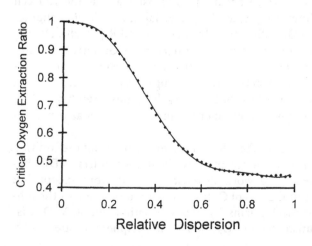

Fig. 4. The effect of increasing heterogeneity of the ratio of microregional oxygen supply to demand. Increased heterogeneity (relative dispersion) theoretically limits the ability of the myocardium to extract oxygen so that the critical oxygen extraction ratio decreases

ical O_2ER [19]. Thus, these data [19, 24] and other observations [30] are consistent with the hypothesis that microregional mismatching of DO_2 to VO_2 contributes substantially to physiologic arterial-venous shunt and therefore may account for the critical O_2ER and the limit to O_2 transport in many tissues. This observation may explain why no evidence of oxygen diffusion limitation is observed in whole body measurements when the O_2-Hb relationship is left-shifted [25].

Capillary and Tissue PO_2

The PO_2 of capillary blood decreases continuously along the length of the capillary [31]. Additionally, O_2 can start to diffuse in reasonable quantities even out of arterioles [32]. In a number of tissues, for example, in the villi of the gut, the perfusing arterioles are anatomically adjacent to draining veins. In these tissues, substantial amounts of O_2 can diffuse from arterioles to venules, bypassing the capillary bed entirely [23, 31, 32]. There is not much evidence for direct anatomic shunting of arterial blood to venules although such shunting would certainly lead to impaired O_2 extraction by the tissues. Diffusional O_2 shunt increases venous PO_2 relative to end-capillary PO_2.

The characteristics of O_2 transport from the capillaries to the tissues, if diffusion were the only mechanism for O_2 transport, would be well described by a Krogh tissue cylinder model [21]. Krogh [33], considering transport by molecular diffusion only, used a theoretical cylindrical model of tissue surrounding a central capillary to describe the tissue distribution of PO_2. Recent use of this theoretical model to predict experimentally measured values of critical O_2ER demonstrated that functional shunting of O_2 past the Krogh tissue cylinder had to be included, or diffusion distances had to be increased, well beyond typical intercapillary distances [21]. Thus, diffusion alone does not account well for experimental observations.

Studies of PO_2 in tissues containing significant quantities of the O_2 carrying molecule, myoglobin, demonstrate that the tissue PO_2 profile predicted by Krogh cylinder models are not found experimentally [34]. Instead, a high PO_2 gradient is found across the capillary wall. As a result, tissue PO_2 has a remarkably flat profile for considerable distances away from capillaries. The high PO_2 gradient across the capillary wall and the relatively uniform tissue PO_2 distribution, are due to the O_2 carrying properties of myoglobin [35]. Tissue myoglobin decreases the tissue PO_2 necessary for high tissue O_2 content (Fig. 1). Tissue myoglobin and other O_2 carrying molecules greatly increase tissue O_2 concentration so that the same flow of O_2 can occur with a greatly reduced driving pressure gradient within the tissues. To better understand this concept, an electrical analogy can be drawn to a resistor described by Ohm's Law:

$$Resistance = Voltage/Current \qquad (4)$$

Flow of electrons through a resistor, which is characterized by relatively few free electrons, requires a high voltage or driving gradient to electron flow. In contrast, the same current flow through a wire with a low resistance, characterized by many free electrons, requires a much lower pressure gradient. Thus, increasing the content of current carrying electrons decreases resistance to total electron flow.

Increasing the O_2 content of tissues is very much analogous to increasing the number of free electrons in a conductor. Increasing O_2 content of tissues greatly reduces the resistance to total O_2 flow. Thus, the PO_2 difference required for O_2 transport is greatly reduced so that, in the presence of O_2 carriers such as myoglobin, tissue PO_2 close to capillaries is not much different from tissue PO_2 far away from capillaries. To maintain normal electron transport, mitochondria require only very low values of PO_2 in the range of 0.25–2 mm Hg, while PO_2 values in the tissues are typically in the range of 4–7 mm Hg. O_2 transport is easily accomplished from the tissues to the mitochondria by using a PO_2 gradient of this magnitude [34, 35].

Physiologic Effects of Hypoxia

In many studies of hypoxic ventilation, the most remarkable finding is the very small physiologic effect of very significant reductions in arterial PO_2 [1, 36]. These observations emphasize the importance of O_2 transport mechanisms that have evolved in order to reduce the importance of PO_2 gradients in diffusive transport of O_2 to the tissues. These mechanisms include the presence of O_2 carrying molecules such as Hb, the curvilinearity of the O_2-Hb dissociation curve, shifts of the O_2-Hb dissociation curve (induced by O_2, CO_2, 2,3-diphosphoglycerate (DPG), and pH), O_2 carrying molecules within tissue such as myoglobin [34, 35], and multiple mechanisms which regulate matching of DO_2 to VO_2 even at the microvascular level [37]. Only when all these systems are taken to their physiologic limit does O_2 diffusion play an important role in limiting O_2 transport. Thus, experimental studies of progressive hypoxia observe relative stability of physiologic function [36] until a precipitous arrest occurs almost coincident with the onset of DO_2 limitation [1]. This observation is in marked contrast to the typical findings in experimental models of progressive hemorrhage, where animals live for much greater periods of time and at much lower whole body DO_2 than that at the onset of anaerobic metabolism [16, 17, 19]. The precipitous arrest during progressive hypoxic hypoxia is consistent with a special role for the heart, as discussed below.

When taken to extreme levels, hypoxic hypoxia decreases central nervous system (CNS) function [38] and results in a specific pattern of neuronal damage [39]. During moderate hypoxia, brain function is relatively preserved with minimal changes in cortical metabolites and high energy phosphate compounds [38]. However, when PaO_2 falls below 40 mm Hg during increased neural activity, brain function decreases [38]. Steps in this process initially include changes in membrane potential and ion concentrations [40]. Later, impaired synaptic transmission occurs, followed by an increase in extracellular concentrations of excitatory amino acid neurotransmitters [40]. Nuclear chromatin clumping, nucleolar condensation and cytoskeletal breakdown are then observed [39]. Ultrastructural changes observed during hypoxic hypoxia that are not observed during ischemic hypoxia, include mitochondrial swelling and microvacuolation, glycogen particles within astroglial processes, and minimal perivascular astroglial swelling despite perineuronal swelling. Chronic hypoxia has an impact on normal brain development [41]. These changes include delay of growth of cholinergic and serotonergic fibers into the hippocampus and neocortex during development, as well as increased neurodegeneration of serotoninergic axons during aging.

There is diversity of vascular smooth muscle responses to hypoxic hypoxia [42]. Hypoxia decreases resistance of systemic arteries so that mean arterial pressure (MAP) usually decreases to some extent even though CO is increased. The mechanism of arterial vasodilation is not dependent on nitric oxide (NO) synthesis [43]. In contrast, systemic veins constrict. This constriction of systemic veins is associated with an increase in mean systemic pressure, the pressure driving venous return to the heart. The changes observed in factors governing venous return are partly due to increased sympathetic tone. The pulmonary vasculature constricts during hypoxic hypoxia in a response termed hypoxic pulmonary vasoconstriction. The pulmonary arteries constrict in response to low alveolar PO_2 and also in response to low SvO_2.

Hypoxic hypoxia results in increased numbers of erythropoietin producing cells in the kidney [44] and increased overall production of erythropoietin. Chronic hypoxia increases erythropoietin messenger ribonucleic acid (mRNA) expression in peritubular cells located in the cortical labyrinth. This response results in increased Hb concentrations in humans exposed to chronic tissue hypoxia of various causes. Erythropoietin production is one compensatory mechanism that improves O_2 transport to tissues. In addition, perfused capillary density increases with acute hypoxic hypoxia to decrease diffusion distances. Chronic hypoxia also results in angiogenesis [45] as an additional long-term mechanism for reducing diffusion distances for O_2 in the tissues. Angiogenesis may depend on chemokine expression [46] and increased expression of other tissue signaling proteins induced by hypoxia.

Hypoxic hypoxia can trigger the synthesis of a set of hypoxia related proteins [47, 48]. Initially, hypoxia can induce increased expression of immediate early genes including c-jun, c-fos, c-myc, and early growth response (egr)-1 [47]. Expression of these genes is observed in all tissues but is most pronounced in the heart and less evident in lung tissue [47]. A set of hypoxic stress proteins are then upregulated, including glyceraldehyde-3-phosphate dehydrogenase (GAPDH) [48], hypoxia inducible factor-1 (HIF-1) [49], vascular endothelial growth factor [50] and interleukin(IL)-6 [50]. These proteins are similar in some respects, but have substantial differences from inflammatory proteins and heat-shock proteins. Interestingly, body temperature decreases during hypoxic hypoxia [51] possibly due to conforming VO_2 [52] where hypoxia results in down-regulation of metabolic processes. Hypoxia down-regulates key ATP dependent metabolic pathways including protein synthesis, protein degradation, gluconeogenesis, urea synthesis, and maintenance of electrochemical gradients [53].

When all compensatory mechanisms are taken to their limit, hypoxic hypoxia results in cell death. A shift to anaerobic metabolic pathways in the absence of adequate O_2 results in an intracellular acidosis. Interestingly, acidosis appears to protect against cell death. Inadequate ATP supplies result in loss of ionic gradients. An important step appears to be induction of the mitochondrial permeability transition (MPT) by hypoxic hypoxia [54], that may be a crucial, relatively irreversible step in the pathway to cell death. The MPT results in uncoupling of oxidative phosphorylation and increased ATP hydrolysis, further compromising cellular energy stores; cell swelling and death follow.

Understanding O_2-sensing mechanisms within cells is an area of considerable recent interest [49, 53]. PO_2 may be sensed in a number of different ways. Heme proteins, including hemokinases, NADH oxidases, cytochromes, and related proteins, appear to be important [53, 55]. Reactive O_2 intermediates (ROI) involved in intracellular signal transduction of acute phase gene expression may play a role [55[. O_2 sensing by ion channels [56], including potassium channels [57] and voltage-gated calcium channels [58], is another likely mechanism of O_2 sensing within cells. Glomus cells within the carotid body are important PaO_2 sensors [59]. Potassium channels appear to be sensitive to hypoxia [57, 59] and modulate the electrical properties of glomus cells that transmit signals to the brainstem via the carotid sinus nerve [59]. Normal O_2 sensing mechanisms that play an important role in responding to change in altitude also include G-protein dependent receptor systems such as cardiac β-receptors, adenosine receptors, and muscarinic receptors [57].

It is unclear how DO_2 can be regulated to meet O_2 demand, when sensing the signal for inadequate DO_2 occurs within the capillary bed yet the regulation of blood flow occurs upstream at the arteriolar level. Tyml and colleagues [60, 61] have shown that the capillary and microvascular endothelium acts to transmit vasoactive signals upstream. A vasoconstrictive stimulus applied to capillaries can be transmitted to upstream arterioles 1000 μm away [62]. Communication from endothelial cell to endothelial cell appears to occur via gap junctions. Endothelial cells also appear to signal underlying smooth muscle, using a similar signal transmission mechanism via gap junctions [63]. In addition, myogenic mechanisms responding to vascular wall strain (responsive to intravascular pressure) and shear stress (responsive to intravascular flow) contribute to microvascular flow regulation [64].

Hypoxemia and the Heart

The multiple compensatory mechanisms that have evolved to avoid diffusion limitation of DO_2 are remarkably effective during progressive hypoxic hypoxia. As a result, progressive hypoxia produces minimal physiologic effects until a critical point at which a precipitous cardiac arrest ensues. The heart plays a central role in determining the limit of hypoxic hypoxia because this organ is particularly dependent upon an adequate DO_2 to maintain aerobic metabolism and function [1, 2]. During progressive hypoxemia, coronary blood flow increases in inverse proportion to the reductions in SaO_2 so that the myocardial O_2ER is maintained relatively constant. During the initial stages of progressive hypoxia, no changes in cardiac contractile function, as measured by the end-systolic pressure-volume relationship, are observed. Likewise, no significant changes in CO or lactate consumption are observed. When SaO_2 is reduced to the extent that increases in coronary blood flow can no longer compensate, then myocardial VO_2 decreases. When myocardial VO_2 decreases, associated physiologic and metabolic effects include: decreased contractile function; ECG changes; and decreases in myocardial lactate consumption [1]. Very soon after the first evidence of myocardial anaerobic metabolism is observed, cardiac arrest occurs. Cessation of myocardial contraction is potentially accounted for by a detrimental positive feedback loop whereby inadequate myocardial DO_2 leads to decreased myocardial contractile function. Decreased myocardial contractile function leads to decreased CO and organ perfusion that then leads to further reductions in cardiac contractile function.

VO_2 by the heart provides approximately 20 J/mL O_2. Suga and colleagues [65–67] and others [68, 69], have shown that there is a close relationship between myocardial VO_2 and the pressure-volume-area (PVA) (Fig. 5) from the pressure-volume loop of a cardiac cycle and the end-systolic pressure-volume relationship. Myocardial VO_2 is linearly related to PVA (Fig. 5) with a significant myocardial VO_2 intercept at zero PVA. The myocardial VO_2 identified by this intercept provides energy used in excitation-contraction coupling and energy to ensure cell viability, for example, by maintaining membrane concentration gradients. Increasing contractility increases the myocardial VO_2 intercept [70]. As external

Fig. 5. A When ventricular pressure-volume trajectories are plotted the area of loops has units of work. End-systolic points from many different contractions (not shown) all lie along the end-systolic pressure-volume relationship (ESPVR). The area enclosed within a cardiac cycle is external mechanical work. Potential mechanical work is the area to the left of pressure-volume loops under the ESPVR. Myocardial oxygen consumption (MVO_2) is found to be closely correlated to pressure-volume-area (shaded area), which is the sum of external mechanical work and potential mechanical work. B MVO_2 is linearly related to pressure-volume-area (PVA). Part of the MVO_2 is used to generate PVA work while part goes to activation, or excitation-contraction coupling, and for basic metabolic processes to maintain cell viability

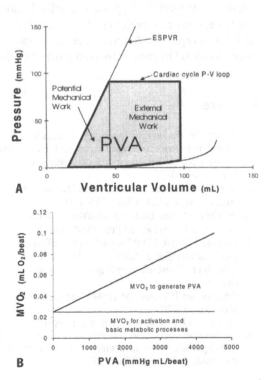

mechanical work and PVA increase, myocardial VO_2 increases. The heart is approximately 40% efficient in generating PVA work from the consumed O_2 [71]. The close relationship between myocardial VO_2 and PVA accounts for the rapid decrease in contractility observed during hypoxic hypoxia [1]. When myocardial VO_2 is limited, PVA must also be limited, either by decreased contractility, afterload, or stroke volume.

Cardiac myocytes demonstrate a critical PO_2 [72]. In a quiescent, state cardiac myocyte VO_2 decreases at PO_2 values less than 1.4 mm Hg. When PO_2 decreases below 1 mm Hg, free ADP and adenosine increase. When cardiac myocytes are stimulated to contract, the critical myocardial PO_2 increases to 10 mm Hg. VO_2 decreases as PO_2 is decreased from 10 to 5 mm Hg, but free ADP and adenosine do not change. Below a PO_2 of 5 mm Hg, free ADP and adenosine increase.

Conclusion

Hypoxic hypoxia refers to limitation of aerobic metabolism due to diffusion limitation of O_2, a phenomenon which in turn is dependent upon PO_2 gradients. In general, diffusion limitation does not occur because of multiple mechanisms. These mechanisms include the presence of O_2 carriers, the non-linear O_2-Hb dissociation curve, tissue myoglobin and other tissue O_2 carriers, and careful matching of capillary DO_2 to microregional VO_2. O_2 diffusion may become the limiting step in working heart and skeletal muscle, but is rarely the limiting step in other organs. In progressive hypoxic hypoxia, the myocardium is generally the first organ to demonstrate evidence of diffusion limitation of DO_2. Diminished myocardial VO_2 is rapidly followed by decreased cardiac function and death because the heart is central to convective transport of O_2 from the lungs to the tissues.

References

1. Walley KR, Becker CJ, Hogan RA, Teplinsky K, Wood LDH (1988) Progressive hypoxemia limits left ventricular oxygen consumption and contractility. Circ Res 63:849–859
2. Coulson RL (1976) Energetics of isovolumic contractions of the isolated rabbit heart. J Physiol 260:45–53
3. Hotchkiss RS, Karl IE (1992) Reevaluation of the role of cellular hypoxia and bioenergetic failure in sepsis. JAMA 267:1503–1510
4. Brooks GA (1986) Lactate production under fully aerobic conditions: the lactate shuttle during rest and exercise. Fed Proc 45:2924–2929
5. Kreuzer F, Hoofd LJ (1976) Facilitated diffusion of CO and oxygen in the presence of hemoglobin or myoglobin. Adv Exp Med Biol 75:207–215
6. West JB (1985) Respiratory Physiology – the essentials. 3rd edition. Williams & Wilkins, Baltimore
7. Schumacker PT, Cain SM (1987) The concept of a critical oxygen delivery. Intensive Care Med 13:223–229
8. Fink M (1997) Cytopathic hypoxia in sepsis. Acta Anaesthesiol Scand 110 (Suppl): 87–95
9. Ogilvie CM, Forster RE, Blakemore WS, Morton JW (1957) A standardized breath-holding technique for the clinical measurement of the diffusing capacity of the lung for carbon monoxide. J Clin Invest 36:1–17

10. Torre-Bueno JR, Wagner PD, Saltzman HA, Gale GE, Moon RE (1985) Diffusion limitation in normal humans during exercise at sea level and simulated altitude. J Appl Physiol 58:989-995
11. Wagner PD, West JB (1972) Effects of diffusion impairment on O_2 and CO_2 time courses in pulmonary capillaries. J Appl Physiol 33:62-71
12. Rossaint R, Hahn SM, Pappert D, Falke KJ, Radermacher P (1995) Influence of mixed venous PO_2 and inspired O_2 fraction on intrapulmonary shunt in patients with severe ARDS. J Appl Physiol 78:1531-1536
13. Melot C (1994) Contribution of multiple inert gas elimination technique to pulmonary medicine. 5. Ventilation-perfusion relationships in acute respiratory failure. Thorax 49:1251-1258
14. Baigorri F, Russell JA (1996) Oxygen delivery in critical illness. Crit Care Clinics 12:971-994
15. Schumacker PT, Samsel RW (1989) Oxygen delivery and uptake by peripheral tissues: physiology and pathophysiology. Crit Care Clinics 5:255-269
16. Nelson DP, King CE, Dodd SL, Schumacker PT, Cain SM (1987) Systemic and intestinal limits of O_2 extraction in the dog. J Appl Physiol 63:387-394
17. Segal JM, Phang PT, Walley KR (1992) Low-dose dopamine hastens onset of gut ischemia in a porcine model of hemorrhagic shock. J Appl Physiol 73:1159-1164
18. Jammes Y, Zattara-Hartmann MC, Badier M (1997) Functional consequences of acute and chronic hypoxia on respiratory and skeletal muscles in mammals. Comp Biochem Physiol A Physiol 118:15-22
19. Humer MF, Phang PT, Friesen BP, Allard MF, Goddard CM, Walley KR (1996) Heterogeneity of gut capillary transit times and impaired gut oxygen extraction in endotoxemic pigs. J Appl Physiol 81:895-904
20. Ronco JJ, Fenwick JC, Tweeddale MG, et al (1993) Identification of the critical oxygen delivery for anaerobic metabolism in critically ill septic and nonseptic humans. JAMA 270:1724-1730
21. Schumacker PT, Samsel RW (1989) Analysis of oxygen delivery and uptake relationships in the Krogh tissue model. J Appl Physiol 67:1234-1244
23. Piiper J, Meyer M, Scheid P (1984) Dual role of diffusion in tissue gas exchange: blood-tissue equilibration and diffusion shunt. Adv Exp Med Biol 180:85-94
24. Walley KR (1996) Heterogeneity of oxygen delivery impairs oxygen extraction by peripheral tissues: theory. J Appl Physiol 81:885-894
25. Schumacker PT, Long GR, Wood LD (1987) Tissue oxygen extraction during hypovolemia: role of hemoglobin P50. J Appl Physiol 62:1801-1807
26. Walley KR, Collins RM, Cooper DJ, Warriner CB (1997) Myocardial anaerobic metabolism occurs at a critical coronary venous PO_2 in pigs. Am J Respir Crit Care Med 155:222-228
27. Gutierrez G, Pohil RJ, Strong R (1988) Effect of flow on O_2 consumption during progressive hypoxemia. J Appl Physiol 65:601-607
28. King CE, Dodd SL, Cain SM (1987) O_2 delivery to contracting muscle during hypoxic or CO hypoxia. J Appl Physiol 63:726-732
29. Rose CP, Goresky CA (1985) Limitations of tracer oxygen uptake in the canine coronary circulation. Circ Res 56:57-71
30. Honig CR, Odoroff CL (1981) Calculated dispersion of capillary transit times: significance for oxygen exchange. Am J Physiol 240:H199-H208
31. Ellis CG, Ellsworth ML, Pittman RN (1990) Determination of red blood cell oxygenation in vivo by dual video densitometric image analysis. Am J Physiol 258:H1216-H1223
32. Ivanov KP, Derii AN, Samoilov MO, Semenov DG (1982) Direct measurements of oxygen tension at the surface of arterioles, capillaries and venules of the cerebral cortex. Pflügers Arch 393:118-120
33. Krogh A (1918) The number and distribution of capillaries in muscles with calculation of the oxygen pressure head necessary for supplying the tissue. J Physiol 52:409-415
34. Gayeski TE, Honig CR (1983) Direct measurement of intracellular O_2 gradients; role of convection and myoglobin. Adv Exp Med Biol 159:613-621
35. Honig CR, Gayeski TE, Federspiel W, Clark A Jr, Clark P (1984) Muscle O_2 gradients from hemoglobin to cytochrome: new concepts, new complexities. Adv Exp Med Biol 169:23-38
36. Engelen M, Porszasz J, Riley M, Wasserman K, Maehara K, Barstow TJ (1996) Effects of hypoxic hypoxia on O_2 uptake and heart rate kinetics during heavy exercise. J Appl Physiol 81:2500-2508

37. Caldwell JH, Martin GV, Raymond GM, Bassingthwaighte JB (1994) Regional myocardial flow and capillary permeability-surface area products are nearly proportional. Am J Physiol 267:H654–H666
38. LaManna JC, Light Al, Peretsman SJ, Rosenthal M (1984) Oxygen insufficiency during hypoxic hypoxia in rat brain cortex. Brain Res 293:313–318
39. Allen A, Yanushka J, Fitzpatrick JH, Jenkins LW, Gilboe DD (1989) Acute ultrastructural response of hypoxic hypoxia with relative ischemia in the isolated brain. Acta Neuropathol 78:637–648
40. Martin RL, Lloyd HG, Cowan AI (1994) The early events of oxygen and glucose deprivation: setting the scene for neuronal death? Trends Neurosci 17:251–257
41. Nyakas C, Buwalda B, Luiten PG (1996) Hypoxia and brain development. Prog Neurobiol 49: 1–51
42. Weir EK, Reeve HL, Cornfield DN, Tristani-Firouzi M, Peterson DA, Archer SL (1997) Diversity of response in vascular smooth muscle cells to changes in oxygen tension. Kidney Int 51:462–466
43. Vallet B, Curtis SE, Winn MJ, King CE, Chapler CK, Cain SM (1994) Hypoxic vasodilation does not require nitric oxide (EDRF/NO) synthesis. J Appl Physiol 76:1256–1261
44. Eckardt KU, Koury ST, Tan CC, Schuster SJ, Kaissling B, Ratcliffe PJ, Kurtz A (1993) Distribution of erythropoietin producing cells in rat kidneys during hypoxic hypoxia. Kidney Int 43:815–823
45. Schaper W, Ito WD (1996) Molecular mechanisms of coronary collateral vessel growth. Circ Res 79:911–919
46. Strieter RM, Polverini PJ, Arenberg DA, Walz A, Opdenakker G, Van Damme J, Kunkel SL (1995) Role of C-X-C chemokines as regulators of angiogenesis in lung cancer. J Leukoc Biol 57:752–762
47. Gess B, Wolf K, Pfeifer M, Riegger GA, Kurtz A (1997) In vivo carbon monoxide exposure and hypoxic hypoxia stimulate immediate early gene expression. Pflügers Arch 434:568–574
48. Graven KK, Farber HW (1995) Hypoxia-associated proteins. New Horizons 3:208–218
49. Bunn HF, Poyton RO (1996) Oxygen sensing and molecular adaptation to hypoxia. Physiol Rev 76:839–885
50. Yan SF, Ogawa S, Stern DM, Pinsky DJ (1997) Hypoxia-induced modulation of endothelial cell properties: regulation of barrier function and expression of interleukin-6. Kidney Int 51:419–425
51. Clark DJ, Fewell JE (1994) Body-core temperature decreases during hypoxic hypoxia in Long-Evans and Brattleboro rats. Can J Physiol Pharmacol 72:1528–1531
52. Schumacker PT, Chandel N, Agusti AG (1993) Oxygen conformance of cellular respiration in hepatocytes. Am J Physiol 265:L395–L402
53. Hochachka PW, Land SC, Buck LT (1997) Oxygen sensing and signal transduction in metabolic defense against hypoxia: lessons from vertebrate facultative anaerobes. Comp Biochem Physiol A Physiol 118:23–29
54. Lemasters JJ, Nieminen AL, Qian T, Trost LC, Herman B (1997) The mitochondrial permeability transition in toxic, hypoxic and reperfusion injury. Mol Cell Biochem 174:159–165
55. Acker H (1996) PO_2 affinities, heme proteins, and reactive oxygen intermediates involved in intracellular signal cascades for sensing oxygen. Adv Exp Med Biol 410:59–64
56. Lopez-Barneo J, Ortega-Saenz P, Molina A, Franco-Obregon A, Urena J, Castellano A (1997) Oxygen sensing by ion channels. Kidney Int 51:454–461
57. Richalet JP (1997) Oxygen sensors in the organism: examples of regulation under altitude hypoxia in mammals. Comp Biochem Physiol A Physiol 118:9–14
58. Franco-Obregon A, Montoro R, Urena J, Lopez-Barneo J (1996) Modulation of voltage-gated Ca^{2+} channels by O_2 tension. Significance for arterial oxygen chemoreception. Adv Exp Med Biol 410:97–103
59. Gonzalez C, Lopez-Lopez JR, Obeso A, Perez-Garcia MT, Rocher A (1995) Cellular mechanisms of oxygen chemoreception in the carotid body. Respir Physiol 102:137–147
60. Dietrich HH, Tyml K (1992) Capillary as a communicating medium in the microvasculature. Microvasc Res 43:87–99

61. Song H, Tyml K (1993) Evidence for sensing and integration of biological signals by the capillary network. Am J Physiol 265: H1235–H1242
62. Dietrich HH, Tyml K (1992) Microvascular flow response to localized application of norepinephrine on capillaries in rat and frog skeletal muscle. Microvasc Res 43: 73–86
63. Little TL, Xia J, Duling BR (1995) Dye tracers define differential endothelial and smooth muscle coupling patterns within the arteriolar wall. Circ Res 76: 498–504
64. Kuo L, Davis MJ, Chilian WM (1988) Myogenic activity in isolated subepicardial and subendocardial coronary arterioles. Am J Physiol 255: H1558–H1562
65. Khalafbeigui F, Suga H, Sagawa K (1979) Left ventricular systolic pressure volume area correlates with oxygen consumption. Am J Physiol 237: H566–H569
66. Suga H (1979) Total mechanical energy of a ventricle model and cardiac oxygen consumption. Am J Physiol 236: H498–H505
67 Suga H, Yamada O, Goto Y, Igarashi Y (1984) Oxygen consumption and pressure-volume area of abnormal contractions in canine heart. Am J Physiol 246: H154–H160
68. Hisano R, Cooper G IV (1987) Correlation of force-length area with oxygen consumption in ferret papillary muscle. Circ Res 61: 318–328
69. Goto Y, Slinker BK, LeWinter MM (1988) Similar normalized Emax and O2 consumption-pressure-volume area relation in rabbit and dog. Am J Physiol 255: H366–H374
70. Suga H, Hisano R, Goto Y, Yamada O, Igarashi Y (1983) Effect of positive inotropic agents on the relation between oxygen consumption and systolic pressure volume area in canine left ventricle. Circ Res 53: 306–318
71. Gibbs CL, Chapman JB (1985) Cardiac mechanics and energetics: chemomechanical transduction in cardiac muscle. Am J Physiol 249: H199–H206
72. Stumpe T, Schrader J (1997) Phosphorylation potential, adenosine formation, and critical PO_2 in stimulated rat cardiomyocytes. Am J Physiol 273: H756–H766

Circulatory Hypoxia

J. Marshall

Introduction

Circulatory hypoxia or systemic hypoxia is characterized by a fall in the arterial partial pressure of oxygen (PaO_2). Acutely, systemic hypoxia can occur as an occupational hazard in healthy individuals who work, for example, as divers or pilots. It can also occur during asthmatic attacks, mild exercise and air travel in those who have respiratory disease, but who manage to maintain a normal PaO_2 so long as they are at rest and at normal atmospheric pressure. Acute hypoxia is also common in the period following anesthesia and surgery. On a more chronic time base, hypoxia occurs in healthy lowlanders who climb to high altitudes, or who travel to high altitude for work or pleasure. Chronic hypoxia may also be present from birth in babies who are born with an under-developed respiratory system or cardiac abnormality, and can occur in adult life in patients with a range of respiratory and cardiovascular disorders.

Despite its prevalence, we know relatively little about the effects of acute systemic hypoxia on the cardiovascular system and are only just beginning to recognize the cellular mechanisms that underlie these effects. As far as chronic systemic hypoxia is concerned, it is becoming increasingly clear that important adaptive changes occur in the cardiovascular system when the hypoxic state is prolonged, but it is not yet known what triggers these changes, nor how the adaptations affect the normal regulation of the cardiovascular system and the ability to respond to other stimuli.

This chapter reviews what is currently known about the reflex and local effects of acute systemic hypoxia on the cardiovascular system of several different species and uses this a background to consider the responses that occur in human infants and adults. The chapter discusses the role of adenosine as a major mediator of the local effects of hypoxia, as well as reviewing some of the recent observations on the adaptations that chronic systemic hypoxia produces, concentrating on the evidence that the balance between neurally-mediated, reflex control and local control mechanisms is changed by chronic hypoxia, so as to favor the dilator influences of substances derived from the endothelium.

Acute Hypoxia

It is generally accepted that acute hypoxia produces vasoconstriction in the pulmonary circulation and vasodilatation in the cerebral circulation and that these changes largely, if not entirely, reflect the local effects of hypoxia upon these circulations. However, the effects that acute hypoxia has on the heart and on the other regional vascular beds of the systemic circulation are far less clear cut. In the heart and other vascular beds, the circulatory effects of acute hypoxia represent a balance among: (1) the primary reflex responses that are produced in the cardiovascular system by hypoxic stimulation of peripheral chemoreceptors; (2) the secondary effects that occur in the cardiovascular system as a consequence of the respiratory changes produced by peripheral chemoreceptor stimulation; (3) the responses that occur as a result of hypoxia of the central nervous system; and (4) the local, or direct influences of hypoxia on the heart and peripheral tissues. The balance among these effects varies between species and with the severity and duration of the period of hypoxia, even within the acute time span of minutes or hours.

The Alerting or Defense Response

It is generally accepted that the primary cardiovascular responses to selective stimulation of peripheral chemoreceptors are bradycardia and peripheral vasoconstriction and that these responses may be overcome by tachycardia and vasodilatation secondary to the chemoreceptor-evoked increase in respiration [1]. However experiments on cats and rats anesthetized with the steroid anesthetic alphaxalone-alphadalone (Saffan or Althesin), which does not depress forebrain influences over the cardiovascular system to the same extent as more commonly used anesthetics, have revealed that selective stimulation of the carotid chemoreceptors can also evoke the pattern of cardiovascular response that is characteristic of the "alerting" or "defense" response [1, 2]. This response includes tachycardia, an increase in cardiac output (CO), vasoconstriction in cutaneous, renal and splanchnic circulations, but vasodilatation in skeletal muscle; these changes generally lead to a rise in systemic arterial pressure. This pattern of response is generally evoked by novel, noxious or painful stimuli and by emotional stress. It is integrated by specific regions of the hypothalamus, midbrain and medulla, traditionally known as the defense areas, in all mammalian species that have been studied including human subjects. The magnitudes of the individual components of the response are graded with the strength of the stimulus, but the pattern of change is consistent. The accompanying behavioural changes range from arousal or increased alertness to overt rage, or aggression [3]. Not surprisingly, the tachycardia and vasoconstrictor components of the response reflect an increase in sympathetic activity. In cats and dogs, the vasodilatation in skeletal muscle has been attributed to the combined effect of a decrease in sympathetic norepinephrine activity and an increase in the activity of sympathetic cholinergic fibres to - this vasculature and to the β-adrenoreceptor-mediated effects of circulating epinephrine [3]. The most recent studies on human subjects suggest that the mechanisms responsible for vasodilatation in skeletal muscle in people are similar although it has been proposed that acetylcholine is not released as a transmitter from a special group of sympathetic fibres but is actually released from the endothelium by some influence, such as shear stress [4]; a similar system might apply in other species as well [3].

The evidence for defense area activation on selective chemoreceptor stimulation in animals anesthetized with alphaxalone-alphadalone has prompted investigation into the effects of systemic hypoxia in anesthetized and conscious animals. There is now strong evidence from experiments on the rat, that systemic hypoxia can evoke episodes of behavioral alerting that are indistinguishable from those evoked by other novel or noxious stimuli and that each of these is accompanied by the full cardiovascular pattern of the alerting response [5–8]. Such detailed investigations have not been made on other species. However, it has been shown that systemic hypoxia induced by breathing 12–6% O_2, can elicit the full cardiovascular pattern of the alerting response in cats anesthetized with alphaxalone-alphadalone [9], while in both conscious dogs and rabbits, systemic hypoxia elicits behavioral alerting, or arousal, that can be prevented by denervating the carotid chemoreceptors [10, 11]. Moreover, volunteers became "restless" when breathing 7.5% O_2 and some individuals feel so anxious or stressed that they cannot continue with the experiment [12, 13]. These findings taken together with the fact that systemic hypoxia increases circulating levels of epinephrine in the conscious rabbit and in at least some human subjects [11–13] are fully consistent with the idea that activation of the brain stem defense areas by peripheral chemoreceptors is an integral part of the response to acute systemic hypoxia in all species.

It seems that the full cardiovascular pattern of the alerting response is more likely to be distinguishable in the first 1–2 minutes of hypoxia when the onset of the hypoxia is sudden; when hypoxia develops gradually or when it is prolonged, the cardiovascular pattern of the alerting response is more likely to be overshadowed by the other reflex and local effects of hypoxia (see below). Nevertheless, even if the characteristic cardiovascular pattern is not immediately apparent, activation of the defense areas may have important functional implications. Firstly, behavioral arousal occurring, for example, in a diver whose O_2 supply begins to fail may improve his chances of resolving the situation, while behavioral arousal triggered by hypoxic stimulation of the peripheral chemoreceptors during sleep might save a baby from "sudden infant death syndrome" (SIDS) and would explain the insomnia that is common in mountaineers at high altitude. Secondly, an increase in defense area activity may explain in whole, or part, reports that the baroreceptor reflex is inhibited during acute systemic hypoxia (see below). Activation of the defense areas either electrically or by selective stimulation of carotid chemoreceptors can suppress the baroreceptor reflex. In fact, when the cardiovascular pattern of the alerting response was evoked by selective chemoreceptor stimulation, then baroreceptor stimulation, even with a pressure in the carotid sinus of 250 mm Hg, had no effect on the cardiovascular system, although the same baroreceptor stimulus in the absence of, or during mild, chemoreceptor stimulation evoked bradycardia and generalized vasodilatation [14]. This observation led to the proposal that peripheral chemoreceptor stimulation may, through the defense areas produce graded suppression of the baroreceptor reflex resulting in complete suppression when the chemoreceptor stimulus is particularly strong [14].

Gradual Effects of Acute Hypoxia

Although acute hypoxia may evoke the pattern of the alerting response, it is clear that this is superimposed upon other, more gradual changes that are graded with the level of hypoxia, but which may change in direction as the period of hypoxia lengthens. It is these gradual changes that vary qualitatively and quantitatively among species due to differences in the balance of effects that determines them (Fig. 1). These differences are explored below.

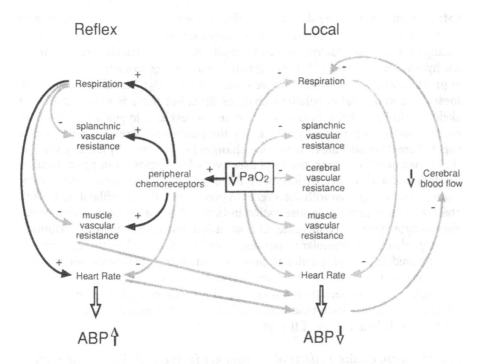

Fig. 1. Schematic diagram showing the roles of reflex and local influences of acute systemic hypoxia and their interactions in determining arterial pressure (ABP). Solid lines and + signs indicate excitatory or positive influences. Stippled lines and − signs indicate inhibitory or negative influences. When the reflex influences predominate, ABP generally rises (*left side*) whereas when the local influences predominate, ABP generally falls (*right side*). Further, if reflex vasodilatation secondary to increased respiration and/or the primary reflex bradycardia of chemoreceptor stimulation (see text) are strong, this may tip the balance towards a fall in arterial pressure. Note, when arterial pressure falls below the cerebral autoregulatory range, cerebral blood flow will fall and may depress respiration by a central neural action

Dog: In the dog, acute systemic hypoxia produces striking hyperventilation, an increase in heart rate, CO and arterial pressure accompanied by a decrease in total peripheral resistance that is largely attributable to vasodilatation in skeletal muscle: all of these changes are graded with the level of hypoxia [10, 15]. When ventilation is held constant, or the lungs are denervated, then the tachycardia is greatly reduced or reversed to bradycardia and the peripheral vasodilatation in skeletal muscle and elsewhere is reversed to vasoconstriction. By contrast, simply preventing the fall in $PaCO_2$ that arises from the hyperventilation has relatively little effect on the cardiovascular changes [10]. Thus, in the dog, the gradual cardiovascular responses to acute hypoxia are heavily dominated by reflex tachycardia and peripheral vasodilatation secondary to hyperventilation-induced stimulation of pulmonary stretch receptors with vagal afferents [10, 15]. When these effects are removed, the bradycardia and peripheral vasoconstriction elicited as the primary response to hypoxic stimulation of peripheral chemoreceptors predominate. It is only when the carotid chemoreceptors are denervated that the local dilator effects of hypoxia are manifest [10].

Cat: By contrast with the dog, the cat shows a weaker respiratory response to acute hypoxia and the cardiovascular changes are much less pronounced, consisting only of a mild tachycardia and a slight increase in arterial pressure when the hypoxia is moderate (15–12% O_2) which may change to a small fall in arterial pressure when the hypoxia is more severe (12–6% O_2). Vascular resistance in mesenteric and renal circulations changes little, but there is vasodilatation in skeletal muscle which is greater at more severe levels of hypoxia [9]. Again, in contrast to the dog, reflexes produced by the pulmonary stretch receptors with vagal afferents contribute little to these changes [9]. However, by holding ventilation constant with a pump, the responses evoked by hypoxia can be changed to bradycardia and vasoconstriction in the mesenteric and renal circulations, changes that are graded with the level of hypoxia while the vasodilatation in skeletal muscle is reduced. This observation indicates that it is the hypocapnia secondary to hypoxia-induced increases in respiration that are the major contribution to the gradual cardiovascular responses evoked in the cat. When these influences are removed, the primary reflex response to peripheral chemoreceptor stimulation becomes more evident [9]. Nevertheless, the fact that vasodilatation in skeletal muscle tends to persist even when the influences of respiration are prevented suggests that the local vasodilator influences of hypoxia are fairly strong, at least in the skeletal muscle of the cat.

Rat: The local, or direct effects of hypoxia are far more obvious in the rat than either the dog or cat. Thus, systemic hypoxia evokes initial hyperventilation and tachycardia, but within 2–3 minutes these changes begin to wane and when the period of hypoxia is prolonged and especially when it is severe, ventilation and heart rate fall below baseline [5, 16, 17]. Moreover, even in mild hypoxia, there is vasodilatation in the mesenteric and renal circulations and particularly in skeletal muscle, such that arterial pressure falls to an extent that is graded with the level of hypoxia [5, 16]. The pulmonary stretch receptors and, to a lesser extent the hypocapnia secondary to hyperventilation, make small contributions to the tachycardia [18, 19], but the remaining tachycardia apparently mainly results from the effects of increased central respiratory drive on cardiac vagal neurones, of central neural hypoxia on cardiac sympathetic activity and of the baroreceptor reflex response to the fall in arterial pressure [5, 17]. The late fall in respiration can be ascribed to the depressive influence of hypoxia on central respiratory neurones [5, 16, 17]. The late bradycardia is partly attributable to gradual predominance of the primary response to peripheral chemoreceptor stimulation in parallel with the waning of the respiratory response, but is largely explained by the local effect of hypoxia on the sinoatrial node [17]. Moreover, the vasodilatation in skeletal muscle and elsewhere is explained by a strong predominance of the local vasodilator influence of hypoxia over the primary vasoconstrictor response to peripheral chemoreceptor stimulation [5, 16, 17].

Adult human subjects: The cardiovascular changes induced by acute hypoxia in healthy adult humans bear little resemblance to those seen in the dog. Rather, they show more in common with those seen in the cat and rat. Thus, heart rate increases by a modest 30 beats/min even in response to the relatively severe stimulus of 7.5% O_2 [12, 20]. Arterial pressure may increase a little with moderate hypoxia, but it generally falls, by $\sim$ 15 mm Hg in severe hypoxia (7.5% O_2) [12, 20]. Meanwhile, splanchnic vascular resistance decreases, indicating vasodilatation in these beds and there is substantial vasodilatation in forearm skeletal muscle which is present even when the sympathetic nerves are blocked [12, 21]. As in the cat, the ventilatory response to acute hypoxia in human subjects is relatively small. There is an initial increase in ventilation, but ventilation then falls back towards the control level during hypoxia lasting 20 minutes [22]; the fall in $PaCO_2$ is only $\sim$ 10 mm Hg when subjects breathe 8% O_2 [23]. Accordingly, the evidence suggests that the pulmonary stretch receptors and hypocapnia secondary to hyperventilation, make only small contributions to the cardiovascular changes evoked in human subjects [23]. In fact, it is generally accepted that pulmonary stretch receptors have little influence in man, at least until tidal volume exceeds $\sim$ 1 liter [1]. Moreover, when CO_2 was added to the inspirate during hypoxia so as to maintain eucapnia at a given level of PaO_2 (40 mm Hg), the tachycardia decreased only by about 7 beats/min, but there was no effect on the forearm vasodilator response to hypoxia [23]. Plasma epinephrine tends to rise at more severe levels of hypoxia, reaching statistical significance after subjects breathe 10% O_2 for 20 mins or 8% O_2 for 8 mins [13]. However, these changes are stronger in some individuals than in others [12, 13] and so the action of epinephrine on β_2 adrenoceptors cannot be held generally responsible for the vasodilatation in forearm skeletal muscle [20]. Thus, in human subjects, as in rats, the tachycardia induced by acute hypoxia largely reflects the effects of central respiratory drive on cardiac vagal activity and the central neural effect of hypoxia on cardiac sympathetic activity and that, as in cats and rats, the peripheral vasodilatation reflects the dominance of the local vasodilator influences of hypoxia over any neurally mediated vasoconstriction [16, 21, 23].

Neonates: It became obvious to us when we were investigating the responses induced by systemic hypoxia in the rat, that they are very similar to those commonly reported in the newborn of many species including human infants. Thus, the characteristic features of the neonatal response are that initial hyperventilation soon turns to respiratory depression, any initial tachycardia gives way to bradycardia, and arterial pressure generally falls due to widespread peripheral vasodilatation [24]. Although the neonatal response has not been investigated to the same extent as that of various adult mammals, the most obvious conclusion to draw is that, as in the rat, the respiratory depression, bradycardia and peripheral vasodilatation largely reflect the predominance of the local effects of hypoxia on central respiratory neurones, the heart and peripheral tissues, over the reflex and neurally-mediated effects of hypoxia [24, 25, Fig. 1]. That effects secondary to hyperventilation are of minimal importance in mediating these responses is consistent with the fact that the bradycardia, peripheral vasodilatation and fall in arterial pressure are most evident in neonates that are under constant artificial ventilation, or in whom the spontaneous increase in ventilation is weak or non-existent [24, 25]. This conclusion is in accord with the knowledge that reflex and neurally mediated cardiovascular and respiratory responses are generally weak or poorly developed in neonates [24]. However, it is also likely that the local effects of hypoxia are generally stronger in small mammals, whether they are newborn or the adults of small mammalian species. Small mammals have a higher rate of O_2 consumption (VO_2) per body mass than larger mammals, and so their tissue VO_2 is more likely to be compromised by systemic hypoxia [5].

Functional Implications

The vasodilatation that occurs in the cerebral circulation during acute systemic hypoxia in several different species, including man, leads to an increase in cerebral blood flow and thereby improves the O_2 supply (DO_2) to the brain. Similarly, it is clear, irrespective of the different explanations for the muscle vasodilator response to acute hypoxia in different mammalian species, that this response tends to increase muscle blood flow [21, 23]. By contrast, the vasodilatation in the splanchnic and renal circulations is generally sufficient to cause only a modest increase in blood flow to these regions [12]. However, when arterial pressure begins to fall as has been reported in severe hypoxia in adult human subjects (see above), then blood flow to all regions particularly that to the brain becomes vulnerable. Indeed, severe hypoxia produced by breathing 7–8% O_2 produces syncope in some human subjects, the syncope being accompanied not only by a pronounced fall in arterial pressure, but also by bradycardia [26, 27].

Hypotension may result, in part, because sympathetic activity is less effective in producing vasoconstriction and because the normal baroreceptor control of blood pressure is impaired during hypoxia. Thus, in one study, the increase in sympathetic activity to skeletal muscle that was evoked by systemic hypoxia in human subjects was accompanied by smaller increases in plasma epinephrine than occurred when similar increases in muscle sympathetic activity were evoked by exercise or the cold pressor test [13]. Hypoxia might presynaptically inhibit the release of norepinephrine from sympathetic fibres or, alternatively, increase the re-uptake of norepinephrine (see below). However, not only did the progressive fall in arterial pressure that occurs in human subjects breathing 7.5% O_2 fail to evoke the progressive tachycardia that would be expected if the baroreceptor reflex were operating normally, but, whereas the pressor response evoked by systemic infusion of norepinephrine evoked a baroreceptor-mediated bradycardia in human subjects breathing air, it did not do so when they breathed 10% O_2 [12]. Moreover, in some human subjects, lower body negative pressure (LBNP) applied during hypoxia (10% O_2) evoked syncope with bradycardia and hypotension, whereas LBNP was well tolerated in these same subjects during normoxia, when they showed the expected tachycardia and maintenance of arterial pressure [26]. These results suggest that there may be a central neural inhibition of the baroreceptor reflex as might be explained, in part, by stimulation of peripheral chemoreceptors and activation of the defense areas (see above). In addition, evidence has been provided that, in some subjects, particularly large increases in plasma epinephrine may contribute to intolerance to orthostatic stress during hypoxia by causing pronounced β-adrenoreceptor-mediated dilatation [26]. However, it is also likely that the hypotension of severe hypoxia results much more directly from the strength of the local influences of hypoxia on the heart and circulation and on their interdependence. Indeed, these influences may contribute to a positive feedback loop such as we have suggested develops in neonates (Fig. 1).

A positive feedback loop: Our finding that the respiratory and cardiovascular changes evoked by acute hypoxia in the rat are very similar to those observed in neonates, led us to investigate the interrelationships between the respiratory and cardiovascular changes in more detail because we suspected a clinical relevance. In experiments on rats, we established that despite the vasodilatation that is induced in the cerebral circulation by acute systemic hypoxia, cerebral blood flow begins to fall when hypoxia-induced arterial hypotension decreases blood pressure below the cerebral autoregulatory range. This observation led us to propose that a positive feedback loop can develop that ultimately leads to death [17, 25]. Thus, when arterial pressure falls below the autoregulatory range, the consequent fall in cerebral blood flow exacerbates the cerebral hypoxia, and accentuates the respiratory depression that is caused by cerebral hypoxia. This, in turn, further exacerbates the fall in PaO_2, and accentuates the bradycardia and peripheral vasodilatation that are caused by tissue hypoxia, leading to an even greater fall in arterial pressure and reduction in cerebral blood flow [17, Fig. 1]. The fact that cerebral blood flow is much better maintained throughout a period of hypoxia when ventilation is maintained constant is fully consistent with this proposal [17].

It is widely held that the respiratory depression that results from the central neural effects of systemic hypoxia is a major contributing factor to SIDS [28]. Our findings have led us to propose that the local effects of hypoxia on the heart and peripheral circulation may be just as important as the respiratory changes because the respiratory and cardiovascular responses are mutually facilitatory. Furthermore, although a positive feedback loop that results in death may be more likely to develop in neonates simply because all of the local effects of hypoxia are stronger in neonates (see above), the interdependence of the fall in PaO_2, peripheral vasodilatation, fall in arterial pressure, reduction in cerebral blood flow and cerebral DO_2, may eventually lead to syncope in adults. It may be that in adults, the stronger central excitatory drive for respiration is normally the ultimate protection against death.

Mediators of the Local Effects of Acute Hypoxia

It should be clear from the above discussion that the local effects of hypoxia are of major importance in systemic hypoxia. Therefore, the identity of the substance(s) that mediate these effects is of considerable interest.

It is well known that adenosine is released by hypoxic tissues, indeed it has been shown to be released under hypoxic conditions in the brain, heart and skeletal muscle. It is also well known that adenosine is a potent vasodilator, that it can decrease heart rate by direct actions on the sinoatrial node, and that it can depress respiration when injected into the cerebral ventricles [29]. The known actions of adenosine led us to hypothesize that this substance may be the major factor responsible for the local effects of systemic hypoxia on respiration, the heart and peripheral circulations. Our studies have fully supported this hypothesis.

We have shown that 8-phenyltheophylline (8-PT) a specific adenosine receptor antagonist, greatly reduces the late respiratory depression, bradycardia, muscle vasodilatation and cerebral vasodilatation evoked in the rat by acute systemic hypoxia [16, 17, Table 1]. Others have shown that adenosine receptor antagonists injected into the cerebral ventricles attenuate hypoxia-induced respiratory depression [30]. Moreover, we found that 8-sulphophenyl-theophylline (8-SPT) or adenosine deaminase which do not cross the blood brain barrier, did not affect the respiratory depression induced by acute hypoxia, but did reduce the muscle vasodilatation and reduced the bradycardia and hypoxia-induced fall in arterial pressure, though to a lesser extent than 8-PT [31]. We have also shown that 8-PT applied directly to the cerebral cortex, or to skeletal muscle, greatly reduces the vasodilatation induced in these beds by hypoxia [32, 33]. Taken together, these results indicate that adenosine contributes independently to the respiratory depression, the bradycardia and to the cerebral and muscle vasodilatation, but they

Table 1. Influences of adenosine during acute systemic hypoxia	Effect	Receptor type
	Respiratory depression	A_1
	Bradycardia	A_1
	Muscle vasodilatation	A_1
	Cerebral vasodilatation	A_{2A}

also add further support to the idea that these responses are connected by a positive feedback loop (see above).

From a therapeutic point of view, these results suggest that an adenosine receptor antagonist might be particularly effective in breaking the positive feedback loop in hypoxic neonates and in preventing severe hypotension in hypoxic adults. It may be noted that theophylline, which is in clinical use and which is an adenosine receptor antagonist, has been shown to reverse hypoxia-induced respiratory depression in human infants as well as the neonates of other species [25] and have a similar effect on the late fall in respiration in adult human subjects [22]. Moreover, theophylline has been shown to have similar effects to 8-PT on the respiratory depression, bradycardia and muscle vasodilatation induced in the rat by systemic hypoxia [16]. However, since theophylline, unlike 8-PT, is also a phosphodiesterase inhibitor [59], some of its effects on cardiac muscle and on the smooth muscle of the respiratory tract and blood vessels may be due to an increase in cyclic adenosine monophosphate (cAMP) levels rather than to blockade of adenosine receptors.

Mechanisms of action of adenosine: It is now generally accepted that adenosine can act via at least four different subtypes of receptors. These receptors have been demonstrated in a range of tissues in many different species including man. There is substantial evidence that adenosine produces bradycardia mainly by acting on the A_1 subtype of the adenosine receptor [34]. Our recent studies on the rat in which we have used selective agonists and antagonists, have shown that the adenosine that is released in acute systemic hypoxia not only acts via A_1 receptors to produce bradycardia, but also acts on A_1 receptors to produce the central respiratory depression and muscle vasodilatation, whereas the cerebral vasodilatation is mediated by the A_{2A} subtype [35, 36, Table 1].

In the heart, adenosine produces bradycardia by acting presynaptically to facilitate vagal, and inhibit sympathetic, influences on the sinoatrial node as well as by directly depressing pacemaker activity [37, 38]. In skeletal muscle, adenosine can also act in several different ways. We have provided evidence that during acute systemic hypoxia adenosine stimulates adenosine receptors on skeletal muscle fibres that are coupled to adenosine triphosphate (ATP) sensitive K^+ (K_{ATP}) channels to cause the efflux of potassium which then acts as a vasodilator [39]. However, most of the hypoxia-induced muscle dilatation that is mediated by adenosine is dependent on the synthesis of nitric oxide (NO) by the endothelium [40]. Our results suggest that adenosine is released from the endothelial cells and acts on A_1 receptors on the endothelium to cause the synthesis of NO which then acts as a vasodilator; these A_1 receptors may be coupled to K_{ATP} channels on the endothelial cells [40–42]. In addition, adenosine and potassium may induce dilatation or, more precisely, antagonize the primary reflex constrictor response to hypoxic stimulation of peripheral chemoreceptors, by pre-synaptically inhibiting the release of norepinephrine from the sympathetic nerve fibres [43].

While adenosine may be the prime mediator of the local effects of hypoxia upon the cardiovascular system, it is not the only mediator, at least of the muscle vasodilatation. The various adenosine receptor antagonists we have used have only been able to reduce the muscle vasodilatation of acute hypoxia by about 50%, even when given at doses sufficient to completely block comparable dilatation produced by exogenous adenosine [31, 39, 40]. It seems likely that other mediators include prostaglandins which have been shown to be released from endothelial cells in response to hypoxia, and which *in vitro*, have been shown to contribute to hypoxia-induced dilatation [44].

Chronic Hypoxia

There is much evidence that chronic hypoxia affects respiratory sensitivity to O_2 and CO_2 as is indicated below. It is also generally accepted that chronic hypoxia leads to an increased hematocrit (Hct) which tends to normalize the arterial O_2 content despite the reduced PaO_2. There is also evidence that angiogenesis occurs, at least in the brain and skeletal muscle; angiogenesis should help to improve the distribution of O_2 to tissue cells [45]. However, despite the pronounced neurally- and locally-mediated effects that acute hypoxia can have on the cardiovascular system, these effects are not apparent in the resting values of cardiovascular variables in individuals who are chronically hypoxic. This finding alone suggests that additional adaptive changes have occurred, but would not necessarily lead one to predict that both reflex and local control of the cardiovascular system have changed.

Chronic Hypoxia from Birth

It is known that chronic hypoxia from birth (CHB) causes a blunting of respiratory sensitivity to hypoxia, mainly because the sensitivity of the peripheral chemoreceptors does not show the usual re-setting from the range of PO_2 values normally experienced in the fetus to the higher values normally found in adult life [46]. We have performed experiments to investigate the parallel effects on the cardiovascular system [47]. We studied rats that were kept in a hypoxic chamber at 12% O_2 from birth until they were 8–9 weeks old (CHB rats) by which time they had reached sexual maturity. They were then experimented upon whilst under anesthesia and were compared with matched controls that had breathed air (normoxia) from birth (NB).

When the CHB rats were breathing 12% O_2, their minute ventilation was raised relative to that of NB rats breathing air. The arterial pressure of the CHB rats was lower than that of the NB rats which was attributable to an increased vascular conductance at least in cerebral and muscle circulation, but the heart rates of the CHB and NB rats were similar [47]. Thus, the CHB rats did not show the tachycardia that would normally be expected as a consequence of the secondary effects of increased respiration, and the baroreceptor reflex response to a reduced arterial pressure (see above). Further, when the CHB rats were subjected to acute hypoxia by changing the inspirate from 12 to 8% O_2 they showed a fall in arterial pressure that was as great as that induced in the NB rats when they experienced the larger change from air to 8% O_2, and this was accompanied by progressive bradycardia, vasodilatation in skeletal muscle and cerebral circulations and a progressive fall in cerebral blood flow; there was no sign of the initial tachycardia or increase in cerebral blood flow that occurred in the NB rats [47]. Thus, the neurally-mediated reflex responses that normally increase heart rate and help to maintain arterial pressure during acute hypoxia were apparently attenuated in the CHB rats, whereas the local effects of acute hypoxia on the cardiovascular system, which we have proposed lead to the development of a positive feedback loop, were accentuated (Fig. 1). According to our hypothesis on the significance of this positive feedback loop (see above), these results suggest that individuals who have been chronically hypoxic from birth would be far more likely to die during an acute hypoxic episode. This is consistent with reports that a high proportion of the victims of SIDS show evidence of chronic hypoxia [28].

As yet, we cannot fully explain this change in the balance between reflex and local control mechanisms. It could be that CHB from birth affects the central nervous system so as to reduce the increase in sympathetic nerve activity to the heart and peripheral circulation that is caused by various afferent inputs and/or that there is a reduction in the cardiac and vascular responses to β and α adrenoreceptor stimulation as has been suggested for the effects of chronic hypoxia in adult life (see below). However, it could also be that the effects of the local influences of hypoxia are increased by chronic hypoxia from birth. In this context, it is interesting that 8-PT virtually abolished the bradycardia that was induced in CHB rats by acute hypoxia suggesting it was mediated by adenosine. But, 8-PT had no effect on the muscle vasodilator response to acute hypoxia in the CHB rats [47]. Since exogenous adenosine was fully capable of evoking muscle vasodilatation, it seems that CHB may lead to a decrease in the importance of adenosine as a vasodilator during acute hypoxia and presumably to an increase in the relative importance of some other dilator factor/s; this contrasts with the changes that occur when chronic hypoxia is imposed in adult life (see below).

Chronic Hypoxia in Adult Life

It is known that chronic hypoxia in adult life causes some blunting of the respiratory sensitivity to hypoxia, probably by an action on the peripheral chemoreceptors, but also leads to a substantial increase in the respiratory sensitivity to CO_2, probably by changes at the level of the central chemoreceptors [48]. On balance, resting ventilation is generally raised in chronic hypoxia. By contrast, reports in the literature on several different mammalian species including man, show variable, but small effects of chronic hypoxia on arterial pressure, whether the chronic hypoxia is produced by high altitude, under laboratory conditions, or by disease. In our own studies on adult rats made chronically hypoxic in a chamber at 12% O_2 for 3–4 weeks (CH rats), their arterial pressure when breathing 12% O_2 was more or less comparable to that of matched controls (N rats) breathing air [49]. Furthermore, although the CH rats breathing 12% O_2 had an increased ventilation relative to that of the N rats breathing air, their heart rates were comparable, suggesting that reflex tachycardia secondary to increased ventilation was impaired in CH rats as in CHB rats (see above). When the CH rats were subjected to acute hypoxia (8% O_2), they showed a very similar pattern of response to N rats in that there was an initial hyperventilation, tachycardia and increase in cerebral blood flow which contrasts with the pattern of response seen in the CHB rats (see above). However, in accord with the CHB rats, the fall in arterial pressure that occurred in the CH rats in acute hypoxia was as large as that seen in N rats when they experienced the larger change from air to 8% O_2 [49]. Thus, it seems that CH rats, like CHB rats, have a reduced ability to maintain arterial pressure by neurally mediated tachycardia and vasoconstriction.

These results are reminiscent of evidence in the literature that patients who were chronically hypoxic because of respiratory disease and healthy human subjects who were made chronically hypoxic in a hypobaric chamber, showed a reduced ability to maintain arterial pressure by tachycardia and peripheral vasoconstriction when they were subjected to lower body negative pressure [27, 50]. These observations are also in accord with reports that healthy human subjects at high altitude show an increased tendency towards postural hypotension and syncope [27].

For chronic hypoxia in adult life, there is evidence that the increase in sympathetic activity to the heart evoked by the baroreceptor reflex is reduced relative to that seen in normoxic subjects [51]. There is also evidence that the heart rate response to sympathetic agonists is reduced in chronically hypoxic individuals of several different species due to down-regulation of cardiac β adrenoreceptors [52, 53], while the influence of the vagus may be increased in part by an increase in the density of cardiac muscarinic receptors [54]. We have concentrated on the mechanisms underlying the change in vascular responsiveness.

In our experiments, the increase in muscle vascular conductance evoked in CH rats by acute hypoxia (8% O_2) was almost as great as that seen in N rats when they were subjected to the larger change from air to 8% O_2 [49]. Further, direct observations on a skeletal muscle preparation made by intravital microscopy showed that the dilator responses evoked in individual arterioles of muscle by 8% O_2 were fully comparable in the CH and N rats and in both cases these dilator responses were reduced by ~ 50% by the adenosine receptor antagonist 8-PT [55]. On the other hand, 8-PT had no effect on the baseline levels of muscle vascular conductance, or arterial pressure in CH rats, implying there was no tonic dilator influence of adenosine in chronic hypoxia [49]. Thus, we conclude that chronic hypoxia in adult life, like CHB, increases the influence of the dilator effects of acute hypoxia and/or reduces the influence of the constrictor effects of acute hypoxia. We also propose that adenosine plays a larger role in this vasodilatation when chronic hypoxia is imposed in adult life than when it is imposed from birth (see above).

Following up these results, we have obtained dose response curves to norepinephrine in the arterioles of skeletal muscle of both CH and N rats and have established that the maximum constrictor response to norepinephrine is greatly reduced in the arterioles of the CH rats relative to that of the N rats, but the curves are not shifted relative to one another [56]. This observation indicates that there is no change in the density, or affinity, of the α adrenoreceptors in the CH rats and suggests that the attenuated response is explained by factors distal to the receptors. These findings are consistent with the reports of others that the aortas of CH rats show a depressed maximum constrictor response to phenylephrine, vasopressin and angiotensin [57]. These results, also, are in accord with the evidence that vasoconstrictor responses evoked in the forearm of chronically hypoxic patients by infusions of norepinephrine were smaller than those evoked in normoxic subjects [50].

To investigate this phenomenon, we performed similar experiments *in vitro* on iliac arteries that were taken from CH and N rats. We found that the responses to norepinephrine were only depressed in the arteries of the CH rats when the endothelium was present. When the endothelium was removed, the iliac arteries of the CH rats showed responses that were fully comparable to those of the N rats [58]. This observation prompted us to test whether NO might be involved. Indeed, we found that the NO synthesis inhibitor L-NAME (nitro-L-arginine methyl ester) substantially increased the basal tone of endothelium-intact arteries from the CH rats, and normalized their responses to norepinephrine to the same extent as removal of the endothelium [59]. Thus, we had a clear indication that the depressed responsiveness to norepinephrine in the CH rats was caused by an accentuated dilator effect of NO released from the endothelium. To establish whether such an interaction also occurs *in vivo* we have tested the effect of L-NAME on the arterioles of CH rats by using intravital microscopy. Topical application of L-NAME reduces baseline diameter and facilitates the maximum constrictor response to norepinephrine so that it equals that seen in N rats (unpublished observations).

Thus, our current hypothesis is that chronic hypoxia in adult life causes upregulation of NO synthesis by the vascular endothelium. A similar phenomenon has been observed as a consequence of exercise training, when it has been proposed that NO synthesis is stimulated by the increased wall shear stress caused by increased blood flow [60]. In chronic hypoxia, there is no evidence that peripheral blood flow is increased significantly. However, wall shear stress must be increased as a consequence of the hypoxia-induced increase in Hct. An increase in NO synthesis would not only be expected to decrease responsiveness to circulating vasoconstrictor hormones and to sympathetic nerve activity, but might also potentiate dilator responses to substances that act in a NO-dependent manner which would, of course, include locally-released adenosine. However, this latter issue is more complex, for there is evidence that long-term exposure to adenosine causes down-regulation of adenosine receptors [60] which may offset any increase in the ability of adenosine to cause dilatation by its post-receptor action on NO synthesis. Indeed, our current evidence leads us to propose that explanation for the greater dilator influence of acute hypoxia in the CH rats may include a greater ability of acute hypoxia to release adenosine from the endothelial, and other, cells of chronically hypoxic individuals. It also may be that there is an increase in the release of other dilator factors such as prostaglandins in chronic hypoxia; it has already been proposed that their synthesis is up-regulated by shear stress during chronic exercise training [59]. It remains to be determined whether or not chronic hypoxia also reduces the increase in sympathetic nerve activity to the vasculature that is evoked by stimuli such as peripheral chemoreceptor stimulation and baroreceptor unloading, and whether or not it reduces the amount of norepinephrine released by a given change in sympathetic activity or increases the rate of re-uptake.

Conclusion

Acute hypoxia may, by stimulating the peripheral chemoreceptors, evoke the characteristic cardiovascular pattern of the alerting response, the response that is evoked by other noxious or stressful stimuli. This response is superimposed upon the other reflex and local effects of hypoxia, including the primary reflex bradycardia and peripheral vasoconstrictor response to chemoreceptor stimulation. The chemoreceptor-evoked increase in ventilation may elicit secondary tachycardia and vasodilatation, particularly in skeletal muscle. On the other hand, the local effects of hypoxia on brain, heart and peripheral tissues cause respiratory depression, bradycardia and vasodilatation; these changes are largely mediated by locally released adenosine. The reflex, or locally-mediated, bradycardia and peripheral vasodilatation may be particularly strong in some individuals leading to syncope. In neonates, the local effects of hypoxia are generally strong and may form part of a positive feedback loop that leads to SIDS.

In chronic systemic hypoxia, the respiratory sensitivity to hypoxia is blunted, sympathetic influences on the heart are reduced, and vagal influences are accentuated. The vasoconstrictor influence of the sympathetic nerve fibers is also depressed, while the dilator influences of tissue hypoxia are facilitated. This latter effect is partly attributable to up-regulation of the dilator influence of endothelially-derived NO. Overall, arterial pressure is less well controlled, such that adults are more susceptible to syncope, and neonates are more at risk of SIDS.

References

1. Marshall JM (1994) Peripheral chemoreceptors and cardiovascular regulation. Physiol Rev 74:543–594
2. Hilton SM, Marshall JM (1982) The pattern of cardiovascular response to carotid chemoreceptor stimulation in the cat. J Physiol 326:495–513
3. Marshall JM (1995) Cardiovascular changes associated with behavioural alerting. In: Jordan D, Marshall JM (eds) Studies in physiology: cardiovascular regulation. Portland Press, London, pp 37–59
4. Halliwill JB, Lawler LA, Eickhoff TD, Dietz NM, Nauss LA, Joyner MJ (1997) Forearm sympathetic withdrawal and vasodilatation during mental stress in humans. J Physiol 504:211–220
5. Marshall JM, Metcalfe JD (1988) Analysis of the cardiovascular changes induced in the rat by graded levels of systemic hypoxia. J Physiol 407:383–403
6. Marshall JM, Metcalfe JD (1990) Effects of systemic hypoxia on the distribution of cardiac output in the rat. J Physiol 426:335–353
7. Louwerse AM, Marshall JM (1996) Behavioural and cardiovascular responses evoked by hypoxia in the unanaesthetised rat. J Physiol 494:P103–104 (Abst)

8. Franchini KG, Kreiger EM (1993) Cardiovascular responses of conscious rats to carotid body chemoreceptor stimulation by intravenous KCN. J Auton Nerv Syst 42:63-69

9. Marshall JM, Metcalfe JD (1989) Analysis of factors that contribute to cardiovascular changes induced in the cat by graded levels of systemic hypoxia. J Physiol 412:429-448

10. Koehler RC, McDonald BW, Krasney JA (1980) Influence of CO_2 on cardiovascular response to hypoxia in conscious dogs. Am J Physiol 239:H545-H558

11. Korner PI, Uther JB, White SW (1969) Central nervous integration of the circulatory and respiratory responses to arterial hypoxia in the rabbit. Circ Res 24:757-776

12. Rowell LR, Blackmon JR (1986) Lack of sympathetic vasoconstriction in hypoxemic humans at rest. Am J Physiol 251:H562-H570

13. Rowell LR, Blackmon JR (1989) Hypoxemia raises muscle sympathetic activity but not norepinephrine in resting humans. J Appl Physiol 66:1736-1743

14. Marshall JM (1981) Interaction between the responses to stimulation of peripheral chemoreceptors and baroreceptors: the importance of chemoreceptor activation of the defence areas. J Auton Nerv Syst 3:389-400

15. Kontos HA, Mauck HP, Richardson DW, Patterson JL (1965) Mechanism of circulatory responses to systemic hypoxia in the anaesthetized dog. Am J Physiol 209:397-340

16. Neylon M, Marshall JM (1991) The role of adenosine in the respiratory and cardiovascular response to systemic hypoxia in the rat. J Physiol 440:529-545

17. Thomas T, Marshall JM (1994) Interdependence of respiratory and cardiovascular changes induced by systemic hypoxia in the rat; the roles of adenosine. J Physiol 480:627-636

18. Marshall JM, Metcalfe JD (1988) Cardiovascular changes associated with augmented breaths in normoxia and hypoxia in the rat. J Physiol 400:15-27

19. Marshall JM, Metcalfe JD (1989) Influences on the cardiovascular response to graded levels of systemic hypoxia of the accompanying hypocapnia in the rat. J Physiol 410:381-394

20. Richardson DW, Kontos HA, Raper AJ, Patterson JL (1967) Modification by beta-adrenergic blockade of the circulatory responses to acute hypoxia in man. J Clin Invest 46:77-85

21. Black JE, Roddie IC (1958) The mechanism of the changes in forearm vascular resistance during hypoxia. J Physiol 143:226-235

22. Easton PA, Anthionsen NR (1988) Ventilatory response to sustained hypoxia after pretreatment with aminophylline. J Appl Physiol 64:1445-1450

23. Richardson DW, Kontos HA, Shapiro W, Patterson JL (1966) Role of hypocapnia in the circulatory responses to acute hypoxia in man. J Appl Physiol 21:22-26

24. Gootman PM, Gootman N, Buckley BJ, Peterson BJ, Steele AM, Sica AL, Gandhi MR (1990) Effects of hypoxia in developing swine. In: Acker H, Trzebski A, O'Regan ARG (eds) Chemoreceptors and chemoreceptor reflexes. Plenum, New York, pp 155-163

25. Elnazir B, Marshall JM, Kumar P (1996) Postnatal development of the pattern of respiratory and cardiovascular response to systemic hypoxia in the piglet – the roles of adenosine. J Physiol 492:573-585

26. Rowell LB, Blackmon JR (1989) Hypotension induced by central hypovolaemia and hypoxaemia. Clin Physiol 9:269-277

27. Heistad DD, Wheeler RC, Aoki VS (1971) Reflex cardiovascular responses after 36 hr of hypoxia. Am J Physiol 220:1673-1676

28. Naeye RL (1980) Sudden infant death. Sci Am 242:56-62

29. Berne RM (1986) Adenosine: an important physiological regulator. NIPS 1:163-167

30. Millhorn DE, Eldridge FL, Kiley JP, Waldrop TG (1984) Prolonged inhibition of respiration following acute hypoxia in glomectomised cats. Resp Physiol 57:331-340

31. Thomas T, Elnazir B, Marshall JM (1994) Differentiation of the peripherally mediated from the centrally mediated influences of hypoxia in the rat during systemic hypoxia. Exp Physiol 79:809-822

32. Mian R, Marshall JM (1991) The role of adenosine in dilator responses induced in arterioles and venules of rat skeletal muscle in systemic hypoxia. J Physiol 443:499-511

33. Coney A, Marshall JM (1995) The role of adenosine in cerebral cortical vasodilatation induced by acute systemic hypoxia in normoxic and chronically hypoxic rats under anaesthesia. J Physiol 487:P174-175 (Abst)

34. Olsson RA, Pearson JD (1990) Cardiovascular purinoceptors. Physiol Rev 70:761–845
35. Bryan PT, Marshall JM (1996) The role of adenosine A_1 receptors in mediating hypoxia-induced vasodilatation in skeletal muscle of the anaesthetised rat. J Physiol 492:P6 (Abst)
36. Coney A, Marshall JM (1996) Effect of ZM241385 on the responses to acute systemic hypoxia and adenosine in the cerebral-cortex of the anaesthetised rat. J Physiol 494:P105–P106 (Abst)
37. Bellardinelli L, Giles WR, West A (1988) Ionic mechanisms of adenosine actions in pacemaker cells from rabbit heart. J Physiol 405:615–633
38. Verlato G, Borgdorff P (1990) Endogenous adenosine enhances vagal negative chronotropic effect during hypoxia in the anaesthetised rabbit. Cardiovasc Res 24:532–540
39. Marshall JM, Thomas T, Turner L (1993) A link between adenosine potassium and ATP-sensitive potassium channels in muscle vasodilatation in the rat in systemic hypoxia. J Physiol 472:1–9
40. Skinner MR, Marshall JM (1996) Studies on the roles of ATP, adenosine and nitric oxide in mediating muscle vasodilatation induced in the rat by acute systemic hypoxia. J Physiol 495:553–560
41. Bryan PT, Marshall JM (1996) Possible mechanisms underlying the vasodilatation induced in skeletal muscle of the rat by stimulation of adenosine A_1 receptors. J Physiol 497:P79 (Abst)
42. Bryan PT, Marshall JM (1997) The role of K_{ATP} channels in adenosine mediated vasodilatation in skeletal muscle of the rat. J Physiol 504:P204–P205 (Abst)
43. Verhaeghe RH, Vanhoutte PM, Shepherd JT (1977) Inhibition of sympathetic neurotransmission in canine blood vessels by adenosine and adenine nucleotides. Circ Res 40:208–215
44. Messina EJ, Sun D, Koller A, Wolin MS, Kaley G (1992) Role of endothelium-derived prostaglandins in hypoxia-elicited arteriolar dilatation in rat skeletal muscle. Circ Res 71:790–796
45. Smith KA, Marshall JM (1997) Does chronic hypoxia induce angiogenesis in skeletal muscle of the rat? J Physiol 499:P118–P119 (Abst)
46. Hanson MA, Kumar P, Williams BA (1989) Effects of chronic hypoxia upon development of respiratory reflexes in newborn kittens. J Physiol 411:563–574
47. Thomas T, Marshall JM (1995) A study on rats of the effects of chronic hypoxia from birth on respiratory and cardiovascular responses evoked by acute hypoxia. J Physiol 487:513–525
48. Dempsey JA, Foster HV (1982) Mediation of ventilation adaptations. Physiol Rev 62:262–346
49. Thomas T, Marshall JM (1997) The roles of adenosine in regulating the respiratory and cardiovascular systems in chronically hypoxic, adult rats. J Physiol 501:439–447
50. Heistad DD, Abboud FM, Mark AL, Schmidt PG (1972) Impaired reflex vasoconstriction in chronically hypoxemic patients. J Clin Invest 51:331–337
51. Farinelli CC, Kayser B, Binzoni T, Cerretelli P, Girardier L (1994) Autonomic nervous control of heart rate at altitude (5050 metres). Eur J Appl Physiol 69:502–507
52. Kacimi R, Richalet J-P, Corsin A, Abousahi E, Crozatier B (1992) Hypoxia-induced down regulation of β adrenoreceptors in rat heart. J Appl Physiol 73:1377–1382
53. Anteza A-M, Kacimi R, Le Trong J-L, Marchal M, Abousahi I, Dubray C (1994) Adrenergic status of humans during prolonged exposure to the high altitude of 6542 m. J Appl Physiol 76:1055–1059
54. Kacimi R, Richalet J-P, Crozatier B (1993) Hypoxia-induced differential modulation of adenosinergic and muscarinic receptors in rat heart. J Appl Physiol 75:1123–1128
55. Mian R, Marshall JM (1995) The role of adenosine in mediating vasodilatation in mesenteric circulation of the rat in acute and chronic hypoxia. J Physiol 489:225–234
56. Mian R, Marshall JM (1994) Effect of chronic hypoxia on microcirculatory responses evoked by noradrenaline. Int J Microcirc 14:244 (Abst)
57. Doyle MP, Walker BR (1991) Alternation of systemic vasoreactivity in chronically hypoxic rats. Am J Physiol 260:R1114–R1122
58. Bartlett IS, Marshall JM (1995) Comparison of the effects of acute hypoxia on iliac artery rings from normal and chronically hypoxic rats. Br J Pharmacol 116:203P

59. Bartlett IS, Marshall JM (1996) Mechanisms underlying the depression of noradrenaline-evoked contractions induced by chronic hypoxia in the rat iliac artery *in vitro*. J Physiol 491:P24-P25 (Abst)

60. Koller A, Huang A, Sun D, Kaley G (1995) Exercise training augments flow-dependent dilation in rat skeletal muscle arterioles-role of endothelial nitric oxide and prostaglandins. Circ Res 76:544-550

Anemic Hypoxia

P. Van der Linden

Introduction

Increasing awareness of transfusion-related infections and immunologic risks has stimulated a re-examination of our transfusion practice. In the perioperative period, experts have for long considered a hematocrit (Hct) of 30% as optimal, but their recommendations were based primarily on theoretical calculations of maximal oxygen delivery (DO_2) to peripheral organs. Clinical studies on Jehovah's Witness patients have reported that, in elective surgery, the hemoglobin (Hb) level alone became a significant predictor of outcome only at levels below 3 g/dl; the strongest independent factors influencing outcome being sepsis and active bleeding [1]. The adequacy of any Hb concentration in a given clinical situation depends on whether a sufficient amount of oxygen (O_2) is carried to the tissues to meet their O_2 requirements. Therefore, the decision to transfuse a given patient cannot be based only on the Hb level [2]. Rather, rigid adherence to an arbitrarily defined transfusion threshold could paradoxically increase homologous blood utilization [3]. Knowledge of the physiologic adjustments occurring during anemia, and of the clinical factors which can limit the ability of the organism to maintain adequate tissue DO_2 in these situations of decreased O_2 carrying capacity will allow the clinician to better define the transfusion trigger for each patient.

Physiologic Response to Acute Reduction in Hemoglobin Concentration

The maintenance of adequate tissue oxygenation during acute anemia depends on both an increase in cardiac output (CO) and an increase in blood O_2 extraction. These compensatory mechanisms require the preservation of an ample circulating blood volume.

Cardiac Output Response to Hemodilution

The most intensively studied compensatory mechanism in acute anemia has been the increase in CO, the magnitude of which seems closely related to the reduction in blood viscosity [4]. This increase in CO is mainly due to an increase in stroke volume but is also dependent on the initial heart rate. The increase in stroke volume is intimately related to the decrease in total peripheral resistance, which reduces afterload and increases venous return [5]. The decrease in total peripheral resistance associated with acute normovolemic hemodilution is essentially related to the reduction in blood viscosity, but might also be related to a decreased scavenging capacity of blood to inactivate nitric oxide (NO) [6]. Enhancement of myocardial contractility, as recently demonstrated by Habler et al. [7] using load-independent variables, could also contribute to the increase in stroke volume observed during acute normovolemic hemodilution. Several experimental investigations indicate that sympathetic innervation of the heart is necessary to achieve, and to maintain, the usual CO response during acute anemia [8, 9]. Other studies demonstrate a reduced CO response during hemodilution after administration of β-adrenergic agents [10–12]. Finally, α-adrenergic tone to capacitance vessels appears essential for the CO increase during anemia [13]. This enhanced venomotor tone, preventing the peripheral pooling of blood, results from the hemodilution-induced stimulation of aortic chemoreceptors [14]. The role of endogenous catecholamines in these compensatory mechanisms remains controversial. While Bowens et al. [15] observed an increased in plasma norepinephrine levels during hemodilution in anesthetized dogs, van Woerkens et al. [16] observed no such increase in pigs using the same anesthetic technique.

Blood Oxygen Extraction Adjustments During Hemodilution

The second compensatory mechanism aims at a better matching of DO_2 to O_2 demand at tissue levels, allowing blood O_2 extraction to increase. This mechanism implies physiologic adjustments at both the systemic and the microcirculatory level.

At the systemic level a better matching of DO_2 to O_2 demand requires redistribution of blood flow to areas of high demand, like the myocardium and the brain. Several experimental studies have demonstrated cerebral and coronary vasodilation so that flow in these areas increases out of proportion to the rise in CO [16–19]. The increase in myocardial blood flow is even more important than the increase in cerebral blood flow as myocardial O_2 demand can increase during anemia [17]. Von Restorff et al. [17] demonstrated that coronary vasodilation becomes nearly maximal at a Hct of 12.5%. Below this value, coronary blood flow can no longer match the enhanced energy of the cardiac pump so that myocardial ischemia can develop, resulting in cardiac failure. This is consistent with experimental data showing a decrease in systemic O_2 uptake (VO_2) at Hct values close to 10% [20, 21].

The excess perfusion of the brain and the heart during anemia occurs at the expense of other organs [16, 18]. Several studies have demonstrated that vasoconstriction develops in some tissues during acute anemia, so that hepatic, renal, mesenteric and splenic blood flows contribute less than other organs to the overall increase in blood flow [22, 23]. This regional response during normovolemic anemia is partly due to α-adrenergic stimulation, but is unaltered in the presence of β-adrenergic blockade [11].

Skeletal muscle is a significant exception to peripheral tissue contributing to the O_2 sparing phenomenon during acute anemia [4]. Cain and Chapler [24] observed that blood flow was not re-directed from hindlimb musculature to other tissues even when anemia was so severe that systemic VO_2 was not maintained. Kubes and Cain [25] demonstrated that the stimulus of anemic hypoxia to resistance vessels in skeletal muscle seemed relatively weak in comparison to other organs. These observations raise interesting questions regarding the neural versus humoral control of skeletal muscle blood flow during acute anemia.

In addition to redistribution of blood flow to areas of high demand, several adjustments occur in the microcirculation, resulting in a more efficient utilization of the remaining red blood cell volume. Several authors have demonstrated, during acute normovolemic anemia, an improvement in DO_2 in the more distal arteriolar branching orders, attributed to an increase in the ratio of microcirculatory to systemic Hct, an increased capillary red cell velocity and a decrease in pre-capillary O_2 loss and diffusional transfer to other microvessels [26–28]. These adjustments result in an improved tissue O_2 extraction as demonstrated in anesthetized dogs undergoing hemorrhagic shock [29]. These microcirculatory compensatory mechanisms allow the maintenance of adequate tissue oxygenation up to a systemic Hct of 10–15%, and recently have been well demonstrated in studies evaluating the effects of acute normovolemic hemodilution on gut oxygenation in the anesthetized pig [30, 31].

Finally, during severe anemia (Hct below 15%), a right shift of the O_2 dissociation curve, related to a rise in 2,3-diphosphoglycerate (2,3 DPG) in the red blood cells, may decrease Hb affinity for O_2, and thereby improve O_2 availability to the cells. However this mechanism takes some time to occur and has been demonstrated only in chronic anemia [32].

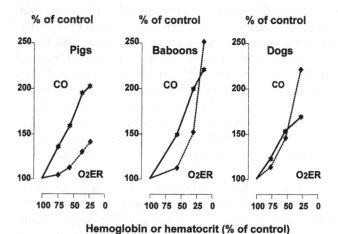

Fig. 1. Respective contribution of cardiac output (CO) and oxygen extraction (O_2ER) in the maintenance of tissue oxygen delivery during progressive hemodilution in different animal species. (Adapted from [63] with permission)

In summary, maintenance of tissue DO_2 at the level of its demand during acute normovolemic anemia depends on physiologic adjustments occurring at both the systemic and the microcirculatory levels, which result in an increase in blood flow and O_2 extraction. The relative contribution of these mechanisms will depend on the ability of the organism to recruit each of them. Several experimental and clinical studies have demonstrated the involvement of both mechanisms even in the early stages of normovolemic anemia (Figs. 1 and 2). These mechanisms allow systemic VO_2 to remain constant until the Hct falls to about 10% at which point it becomes dependent on DO_2. Experimental studies in dogs [33], pigs [34] and baboons [35] have demonstrated this "critical" Hb value to be around 4 g/dl. Corresponding values are obviously difficult to obtain in man. Van Woerkens et al. [36] studied a Jehovah's Witness patient who died from extreme hemodilution, and observed a critical Hb level of 4 g/dl. The critical value of Hb not only depends on the integrity of the compensatory mechanisms described above, but also on the level of tissue O_2 demand. For a given CO and O_2 extraction response, any decrease in tissue O_2 demand will result in a decrease in the critical Hb level and *vice versa*.

Finally, the inspired fraction of O_2 (FiO_2) might also influence the critical Hb level, as the contribution of the dissolved O_2 in the plasma increases markedly during hemodilution. Schou et al. [37] recently reported in anesthetized pigs that dissolved O_2 at $FiO_2 = 1.0$ and $FiO_2 = 0.35$ constituted 25.4 and 10.1% respectively, of systemic DO_2 after hemodilution (Hct 10%), compared with 10.7 and 3.9% before hemodilution (Hct 33%). This effect could be magnified by the use of O_2 carriers, like fluorocarbons, as plasma substitutes, which markedly increase the amount of O_2 carried by the plasma, and might promote the diffusion of O_2 between the tissue site of use and the red blood cells [38]. An indirect argument in favor of this hypothesis is found in the study by Spence et al. [1] reporting that, in elective surgery, the Hb level alone became a significant predictor of outcome

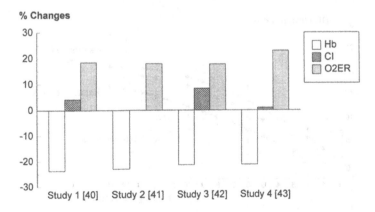

Fig. 2. Respective contribution of cardiac index (CI) and oxygen extraction (O_2ER) in the maintenance of tissue oxygen delivery during progressive hemodilution in humans. (Data from [40–43])

only at levels below 3 g/dl. In this study [1] all patients received a fluorocarbon solution as a volume substitute in the perioperative period.

Effects of Anesthesia on the Physiologic Adjustments Occurring During Acute Anemia

Anesthesia can alter the physiologic adjustments occurring during anemia at different levels (Table 1). The more important observation is related to the fact that anesthetic agents can blunt the CO increase associated with normovolemic hemodilution [27, 39–43]. A remarkable finding is that in most of these studies, hemodilution was associated with a moderate increase in stroke volume, but a decrease in heart rate so that CO did not increase or increased only slightly [40–43]. As a consequence, DO_2 decreased even for mild degrees of hemodilution (Hct 27–30%) and O_2 extraction had to increase in order to maintain tissue VO_2 [40–43]. Decreased venomotor tone, direct negative inotropic and chronotropic effects and reduced sympathetic activity are the main mechanisms responsible for this altered CO response. This effect of anesthetic agents seems to be dose-dependent and has been associated with an increase in the critical value of Hb [44]. DO_2 decreases progressively along with the hemodilution, and the typical Hb-DO_2 relationship described by Messmer et al. [45] showing a peak DO_2 value of about 110% of the pre-anemic control at a Hct of 30% is not observed [44] (Fig. 3).

The vasodilating properties of some anesthetic agents altering the regional distribution of blood flow, have been implicated in the development of tissue hypoxia during hemodilution [39, 46].

Another interesting point is related to the effects of anesthesia on systemic VO_2. Anesthetic agents decrease VO_2 by reducing sympathetic activity but also

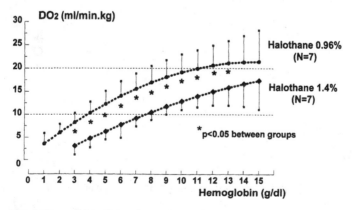

Fig. 3. Hemoglobin-DO_2 relationship in dogs anesthetized with a low dose of halothane (0.96% end-tidal; N = 7, closed circles) and in dogs anesthetized with a high dose of halothane (1.4% end-tidal; N = 7, closed diamonds)

Table 1. Major effects of anesthesia on physiologic adjustments occurring during anemia

Effects on cardiac output response
- Decreased venomotor tone
- Decreased myocardial contractility
- Decreased sympathetic activity

Effects on O_2 extraction response
- Direct vasodilating properties
- Decreased sympathetic activity

Effects on tissue O_2 demand
- Abolition of pain and stress
- Decreased muscular activity
- Decreased myocardial VO_2
- Hypothermia

Effects on gas exchange
- Decreased functional residual capacity

by a direct effect on some organs like the myocardium. Indeed, the effects of some anesthetic agents, and in particular of the halogenated agents, on the heart rate and myocardial contractility have been associated with a decrease of 10–20% in VO_2 [47]. This could explain why the increased VO_2 observed by some authors [17] during progressive normovolemic hemodilution is not always observed [18].

Finally, the use of mechanical ventilation during anesthesia not only participates to the decreased tissue O_2 metabolism but also allows the maintenance of a relatively high FiO_2, increasing the amount of O_2 carried by the plasma.

Clinical Limits of Anemia

Any factor altering either the CO response or (and) the O_2 extraction response will reduce a patient's tolerance to acute anemia (Table 2). The efficacy of the mechanisms preserving tissue DO_2 when the blood O_2 carrying capacity is reduced depends primarily on the maintenance of an adequate blood volume. Indeed hypovolemia blunts the effects of decreased blood viscosity on venous return [48]. Although "normovolemic" conditions are difficult to define, replacement of blood losses by at least a quantity of plasma substitute having the same expanding effect on the intravascular volume is required. The CO response to hemodilution could also be reduced in the presence of altered myocardial contractility. Administration of negative inotropic agents like disopyramide, resulted in a dose-dependent decrease in CO response during hemodilution [49]. Acute administration of β-blocking agents also tends to decrease the CO response to hemodilution [10–12]. However, Spahn et al. [43] recently observed during moderate hemodilution in coronary artery disease (CAD) patients that chronic β-blockade patients slightly, but significantly, increased their CO, while non β-blockade patients did not increase CO. This observation has been attributed to the increased response to endogenous sympathetic stimulation in chronic β-blocked patients related to a rise in the number of myocardial β-adrenergic receptors. Nevertheless, in both groups, systemic DO_2 decreased significantly after hemodilution and O_2 extraction increased to maintain a stable VO_2. This study [43] highlights once again the ability of the organism to recruit CO and/or O_2 extraction to maintain tissue DO_2, depending on the basal conditions of the patient. Before hemodilution, chronically β-blocked patients had a lower CO and a higher O_2 extraction ratio than non β-blockade patients.

CAD will obviously limit the tolerance of the heart to normovolemic hemodilution. As myocardial O_2 extraction is already nearly maximal in resting conditions, the maintenance of myocardial VO_2 depends essentially on the increase in coronary blood flow. Therefore, the coronary reserve (the ratio between maximal coronary blood flow and resting coronary blood flow) is significantly reduced during hemodilution [50, 51], especially in CAD patients who already have a decreased maximal coronary blood flow. The lowest tolerable Hct in CAD patients is not known but experimental data on animals with extrinsically applied coronary stenosis has demonstrated a significant increase in the critical Hct level to 17–18% [51, 52]. Based on theoretical analysis, Kettler [53] recently estimated that CAD patients may tolerate some degree of hemodilution intraoperatively but require a higher Hct in the early postoperative period to meet the increased tissue, and especially cardiac, O_2 demand. These observations have been confirmed by the study of Nelson et al. [54], showing that a postoperative Hct below 28% was significantly associated with increased myocardial ischemic episodes and morbid cardiac events. Cardiovascular disease patients having a lower preoperative Hct have an increased risk of death when compared to non-cardiovascular disease patients with the same preoperative Hct [55].

Table 2. Clinical events altering physiologic adjustments occurring during anemia

Factors associated with decreased cardiac output response
- Hypovolemia
- Coronary artery disease
- Valvular disease
- Cardiac failure
- Negative inotropic agents
- Sedative/anesthetic agents

Factors associated with decreased O_2 extraction response
- Acute respiratory distress syndrome (ARDS)
- Sepsis/systemic inflammatory response syndrome (SIRS), traumatic injury
- Ischemia-reperfusion syndromes
- Alpha-blocking agents
- Sedative/anesthetic agents
- Hypothermia

Factors associated with increased oxygen consumption
- Fever, pain, stress, anxiety
- Sepsis, SIRS
- Hyperventilation syndromes

Factors associated with altered gas exchange
- Chronic pulmonary obstructive disease
- ARDS

In patients with no evidence of cardiovascular disease, age alone does not seem to be a major factor in determining tolerance to anemia [42], although compensatory mechanisms to an acute reduction in blood O_2 content could be less efficient [2].

Controlled hypotension is frequently used during surgical procedures to decrease peroperative blood loss. However, the use of vasodilating agents and, in particular, α-blocking agents, could interfere with the normal regional redistribution of blood flow occurring during hemodilution. Several experimental studies have demonstrated impaired renal and splanchnic tissue oxygenation when controlled hypotension is superimposed on normovolemic hemodilution [18, 46].

Respiratory insufficiency will also limit the physiologic adjustment to acute anemia. On the one hand, altered arterial oxygenation will participate in the decreased O_2 carrying capacities of the blood, and on the other hand, hemodilution could have a deleterious effect on pulmonary gas exchange, possibly through attenuation of hypoxic pulmonary vasoconstriction [56]. Although the optimal Hct during respiratory insufficiency is not known, patients with chronic respiratory failure develop polycythemia in an attempt to maintain adequate tissue DO_2.

In critical illness, most of the compensatory mechanisms for anemia are reduced by the presence of hypovolemia, hypoxemia, depressed myocardial function and/or altered tissue O_2 extraction capabilities. In addition, tissue O_2 demand is often increased in these situations, due to fever, pain, stress and increased respiratory work. The current clinical guidelines recommend maintaining a Hb level between 7.0 and 10.0 g/dl in the patient "at risk" [2, 57] and greater than 10.0 g/dl in the septic patient [58].

Monitoring Tissue Oxygenation During Normovolemic Anemia

The adequacy of any Hb concentration in a given clinical situation depends on whether a sufficient amount of O_2 is carried to the tissues to meet their O_2 requirements. Clinical signs of inadequate tissue oxygenation during anemia (e.g., tachycardia, postural hypotension dizziness, etc.) are very sensitive, but non-specific. Moreover they are usually absent in sedated or anesthetized patients. In critically ill patients, the mixed venous O_2 saturation (SvO_2) is frequently used to detect the development of an imbalance between DO_2 and VO_2. Several authors have assessed the potential value of monitoring SvO_2 as an indicator of tissue oxygenation during progressive acute hemodilution in anesthetized pigs. In these conditions, Trouwborst et al. [59] and Räsänen [34] determined that the critical value of Hb was around 4 g/dl, corresponding to a SvO_2 of 44% and an O_2 extraction ratio of 57%. However, when profound hemodilution is combined with progressive hypoxemia, SvO_2 may be a less reliable indicator of inadequate tissue DO_2 [60]. In anesthetized animals with or without limited coronary reserve, significant myocardial production reflecting anaerobic metabolism occurred only when the systemic O_2 extraction ratio exceed 50% [21]. In a Jehovah's Witness patient dying from extreme hemodilution, the critical Hb level was reached at a SvO_2 value of 56% and an O_2 extraction ratio of 44% [36]. Several clinical observations tend to indicate that the SvO_2 (or the O_2 extraction ratio) could be a reliable physiologic guide to transfusion. In eight ASA class I patients undergoing orthopedic surgery, Fontana et al. [61] performed profound intraoperative normovolemic hemodilution, using a SvO_2 of 60% as a "transfusion trigger". In their patients breathing 100% O_2, Hb decreased from 10.0 to a nadir of 3.0 g/dl while SvO_2 decreased from 91 to 72% and O_2 extraction ratio increased from 17 to 44%. No patient suffered any clinically adverse outcome. Using a SvO_2 of 55% as the transfusion trigger during hypothermic cardiopulmonary bypass in 100 CAD patients, Paone and Silverman [3] observed a significant reduction in the use of allogeneic blood with no increase in postoperative morbidity or mortality. Although SvO_2 presents some limitations, in particular during cardiopulmonary bypass [62], these studies suggest that the transfusion threshold requires consideration of the Hct in conjunction with clinical judgment and other factors like SvO_2 and the overall hemodynamic status of the patient.

Conclusion

An acute decrease in blood O_2 carrying capacities during anemia elicits physiologic adjustments at both the systemic and the microcirculatory level, resulting in an increased CO and an increased O_2 extraction ratio. In physiologic situations, these adjustments are very efficient as they allow the maintenance of tissue DO_2 up to a systemic Hct of 10–15% in resting conditions. In pathophysiologic situations, tolerance to acute anemia will depend on the ability of the organism to recruit each mechanism, and on the level of tissue O_2 demand. In any case, maintenance of adequate volume replacement is of paramount importance. Anesthesia has complex effects on the physiologic adjustments associated with acute normovolemic anemia. On one hand, it decreases the CO response; on the other hand it decreases tissue VO_2. In these conditions, SvO_2, usually used to detect the development of an imbalance between DO_2 and VO_2, could be a reliable physiologic guide to transfusion. The decision to transfuse a given patient cannot be based only on the Hb level.

References

1. Spence RK, Costabile JP, Young GS, et al (1992) Is hemoglobin level alone a reliable predictor of outcome in the severely anemic surgical patient? Am Surg 58:92–95
2. Janvier G, Annat G (1995) Are there any limits to hemodilution? Ann Fr Anesth Reanim 14 (suppl 1):9–20
3. Paone G, Silverman NA (1997) The paradox of on-bypass transfusion thresholds in blood conservation. Circulation 96 (suppl II):II 205–II 209
4. Chapler CK, Cain SM (1986) The physiologic reserve in oxygen carrying capacity: studies in experimental circulation. Can J Physiol Pharmacol 64:7–12
5. Fowler NO, Holmes JC (1975) Blood viscosity and cardiac output in acute experimental anemia. J Appl Physiol 39:453–456

6. Doss DN, Estafanous FG, Ferrario CM, Brum JM, Murray PA (1995) Mechanism of systemic vasodilation during normovolemic hemodilution. Anesth Analg 81:30–34
7. Habler OP, Kleen MS, Podtschaske AH, et al (1996) The effect of acute normovolemic hemodilution (ANH) on myocardial contractility in anesthetized dogs. Anesth Analg 83: 451–458
8. Hatcher J, Sadik N, Baumber J (1959) The effect of sympathectomy (Stellate-T5) on cardiovascular responses to anemia produced by dextran-for-blood exchange. Proc Can Fed Biol Soc 2:28 (Abst)
9. Glik G Jr, Plauth WH, Braunwald E (1964) Role of the autonomic nervous system in the circulatory response to acutely induced anemia in unanesthetized dogs. J Clin Invest 43: 2112–2124
10. Escobar E, Jones NL, Rapaport E, Murray JF (1966) Ventricular performance in acute normovolemic anemia and effects of beta-blockade. Am J Physiol 211:877–884
11. Crystal GJ, Ruiz JR, Rooney MW, Salem RM (1988) Regional hemodynamics and oxygen supply during isovolemic hemodilution in the absence and presence of high-grade beta-adrenergic blockade. J Cardiothorac Vasc Anesth 2:772–780
12. Shinoda T, Smith CE, Khairallah PA, Fouad-Tarazi FM, Estafanous FG (1991) Effects of propranolol on myocardial performance during acute normovolemic hemodilution. J Cardiothorac Vasc Anesth 5:15–22
13. Chapler CK, Cain SM (1982) Effects of alpha-adrenergic blockade during acute anemia. J Appl Physiol 52:16–20
14. Szlyk PC, King C, Jennings B, Cain SM, Chapler CK (1984) The role of the aortic chemoreceptors during acute anemia. Can J Physiol Pharmacol 62:519–523
15. Bowens C Jr, Spahn DR, Frasco PE, Smith R, McRae RL, Leone BJ (1993) Hemodilution induces stable changes in global cardiovascular and regional myocardial function. Anesth Analg 76:1027–1032
16. Van Woerkens ECSM, Trouwborst A, Duncker JGM, Koning MMG, Boomsma F, Verdouw PD (1992) Catecholmines and regional hemodynamics during isovolemic hemodilution in anesthetized pigs. J Appl Physiol 72:760–769
17. Von Restorff W, Hofling B, Holtz J, Bassenge E (1975) Effect of increased blood fluidity through hemodilution on coronary circulation at rest and during exercise in dogs. Pflugers Arch 35:15–24
18. Crystal GJ, Rooney MW, Salem MR (1988) Regional hemodynamics and oxygen supply during isovolemic hemodilution alone or in combination with adenosine-induced controlled hypotension. Anesth Analg 67:211–218
19. Crystal GJ, Salem MR (1991) Myocardial and systemic hemodynamics during isovolemic hemodilution alone and combined with nitroprusside-induced controlled hypotension. Anesth Analg 72:227–237
20. Cain SM (1977) Oxygen delivery and uptake in dogs during anemic and hypoxic hypoxia. J Appl Physiol 42:228–234
21. Levy PS, Chavez RP, Crystal GJ, et al (1992) Oxygen extraction ratio: a valid indicator of transfusion need in limited coronary vascular reserve? J Trauma 32:769–774
22. Race D, Dedichen H, Schenk W (1967) Regional blood flow during dextran-induced normovolemic hemodilution in the dog. J Thorac Cardiovasc Surg 53:578–586
23. Fan FC, Chen RYZ, Schuessler GB, Chien S (1980) Effects of hematocrit variations on regional hemodynamics and oxygen transport in the dog. Am J Physiol 238:H545–H552
24. Cain SM, Chapler CK (1978) O_2 extraction by hindlimb versus whole dog during anemic hypoxia. J Appl Physiol 45:966–970
25. Kubes P, Cain SM, Chapler CK (1988) Hindlimb skeletal muscle blood flow during sympathetic nerve block before and during acute anemia. Can J Physiol Pharmacol 66: 1148–1153
26. Lipowski HH, Firrell JC (1986) Microvascular hemodynamics during systemic hemodilution and hemoconcentration. Am J Physiol 250:H908–H922
27. Kuo L, Pittman RN (1988) Effect of hemodilution on oxygen transport in arteriolar networks of hamster striated muscle. Am J Physiol 254:H331–H339

28. Lindbom L, Mirhashemi S, Intaglietta M, Arfors KE (1988) Increase in capillary blood flow and relative haematocrit in rabbit skeletal muscle following acute normovolaemic anaemia. Acta Physiol Scand 134:503–513

29. Van der Linden P, Gilbart E, Pâques P, Simon C, Vincent JL (1993) Influence of hematocrit on tissue O_2 extraction capabilities during acute hemorrhage. Am J Physiol 264:H942–H947

30. Nöldge GFE, Priebe HJ, Bohle W, Buttler KJ, Geiger K (1991) Effects of acute normovolemic hemodilution on splanchnic oxygenation and on hepatic histology and metabolism in anesthetized pigs. Anesthesiology 74:908–918

31. Haisjackl M, Luz G, Sparr H, et al (1997) The effects of progressive anemia on jejunal mucosal and serosal tissue oxygenation in pigs. Anesth Analg 84:538–544

32. Rodman T, Close HP, Purcell MK (1960) The oxyhemoglobin dissociation curve in anemia. Ann Intern Med 52:295–301

33. Schmartz D, Van der Linden P, Mathieu M, De Groote F, Vincent JL (1994) Critical hemoglobin level in anesthetized dogs:comparative effects of HES 200/05 and Gelatin. Anesthesiology 81:A725 (Abst)

34. Räsänen J (1992) Supply-dependent oxygen consumption and mixed venous oxyhemoglobin saturation during isovolemic hemodilution in pigs. Chest 101:1121–1124

35. Wilkerson DK, Rosen AL Seghal LR (1988) Limits of cardiac compensation in anemic baboons. Surgery 103:665–671

36. Van Woerkens ECSM, Trouwborst A, van Lanschot JJB (1992) Profound hemodilution:what is the critical level of hemodilution at which oxygen delivery-dependent oxygen consumption starts in an anesthetized human? Anesth Analg 75:818–821

37. Schou H, Perez de Sa V, Roscher R, Larsson A (1997) Nitrous oxide reduces inspired oxygen fraction but does not compromise circulation and oxygenation during hemodilution in pigs. Acta Anaesthesiol Scand 41:923–930

38. Faithfull NS, Cain SM (1988) Critical levels of O_2 extraction following hemodilution with dextran or fluosol-DA. J Crit Care 3:14–18

39. Schou H, Perez de Sa V, Larsson A, Roscher R, Kongstad L, Werner O (1997) Hemodilution significantly decreases tolerance to isoflurane-induced cardiovascular depression. Acta Anaesthesiol Scand 41:218–228

40. Van der Linden P, Wathieu M, Gilbart E, et al (1994) Cardiovascular effects of moderate normovolemic hemodilution during enflurane-nitrous oxide anesthesia in man. Acta Anaesthesiol Scand 38:490–498

41. Biboulet P, Capdevila X, Benetreau D, Aubas P, D'Athis F, Du Cailar J (1996) Haemodynamic effects of moderate normovolaemic haemodilution in conscious and anaesthetized patients. Br J Anaesth 76:81–84

42. Spahn DR, Zollinger A, Schlumpf RB, et al (1996) Hemodilution tolerance in elderly patients without known cardiac disease. Anesth Analg 82:681–686

43. Spahn DR, Seifert B, Pasch T, Schmid ER (1997) Effects of chronic beta-blockade on compensatory mechanisms during acute isovolaemic haemodilution in patients with coronary artery disease. Br J Anaesth 78:381–385

44. Mathieu M, Rausin I, Schmartz D, Willaert P, Van der Linden P (1996) Critical hemoglobin level in dogs: effects of halothane anesthesia. Anesth Analg 82:S304 (Abst)

45. Messmer K, Lewis DH, Sunder-Plassmann L, Kloverkorn WP, Mendler N, Hopler K (1972) Acute normovolemic hemodilution. Eur Surg Res 4:55–70

46. Nöldge GFE, Priebe HJ, Geiger K (1992) Splanchnic hemodynamics and oxygen supply during acute normovolemic hemodilution alone and with isoflurane-induced hypotension in the anesthetized pig. Anesth Analg 75:660–674

47. Benhamou D, Desmonts JM (1984) La consommation d'oxygène per et post-anesthésique. Ann Fr Anesth Reanim 3:205–211

48. Chien S (1987) Physiological and pathophysiological significance of hemorheology. In: Chien S, Dormandy J, Ernst E, Matrai A (eds) Clinical hemorheology. Nijhoff, Boston, pp 125–163

49. Estafanous FG, Smith CE, Selim WM, Tarazi RC (1990) Cardiovascular effects of acute normovolemic hemodilution in rats with disopyramide-induced myocardial depression. Basic Res Cardiol 85:227–236

50. Geha AS (1976) Coronary and cardiovascular dynamics and oxygen availability during acute normovolemic anemia. Surgery 80:47–53
51. Levy PS, Kim SJ, Eckel PK, et al (1993) Limit to cardiac compensation during acute isovolemic hemodilution: influence of coronary stenosis. Am J Physiol 265:H340–H349
52. Spahn DR, Smith LR, Veronee CD, et al (1993) Acute isovolemic hemodilution and blood transfusion: Effects on regional function and metabolism in myocardium with compromised coronary blood flow. J Thorac Cardiovasc Surg 105:694–704
53. Kettler D (1994) "Permissive anemia" compared with blood transfusion in patients with cardiac disease: another point of view. Curr Opin Anesth 7:1–4
54. Nelson AH, Fleisher LA, Rosenbaum SH (1993) Relationship between postoperative anemia and cardiac morbidity in high-risk vascular patients in the intensive care unit. Crit Care Med 21:860–866
55. Carson JL, Duff A, Poses RM, et al (1996) Effect of anaemia and cardiovascular disease on surgical mortality and morbidity. Lancet 348:1055–1060
56. Deem S, Bishop MJ, Alberts MK (1995) Effect of anemia on intrapulmonary shunt during atelectasis in rabbits. J Appl Physiol 79:1951–1957
57. Welch GH, Meehan KR, Goodnough LT (1992) Prudent strategies for elective red blood cell transfusion. Ann Intern Med 117:441–442
58. Sibbald WJ, Doig GS, Morisaki H (1995) Role of RBC transfusion therapy in sepsis. In: Sibbald WJ, Vincent JL (eds) Clinical trials for the treatment of sepsis. Springer-Verlag, Berlin, Heidelberg, New York, pp 191–206
59. Trouwborst A, Tenbrinck R, Van Woerkens ECSM (1990) Blood gas analysis of mixed venous blood during normoxic acute isovolemic hemodilution in pigs. Anesth Analg 70:523–529
60. Shou H, Perez de Sa V, Sigurdardottir M, Roscher R, Jonmarker C, Werner O (1996) Circulatory effects of hypoxia, acute normovolemic hemodilution and their combination in anesthetized pigs. Anesthesiology 84:1443–1454
61. Fontana JL, Welborn L, Mongan PD, Sturm P, Martin G, Bünger R (1995) Oxygen consumption and cardiovascular function in children during profound intraoperative normovolemic hemodilution. Anesth Analg 80:219–225
62. McDaniel LB, Zwischenberger JB, Vertrees RA, et al (1995) Mixed venous oxygen saturation during cardiopulmonary bypass poorly predicts regional venous saturation. Anesth Analg 80:466–472
63. Spahn DR, Leone BJ, Reves JG, Pasch T (1994) Cardiovascular and coronary physiology of acute isovolemic hemodilution: a review of nonoxygen-carrying and oxygen carrying solutions. Anesth Analg 78:1000–1021

Cytopathic Hypoxia: Mitochondrial Dysfunction as a Potential Mechanism Contributing to Organ Failure in Sepsis

M. P. Fink

Introduction

According to Barcroft's classic analysis [1], diminished availability of oxygen (O_2) at the cellular level can result via three main mechanisms:
1) inadequate arterial O_2 tension ("hypoxic hypoxia");
2) inadequate circulating hemoglobin (Hb) concentration ("anemic hypoxia");
3) inadequate blood flow ("stagnant hypoxia").

Increasingly, it is apparent that there is a fourth way that cellular aerobic metabolism can be deranged under pathologic conditions, a mechanism we might denote "cytopathic hypoxia" to indicate impaired production of adenosine triphosphate (ATP) despite adequate availability of O_2 in the vicinity of mitochondria within cells.

A number of different, but mutually compatible mechanisms, might foster the development of cytopathic hypoxia under pathological conditions. These mechanisms include: diminished delivery of pyruvate into the mitochondrial tricarboxylic acid (TCA) cycle, inhibition of key mitochondrial enzymes involved in either the TCA cycle (*cis*-aconitase) or the electron transport chain (NADH-ubiquinone oxidoreductase, succinate-ubiquinone oxidoreductase); activation of the enzyme, poly-(ADP)-ribosylpolymerase (PARP); or collapse of the protonic gradient across the inner mitochondrial membrane leading to uncoupling of oxidative phosphorylation.

Tissue Oxygen Tension in Sepsis

Several investigators have reported that tissue oxygenation is impaired in experimental models of sepsis. For example, Vallet et al. [2] investigated the effects of acute endotoxemia on skeletal muscle and ileal tissue O_2 tension (PO_2) values. Sequential measurements were obtained in a single group of dogs at baseline, during a one-hour infusion of lipopolysaccharide (LPS), and then during a two-hour infusion of dextran solution. Infusion of LPS resulted in a marked decrease in systemic O_2 delivery (DO_2), but this parameter was normalized by resuscitating the animals with the colloid solution. The skeletal muscle PO_2 distribution shifted toward the left (i.e., to lower than normal values) after the induction of endotoxemic shock, but shifted back toward the right (i.e., to higher than normal values) following resuscitation. The distribution of intestinal mucosal PO_2 also shifted to the left during the first hour of the protocol, but the mean mucosal PO_2 remained low during the resuscitation period despite a marked increase in mesenteric DO_2. These findings were reproduced in a subsequent study by Hasibeder et al. [3], who showed that jejunal mucosal PO_2 decreased in a hypodynamic model of endotoxemia in anesthetized pigs. Similarly, Sair and colleagues [4] recently reported that skeletal muscle PO_2 decreased markedly in a rat model of endotoxemia. Interestingly, in this study [4], there was no difference between endotoxemic animals and controls with respect to skeletal muscle perfusion as assessed by measuring inert gas (N_2O or H_2) washout curves. Therefore, the development of tissue hypoxia following the injection of LPS was attributed to impaired microvascular control of nutritive flow.

Astiz and colleagues [5] studied three groups of animals: rats rendered septic by cecal ligation and puncture; rats made septic and resuscitated with intravenous albumin solution; and control rats subjected to a sham procedure. Similar to the observations obtained in endotoxemic dogs [2], bacterial peritonitis in rats was associated with significant decreases in both systemic DO_2 and mean skeletal muscle PO_2. Moreover, infusion of albumin restored both of these parameters to values not different from non-septic controls. It is noteworthy, however, that tissue ATP levels were low and tissue lactate concentrations were high (relative to non-septic controls) in both albumin-resuscitated and non-resuscitated septic rats. Taken together, the data obtained by Vallet et al. [2] and Astiz et al. [5] support two important conclusions. First, skeletal muscle PO_2 decreases in unresuscitated sepsis on the basis of inadequate perfusion, but stagnant hypoxia due to sepsis can be ameliorated by increasing systemic DO_2. Second, tissue ATP stores are diminished and tissue lactate levels are increased in sepsis as a consequence of some mechanism other than tissue hypoxia.

In contrast to the data just cited, a number of studies suggest that tissue PO_2 values are normal or even elevated in endotoxemia or sepsis. For example, Hotchkiss et al. [6] estimated tissue PO_2 values in a number of organs in rats rendered septic by cecal ligation and perforation. Tissue PO_2 values were estimated by measuring retention of [18F]-fluoroisonidazole, a lipophilic 2-nitroimidazole derivative that is irreversibly bound to intracellular macromolecules under hypoxic, but not normoxic, conditions. As a positive control, these investigators showed that retention of [18F]-fluoroisonidazole was increased in the ipsilateral gastrocemius of rats subjected to reversible hind limb ischemia induced by application of a rubber tourniquet. However, retention of [18F]-fluoroisonidazole in skeletal muscle, cardiac muscle, liver, and kidney was similar in septic rats and non-septic controls; i.e., sepsis was not associated with the development of tissue hypoxia.

Our laboratory investigated the effects of endotoxemia on intestinal mucosal PO_2 [7]. In these studies, anesthetized pigs were infused with LPS and simultaneously resuscitated to maintain normal cardiac output (CO). In marked contrast to the findings of Vallet et al. [2] and Hasibeder et al. [3], mean mucosal PO_2 did not decrease, but rather increased significantly. Although endotoxemia was not associated with mucosal hypoxia, mucosal hydrogen ion concentration increased significantly, suggesting that the development of tissue acidosis in this model was not the result of tissue hypoxia. Although inconsistent with the findings of Vallet et al. [2] and Hasibeder et al. [3], our observations are consistent with recently published data obtained by Rosser et al. [8, 9], who have demonstrated that PO_2 increases in the bladder epithelium of endotoxic rats. Interestingly, Boekstegers and colleagues [10, 11] have documented that skeletal muscle PO_2 decreases (relative to normal values) in patients with cardiogenic shock, but increases in patients with sepsis.

Evidence for Impaired Mitochondrial Function in Sepsis

Data showing that tissue PO_2 increases in sepsis or endotoxemia can be cited as evidence that O_2 utilization by tissues is deranged under these conditions. However, much more direct evidence of impaired cellular respiration (i.e., cytopathic hypoxia) has been obtained in several experimental studies. For example, Simonson et al. [12] have obtained evidence that cellular respiration is impaired in sepsis. These investigators used near-infrared spectroscopy (NIR) to monitor the redox state of cytochrome aa_3 in skeletal muscle cells of baboons rendered septic by an infusion of viable *Escherichia coli*. The functional status of cytochrome aa_3 was monitored by periodically causing temporary skeletal muscle ischemia using a proximally placed tourniquet. Inflating the tourniquet caused a decrease in the signal from oxided cytochrome aa_3, whereas deflating the tourniquet resulted in an increase in the NIR signal from the reoxided enzyme. Early in the sepsis protocol (i.e., at 6 hours), the rate of cytochrome aa_3 reduction following tourniquet ischemia was the same as at baseline, although the rate of reoxidation following the release of ischemia was slowed. These data can be interpreted as showing decreased DO_2 to the tissue. Later in the sepsis protocol (e.g., at 18 hours), the rate of cytochrome aa_3 reduction during tourniquet ischemia was markedly slowed, a finding that suggests the presence of either a defect in the ability of the enzyme to accept electrons from O_2 or a limitation in the availability of NADH.

Recently, our laboratory has obtained further evidence that O_2 utilization by at least one tissue, the intestinal mucosa, is impaired in sepsis. Rats were injected with saline or LPS (5 mg/kg) [13]. Twenty-four hours later, ileal mucosal cellular respiration was assessed by measuring the mitochondrial-dependent reduction of 3-(4,5-dimethylthiazol-2-yl)-2,5-diphenyltetrazolium bromide (MTT) to its formazan derivative (MTT-FZ). The lumen of the intestine was loaded with a solution of MTT, and then the concentration of the reduced formazan form of the compound was measured in enterocytes (normalized to DNA content) after 30 min of incubation. Mitochondrial respiration was significantly impaired in enterocytes from endotoxemic rats as compared to enterocytes from non-endotoxemic controls; MTT-FZ concentrations were 34.5 ± 7.1 and 84.6 ± 9.1 µg/mg DNA, respectively ($p < 0.01$). Interestingly, LPS-induced intestinal epithelial mitochondrial dysfunction was significantly ameliorated in endotoxemic rats treated with aminoguanidine, an inhibitor of nitric oxide (NO) biosynthesis. The

MTT-FZ concentration in enterocytes was 74.9 ± 9.6 µg/mg DNA in enterocytes from rats challenged with LPS and treated with aminoguanidine ($p < 0.01$ vs enterocytes from endotoxemic controls). These data support two conclusions: mitochondrial respiration is impaired following the administration of LPS to rats; and this phenomenon is mediated, at least in part, by upregulation of NO synthesis.

In a series of preliminary studies, our laboratory now has obtained even more direct evidence that intestinal O_2 utilization is impaired in endotoxemic rats. Rats were injected with saline or LPS (5 mg/kg). Eight hours later, the animals were anesthetized and the ileum exteriorized. A small segment of ileal tissue was sutured to an O-ring, and then excised. The piece of tissue, supported by the O-ring, was then mounted in a polarimeter and incubated at $37\,°C$ in oxygenated glucose-containing buffer. Oxygen consumption (VO_2) was measured directly and normalized to the subsequently determined dry weight of the tissue. Using this methodology, we have shown that endotoxemia is associated with a small, but statistically significant, decrease in the rate of *ex vivo* VO_2 by ileal tissue samples from rats.

Uncoupling is a special form of mitochondrial dysfunction. The term "mitochondrial uncoupling" implies that the utilization of O_2 (as the final electron acceptor for the oxidation of reducing equivalents in the form of NADH and FADH) is not tightly linked to the phosphorylation of ADP to form ATP. Uncoupled respiration is manifested by an increase in the ratio of VO_2 under *State 4* conditions (excess substrate, ADP absent) to VO_2 under *State 3* conditions (excess substrate, ADP present). Like measurements of cellular energy charge, data regarding the adequacy of mitochondrial coupling in sepsis or endotoxemia tend to be confusing and conflicting. In one early study, Decker et al. [14] evaluated hepatic mitochondrial function in rats with peritonitis caused by *Klebsiella pneumoniae*. Although ATP levels were decreased in samples of liver tissue obtained 18 hours after the induction of sepsis, the function of isolated mitochondria, as assessed by measuring O_2 utilization following addition of appropriate substrates in the presence (*State 3*) or absence (*State 4*) of ADP, was entirely normal. Similar findings have been reported by other investigators [15, 16]. In contrast, Mela et al. [17] found evidence of uncoupling of hepatic mitochondrial respiration in endotoxemic rats. Similarly, Tavakoli and Mela [18] showed that although oxygen utilization by isolated muscle and liver mitochondria from septic rats was normal under *State 3* conditions, VO_2 under *State 4* conditions was markedly increased, a finding indicative of a loss of the normal coupling between substrate oxidation and phosphorylation of ADP.

A number of studies have shown that endotoxin and various pro-inflammatory cytokines are capable of causing hepatic mitochondrial dysfunction *in vitro* by means of a mechanism dependent upon the production of NO and/or other related reactive nitrogen metabolites. In various *in vitro* systems, these compounds have been shown to inhibit *cis*-aconitase (the rate-limiting enzyme in the TCA cycle) as well as two key enzymes in the mitochondrial electron transport chain, NADH-ubiquinone oxidoreductase and succinate-ubiquinone oxidoreductase [19, 20]. These *in vitro* phenomena are associated with inhibition of mitochondrial energization [21] as well as partial uncoupling of mitochondrial oxidative-phosphorylation [19]. Interestingly, recently obtained data suggest that these effects may be artifacts of the *in vitro* conditions employed, because under normal *in vivo* conditions, Hb in the hepatic sinusoid effectively scavenges NO before it can impair mitochondrial performance [20].

Recently, another form of NO-dependent mitochondrial dysfunction has been postulated to occur in endotoxemia [22]. According to this hypothesis, increased production of NO by a variety tissues during endotoxemia leads, via indirect means, to activation of the enzyme PARP. NO can react with superoxide radical anion to form the versatile and potent oxidizing agent, peroxynitrite, or its protonated form, peroxynitrous acid ($ONOO^-$ and ONOOH, respectively) [23]. An accumulating body of data suggest that $ONOO^-$ (or, perhaps, ONOOH) is capable of causing single-strand breaks in the DNA of various cell types [24–27] and thereby activating the nuclear repair enzyme, PARP [25–27]. Upon activation, PARP catalyzes the poly-ADP-ribosylation of proteins, a reaction which consumes NAD^+ and ATP, leading to energetic failure in cells [26, 28, 29]. Using the reduction of MTT to assess mitochondrial respiration, Zingarelli et al. [22] have documented that mitochondrial respiration is impaired in peritoneal macrophages harvested from endotoxemic rats [22]. Moreover, these investigators have demonstrated that this phenomenon can be blocked using an agent, nicotinamide, which inhibits PMP [22].

NO also appears to be able to inhibit mitochondrial respiration in a completely reversible fashion. Work from several laboratories shows that physiologically relevant concentrations of NO bind to and inhibit cytochrome aa_3, resulting in diminished respiration and ATP biosynthesis [30–32]. Inhibition of cytochrome aa_3 via this mechanism could account for the findings noted by Simonson et al. [12] cited previously. Alternatively, NAD^+ depletion caused by PARP activation could also explain the findings reported by Simonson et al. [12].

There are at least two other potential causes of mitochondrial dysfunction in sepsis. One is increased expression of various mitochondrial uncoupling proteins. These are molecules that promote the entry of protons into the mitochondrial matrix independent of the ATP synthetase, and thereby dissipate the mitochondrial protonic gradient. At least three different uncoupling proteins have been described (UCP1, UCP2 and UCP3) [33, 34]. It is possible, although unproved, that sepsis leads to upregulation of the expression of one or more of these uncoupling proteins, thereby leading to functional dissociation of respiration from phosphorylation of ADP.

Another potential mechanism for mitochondrial dysfunction in sepsis is the mitochondrial permeability transition (MPT). The MPT is caused by opening of a non-specific channel in the inner mitochondrial membrane under conditions of mitochondrial overload with ionized calcium (Ca^{2+}) [35]. The MPT has been implicated in the pathogenesis of myocardial ischemia/reperfusion injury [36], although the role of this phenomenon in sepsis or endotoxemia remains to be explored.

Lactic Acidosis in Sepsis

During anaerobiosis, pyruvate accumulates within the cytosol, since consumption of this partially oxidized metabolic fuel via the TCA cycle is blocked by the absence of mitochondrial oxidative metabolism. During anaerobic glycolysis, NAD^+ is reduced to NADH as a consequence of the reaction catalyzed by glyceraldehyde-3-phosphate dehydrogenase. In order to regenerate NAD^+ under anaerobic conditions, cells convert pyruvate to lactate in the reaction catalyzed by lactate dehydrogenase. Thus, accumulation of lactate in cells and blood is a characteristic feature of anaerobic metabolism. Hyperlactatemia is also a common finding in patients with sepsis. Indeed, the presence of elevated circulating lactate levels is commonly cited as evidence that sepsis is associated with inadequate perfusion leading to cellular hypoxia [37]. This notion, however, is poorly supported by the available data. In septic patients, systemic DO_2 correlates poorly with circulating concentrations of lactate [38]. Furthermore, in a study of endotoxemic dogs, Bellomo et al. [39] found that transvisceral lactate fluxes across several organs (skeletal muscle, liver, gut, kidney) were either neutral or were indicative of net uptake. In contrast, lactate flux across the pulmonary vascular bed was positive, suggesting that the lung is a major source of lactate in this model.

Another key study lends support to the notion that elevated lactate levels in sepsis reflect factors other than (or in addition to) stagnant hypoxia in tissues. Hurtado et al. [40] compared a number of parameters in two groups of rabbits. One group developed a low CO state after being challenged with an intravenous bolus of LPS. The other group was subjected to a comparable decrease in CO (and, therefore, systemic DO_2) by inflating a balloon in the right ventricle. In both groups, mean skeletal muscle PO_2 decreased relative to the baseline value. Despite similar decrements in systemic DO_2, arterial lactate concentrations were significantly higher in the endotoxemic as compared to the control rabbits. In other words, tissue hypoperfusion is insufficent by itself to explain the apparent increase in anaerobic metabolism characteristic of sepsis.

One possible explanation for increased lactate production in sepsis is downregulation of the activity of the enzyme complex, pyruvate dehydrogenase (PDH), which regulates the intramitochondrial oxidation of pyruvate to acetyl-CoA. PDH can exist in enzymatically active (dephosphorylated) and inactive (phosphorylated) forms. Interconversion between the two forms of PDH is catalyzed by a PDH kinase and PDH phosphatase. Over the past several years, Vary and colleagues [41–43] have accumulated data suggesting that the total concentration of PDH in liver and muscle tissue in sepsis is unchanged, but the fraction in the active form is decreased. Predictable consequences of diminished PDH activity would be a decrease in the flux of glucose through the mitochondrial TCA cycle and an increase in the production of lactate [41–43]. Conversion of PDH to its inactive form, therefore, is one potential mechanism leading to the development of cytopathic hypoxia in sepsis.

Cellular ATP Levels in Sepsis

Data regarding the effects of sepsis on tissue levels of adenine nucleotides are plentiful but, largely because of conflicting findings, remarkably difficult to interpret. Many investigators have documented diminished concentrations of ATP (and/or reduced ATP/ADP ratios) in at least some organs in experimental animals with sepsis [5, 41, 44–47] or endotoxemia [48–52]. Other studies have determined that cellular ATP levels are well preserved in septic or endotoxemic animals [53–57]. Some studies have determined that skeletal muscle concentrations of creatine phosphate, a buffer of the high energy phosphate pool in skeletal and cardiac muscle, are diminished in septic or endotoxemic animals, whereas ATP levels are normal [58–60]. One study found that although basal skeletal muscle concentrations of high energy phosphates (creatine phosphate and ATP) are normal in endotoxemic rats, the ability of the tissue to restore normal energy levels after a brief period of ischemia is compromised following injection of LPS [61].

Data regarding tissue ATP levels in human sepsis are necessarily much more limited than are results from animal studies. In two studies with small sample sizes, Bergstrom et al. [62] and Liaw et al. [63] reported that skeletal muscle ATP and creatine phosphate levels are decreased in patients with sepsis. In a larger study, Tresadern et al. [64] found that skeletal muscle ATP, but not creatine phosphate, concentrations were decreased in septic patients, although these authors noted that skeletal muscle ATP levels also were decreased in patients with malnutrition in the absence of sepsis. Furthermore, Tresadern et al. [64] found that the overall "energy charge" defined as $([ATP] + 0.5[ADP])/([ATP] + [ADP] + [AMP])$ was normal in skeletal muscle samples from patients with sepsis or malnutrition, suggesting that these conditions deplete the total adenine nucleotide pool but do not affect cellular bioenergetics.

Conclusion

Several lines of evidence support the notion that cellular energetics are deranged in sepsis, not on the basis of inadequate tissue perfusion, but rather on the basis of impaired mitochondrial respiration and/or coupling; i.e., organ dysfunction in sepsis may occur on the basis of cytopathic hypoxia. If this concept is correct, then the therapeutic implications are enormous. Efforts to improve outcome in septic patients by monitoring and manipulating CO, systemic DO_2, and regional blood flow are doomed to failure. Instead, our focus should be on developing pharmacological strategies to restore normal mitochondrial function and cellular energetics.

Acknowledgements. Preparation of this manuscript was supported in part by NIH grant GM37631. The concepts presented herein are based upon the work and ideas of some of the research fellows, who have participated in our laboratory's efforts over the past few years. Among these fellows are the following very talented and creative individuals: Tom VanderMeer MD, Andy Salzman MD, Naoki Unno PhD MD, and Stephan Tytgaat MD.

References

1. Barcroft J (1920) On anoxaemia. Lancet ii:485
2. Vallet B, Lund N, Curtis SE, et al (1994) Gut and muscle tissue PO_2 in endotoxemic dogs during shock and resuscitation. J Appl Physiol 76:793–800
3. Hasibeder W, Germann R, Wolf HJ, et al (1996) Effects of short-term endotoxemia and dopamine on mucosal oxygenation in porcine jejunum. Am J Physiol 270:G667–G675
4. Sair M, Etherington PJ, Curzen NP, et al (1996) Tissue oxygenation and perfusion in endotoxemia. Am J Physiol 271:H1620–H1625
5. Astiz M, Rackow EC, Weil MH, et al (1988) Early impairment of oxidative metabolism and energy production in severe sepsis. Circ Shock 26:311–320
6. Hotchkiss RS, Rust RS, Dence CS, et al (1991) Evaluation of the role of cellular hypoxia in sepsis by the hypoxic marker [^{18}F]fluoroisonidazole. Am J Physiol 261:R965–R972
7. VanderMeer TJ, Wang H, Fink MP (1995) Endotoxemia causes ileal mucosal acidosis in the absence of mucosal hypoxia in a normodynamic porcine model of septic shock. Crit Care Med 23:1217–1226
8. Rosser DM, Stidwill RP, Jacobson D, et al (1995) Oxygen tension in the bladder epithelium rises in both high and low cardiac output endotoxemic sepsis. J Appl Physiol 79:1878–1882
9. Rosser DM, Stidwill RP, Jacobson D, et al (1996) Cardiorespiratory and tissue oxygen dose response to rat endotoxemia. Am J Physiol 271:H891–H895
10. Boekstegers P, Weidenhofer S, Pilz G, et al (1991) Peripheral oxygen availability within skeletal muscle in sepsis and septic shock: comparison to limited infection and cardiogenic shock. Infection 19:317–323
11. Boekstegers P, Weidenhofer S, Kapsner T, et al (1994) Skeletal muscle partial pressure of oxygen in patients with sepsis. Crit Care Med 22:640–650
12. Simonson SG, Welty-Wolf K, Huang Y-CT, et al (1994) Altered mitochondrial redox responses in Gram negative septic shock in primates. Circ Shock 43:34–43
13. Unno N, Wang H, Menconi MJ, et al (1997) Inhibition of inducible nitric oxide synthase ameliorates lipopolysaccharide-induced gut mucosal barrier dysfunction in rats. Gastroenterology 113:1246–1257
14. Greer GG, Milazzo FH (1975) *Pseudomonas aeruginosa* lipopolysaccharide: an uncoupler of mitochondrial oxidative phosphorylation. Can J Microbiol 21:877–883
15. Geller ER, Jankauskas S, Kirkpatrick J (1986) Mitochondrial death in sepsis: a failed concept. J Surg Res 40:514–517
16. Fry DE, Silva BB, Rink RD, et al (1979) Hepatic cellular hypoxia in murine peritonitis. Surgery 85:652–661
17. Mela L, Bacalco LV Jr, Miller LD (1971) Defective oxidative metabolism of rat liver mitochondria in hemorrhagic and endotoxin shock. Am J Physiol 220:571–577
18. Tavakoli H, Mela L (1982) Alterations of mitochondrial metabolism and protein concentrations in subacute septicemia. Infect Immun 38:536–541
19. Stadler J, Billiar TR, Curran RD, et al (1991) Effect of exogenous and endogenous nitric oxide on mitochondrial respiration rat hepatocytes. Am J Physiol 260:C910–C916
20. Fisch C, Robin A-M, Letteron P, et al (1996) Cell-generated nitric oxide inactivates rat hepatocyte mitochondria in vitro but reacts with hemoglobin in vivo. Gastroenterol 110:210–220
21. Kurose I, Kato S, Ishii H, et al (1993) Nitric oxide mediates lipopolysaccharide-induced alteration of mitochondrial function in cultured hepatocytes and isolated perfused liver. Hepatology 18:380–388
22. Zingarelli B, Salzman AL, Szabó C (1996) Protective effects of nicotinamide against nitric oxide-mediated delayed vascular failure in endotoxic shock: potential involvement of poly-ADP ribosyl synthetase. Shock 5:258–264
23. Pryor WA, Squadrito GL (1995) The chemistry of peroxynitrite: a product from the reaction of nitric oxide with superoxide. Am J Physiol 268:L699–L722
24. Salgo MG, Bermudez G, Squadrito G, et al (1995) Peroxynitrite causes DNA damage and oxidation of thiols in rat thymocytes. Arch Biochem Biophys 322:500–505

25. Szabó C, Zingarelli B, O'Connor M, et al (1996) DNA strand breakage, activation of poly-ADP ribosyl synthetase, and cellular energy depletion are involved in the cytotoxicity in macrophages and smooth muscle cells exposed to peroxynitrite. Proc Natl Acad Sci USA 93: 1753-1758

26. Szabó C, Saunders C, O'Connor M, et al (1997) Peroxynitrite causes energy depletion and increases permeability via activation of poly (ADP-ribose) synthetase in pulmonary epithelial cells. Am J Respir Cell Mol Biol 16:105-109

27. Szabó C, Zingarelli B, Salzman AL (1996) Role of poly-ADP ribosyltransferase activation in the vascular contractile and energetic failure elicited by exogenous and endogenous nitric oxide and peroxynitrite. Circ Res 78:1051-1063

28. Szabó C, Zingarelli B, Salzman AL (1996) Role of poly-ADP ribosyltransferase activation in the vascular and energetic failure elicited by exogenous and endogenous nitric oxide and peroxynitrite. Circ Res 78:1051-1063

29. Schraufstatter IU, Hinshaw DB, Hyslop PA, et al (1986) Oxidant injury of cells. DNA strand-breaks activate polyadenosine diphosphate-ribose polymerase and lead to depletion of nicotinamide adenine dinucleotide. J Clin Invest 77:1312-1320

30. Lizasoain I, Moro MA, Knowles RG, et al (1996) Nitric oxide and peroxynitrite exert distinct effects on mitochondrial respiration which are differentially blocked by glutathione or glucose. Biochem J 314:877-880

31. Borutaité V, Brown GC (1996) Rapid reduction of nitric oxide by mitochondria, and reversible inhibition of mitochondrial respiration by nitric oxide. Biochem J 315:295-299

32. Schweizer M, Richter C (1994) Nitric oxide potently and reversibly deenergizes mitochondria at low oxygen tension. Biochem Biophys Res Commun 204:169-175

33. Casteilla L, Blondel O, Klaus S, et al (1990) Stable expression of functional mitochondrial uncoupling protein in Chinese hamster ovary cells. Proc Natl Acad Sci USA 87:5124-5128

34. Vidal-Puig A, Solanes G, Grujic D, et al (1997) UCP3: an uncoupling protein homologue expressed preferentially and abundantly in skeletal muscle and brown adipose tissue. Biochem Biophys Res Commun 235:79-82

35. Zoratti M, Szabo I (1995) The mitochondrial permeability transition. Biochem Biophys Acta 1241:139-176

36. Griffiths EJ, Halestrap AP (1993) Protection by cyclosporin a of ischemia reperfusion-induced damage in isolated rat hearts. J Mol Cell Cardiol 25:1461-1469

37. Mizock BA, Falk JL (1992) Lactic acidosis in critical illness. Crit Care Med 20:80-93

38. Ronco JJ, Fenwick JC, Tweeddale MG, et al (1993) Identification of the critical oxygen delivery for anaerobic metabolism in critically ill septic and nonseptic humans. JAMA 270: 1724-1730

39. Bellomo R, Kellum JA, Pinsky MR (1996) Transvisceral lactate fluxes during early endotoxemia. Chest 110:198-204

40. Hurtado FJ, Gutierrez AM, Silva N, et al (1992) Role of tissue hypoxia as the mechanism of lactic acidosis during E. coli endotoxemia. J Appl Physiol 72:1895-1901

41. Vary TC, Siegel JH, Nakatani T, et al (1986) Effect of sepsis on activity of pyruvate dehydrogenase complex in skeletal muscle and liver. Am J Physiol 250:E634-E640

42. Vary TC, Siegel JH, Tall BD, et al (1988) Metabolic effects of partial reversal of pyruvate dehydrogenase activity by dichloroacetate in sepsis. Circ Shock 24:3-18

43. Vary TC, Drnevich D, Jurasinski C, et al (1995) Mechanisms regulating skeletal muscle glucose metabolism in sepsis. Shock 3:403-410

44. Chaudry IH, Wichterman KA, Baue AE (1979) Effect of sepsis on tissue adenine nucleotide levels. Surgery 85:205-211

45. Haybron DM, Townsend MC, Hampton WW, et al (1987) Alterations in renal perfusion and renal energy charge in murine peritonitis. Arch Surg 122:328-331

46. Shimahara Y, Kono Y, Tanaka J, et al (1987) Pathophysiology of acute renal failure following living Escherichia coli injection in rats: high-energy metabolism and renal functions. Circ Shock 21:197-205

47. Angerås U, Hall-Angerås M, Wagner KR, et al (1991) Tissue metabolite levels in different types of skeletal muscle during sepsis. Metabolism 40:1147-1151

48. van Lambalgen AA, van Kraats AA, Mulder MF, et al (1994) High-energy phosphates in heart, liver, kidney, and skeletal muscle of endotoxemic rats. Am J Physiol 266:H1581-H1587
49. Pelias ME, Townsend MC (1992) In vivo [^{31}P]NMR assessment of early hepatocellular dysfunction during endotoxemia. J Surg Res 52:505-509
50. Raymond RM, Gordey J (1989) The effect of hypodynamic endotoxin shock on myocardial high energy phosphates in the rat. Cardiovasc Res 23:200-204
51. Koprach S, Hörkner U, Orlik H, et al (1989) Energy state, glycolytic intermediates and mitochondrial function in the liver during reversible and irreversible endotoxin shock. Biochem Biophys Acta 9:653-659
52. Jabs CM, Neglen P, Eklof B (1995) Breakdown of adenine nucleotides, formation of oxygen free radicals, and early markers of cellular injury in endotoxic shock. Eur J Surg 161:147-155
53. Jepson MM, Cox M, Bates PC, et al (1987) Regional blood flow and skeletal muscle energy status in endotoxemic rats. Am J Physiol 252:E581-E587
54. Deaciuc IV, Spitzer JA (1988) Further characterization of a model of chronic endotoxemia in the rat: adenine nucleotide content in liver. Circ Shock 25:1-7
55. Gitomer WL, Miller BC, Cottam GL (1995) In vivo effects of lipopolysaccharide on hepatic free-NAD(P)$^+$-linked redox states and cytosolic phosphorylation potential in 48-hour-fasted rats. Metabolism 44:1170-1174
56. Pedersen P, Saljo A, Hasselgren P-O (1987) Protein and energy metabolism in liver tissue following intravenous infusion of live E. coli bacteria in rats. Circ Shock 21:59-64
57. Hotchkiss RS, Song SK, Neil JJ, et al (1991) Sepsis does not impair tricarboxylic cycle in the heart. Am J Physiol 260:C50-C57
58. Jacobs DO, Kobayashi T, Imagire J, et al (1991) Sepsis alters skeletal muscle energetics and membrane function. Surgery 110:318-326
59. Mitsuo T, Rounds J, Prechek D, et al (1996) Glucocorticoid receptor antagonism by mifepristone alters phosphocreatine breakdown during sepsis. Arch Surg 131:1179-1185
60. Song SK, Hotchkiss RS, Karl E, et al (1992) Concurrent quantification of tissue metabolism and blood flow via ^{2}H/^{31}P NMR in vivo, III: alterations in muscle blood flow and metabolism during sepsis. Magn Reson Med 25:67-77
61. Gilles RJ, D'Orio V, Ciancabilla F, et al (1994) In vivo ^{31}P nuclear magnetic resonance spectroscopy of skeletal muscle energetics in endotoxemic rats: a prospective, randomized study. Crit Care Med 22:499-505
62. Bergstrom J, Bostrom H, Furst P, et al (1976) Preliminary studies of energy-rich phosphagens in muscle from severely ill patients. Crit Care Med 4:197-204
63. Liaw KY, Askanazi J, Michelson CB, et al (1980) Effect of injury and sepsis on high-energy phosphates in muscle and red cells. J Trauma 20:755-759
64. Ohrui T, Yamauchi K, Sekizawa K, et al (1992) Histamine N-methyltransferase controls the contractile response of guinea pig trachea to histamine. J Pharmacol Exp Ther 261:1268-1272

Poly (ADP-ribose) Synthetase Activation in Circulatory Shock

A. L. Salzman

Introduction

Tissue injury in circulatory shock is mediated in part by the end-organ loss of effective mitochondrial respiration, resulting in an inadequate production of high energy phosphates and the ultimate loss of cellular function. The depletion of intracellular energetics in various shock states has been ascribed to inadequate oxygen delivery (DO_2) to tissues, secondary to macrovascular and microcirculatory ischemia. The development of ischemia in shock has a multifactorial basis, and reflects impaired cardiac function, vascular hypocontractility, and capillary leak, leading to intravascular volume depletion and inadequate preload. More recent evidence suggests that end-organ energetic depletion in shock may also be caused by a failure at the cellular level to adequately utilize ambient cellular O_2. A variety of cytotoxic species generated by shock, including free radicals and oxidants, appear to directly impair respiration via their effects on critical enzymes involved in adenosine triphosphate (ATP) formation as well as indirectly via an effect on intracellular ionic composition, membrane stability, and induction of apoptosis. Substantive evidence now supports a role for both ischemia and O_2 dysutilization as primary factors in the loss of effective mitochondrial respiration in shock and the consequent development of tissue dysfunction and organ failure.

Although it is overly reductive to assign a single mechanism to the development of ischemia and O_2 dysutilization in circulatory shock, increasing evidence supports a major role for a novel mechanism of injury mediated by the action of poly (adenosine diphosphate-ribose) synthetase (PARS) in both of these pathologic developments [1–3]. PARS is an abundant nuclear enzyme which is present under constitutive conditions in eukaryotic cells throughout the phylogenetic spectrum [4]. The precise physiologic function of PARS is uncertain; at low basal levels it may play a role in desoxyribonucleic acid (DNA) repair [5, 6], chromatin relaxation [7], cell differentiation [8], DNA replication [9], transcriptional regulation [10], control of cell cycle [11], p53 expression and apoptosis [12], and transformation [13]. Under pathologic conditions, including radiation injury, circulatory shock, and regional inflammation, PARS activity may be upregulated substantially [3, 14–16]. Pathologic activation of PARS has been associated with many of the fundamental derangements of septic shock, including impairment of mitochondrial respiration, loss of vascular contractility, and reduction of myocardial function [1-3,17-25]. Inhibition of PARS activity, therefore, may represent a novel means of improving tissue oxygenation and respiration in circulatory shock.

Structure-Function of PARS

The tertiary structure of PARS is organized into three principal domains which serve distinct functions. The N-terminal domain has two zinc-finger structures which specifically recognize and bind DNA single strand breaks [26], inducing a conformational change in the protein which activates a C-terminal catalytic domain [4]. The presence of DNA with strand termini is an absolute requirement for PARS activation [27]. Moreover, removal of the N-terminal DNA binding domain abolishes PARS activity [26]. Both zinc fingers are required for recognition of DNA single-strand breaks, as evidenced by the absence of activity of PARS proteins in which either of the zinc fingers has been inactivated by deletion or mutagenesis [26]. Footprinting studies demonstrate that PARS specifically recognizes DNA nicks and protects about 14 nucleotides around a nick [28]. Beyond the requirement for DNA strand termini, PARS does not appear to have a preferred consensus sequence, as is the case for most DNA-binding proteins.

Once activated, the C-terminal domain of PARS catalyzes the cleavage of NAD^+ into ADP-ribose and nicotinamide and generates a covalent bond between ADP-ribose and various acceptor proteins [1, 14, 29-31]. The intramolecular mechanism by which N-terminal DNA binding activates the C-terminal catalytic domain is not well worked out. In contrast to mono ADP-ribosyl transferases, PARS attaches successive ADP-ribose moieties via O-glycosidic linkages to form a nucleic acid homopolymer attached to the initial ADP-ribose group, ultimately forming a highly charged poly (ADP) ribose polymer [32]. Poly ADP-ribose, which represents the third class of nucleic acids in the cell (in addition to DNA and RNA), may range in length from a few residues to polymers of several hundred subunits [33]. PARS is able to form both linear chains, via a ribosyl $(1'' \rightarrow 2')$ ribose bond, as well as branched structures, via a ribosyl$(1'' \rightarrow 2'')$ ribose bond, although the latter is decidedly less frequent [32]. A growing list of proteins that undergo this process of post-translational modification have been identified, including histones, transcription factors, cell cycle associated proteins, an auto-modification domain of PARS itself, and proteins involved in breaking or joining of DNA strands, such as ligase II, topoisomerases I and II, and endonucleases [28, 34]. The functional consequences of these alterations are, however, unknown. It is tempting to speculate that the highly charged nature of poly(ADP-ribose) confers electrostatic properties on the proteins it modifies, altering their binding to DNA. Such a phenomenon might be important, for instance, in the regulation of gene transcription and DNA folding.

Poly(ADP-ribose), formed by PARS, is subject to degradation by three enzymes:
1) Poly(ADP-ribose) glycohydrolase, which is the principal mechanism of polymeric degradation, reduces the polymer via an exoglycosidic activity, leaving

a mono-ribosylated acceptor protein. The time course of polymer degradation by this enzyme is extremely rapid, starting less than 2 minutes after poly(ADP-ribose) formation [28].

2) ADP-ribosyl protein lyase cleaves mono-ribosylated proteins and is considered the rate-limiting step in polymeric degradation.

3) An unspecified phosphodiesterase is activated several minutes later, completing the degradation of poly(ADP-ribose) via a cleavage of pryophosphate linkages [28]. The regulatory aspects of poly(ADP-ribose) catabolism are little understood, but clearly play a critical role in determining the size and duration of the polymer. Aberrant degradation of poly(ADP-ribose) might be expected to have pathologic consequences, decreasing the threshhold for PARS-mediated injury, but there are currently no existing reports examining the relationship between poly(ADP-ribose) degradation and the inflammatory response. The recent description of a macrocircular ellagitannin oenothein B as a PARS glycohydrolase inhibitor may help to resolve this question in future *in vivo* studies [35].

Regulation of PARS Activity

PARS is expressed constitutively at low basal levels in nearly all cells. The 5′ flanking region of the human PARS gene has been cloned and sequenced, revealing numerous putative sites for activator protein (AP)-2 binding. Reporter assays suggest that the proximal promoter contained within 99 bp upstream of the transcription initiation site is sufficient for transcriptional activation [36]. Expression of PARS reporter constructs is upregulated in response to cellular stimulation by phorbol ester, implying a role for protein kinase C activation, and by cyclic AMP. Suppression of PARS expression in several cell lines has also been observed in response to differentiating agents, including retinoic acid [37] and nerve growth factor [38].

Under pathologic conditions in which high levels of DNA single strand breakage occur, PARS activity may increase substantially, without an alteration in the level of expression of PARS mRNA or protein. Increased activation of PARS activity is associated with high levels of poly(ADP-ribose) formation [4]. A variety of cytotoxic agents are associated with the *in vitro* and *in vivo* development of DNA strand breaks, including oxidants, radiation, and mutagens. In circulatory shock of various etiologies, oxidant formation is greatly increased; thus, shock of all types is a potent trigger of PARS activation.

Oxidants may be generated during reperfusion in shock via the activation of xanthine oxidase, a purine metabolizing enzyme which is present in low concentrations in healthy tissues, but is markedly increased in shock due to the proteolytic cleavage of its precursor, xanthine dehydrogenase [39]. In the presence of O_2, which is restored during reperfusion, xanthine oxidase forms superoxide anion from xanthine, a breakdown product of ATP formed in ischemic tissues [39]. Xanthine oxidase may also be activated from xanthine dehydrogenase by cytokine stimulation [39], and is markedly upregulated during viral and bacterial infection [39, 40]. Superoxide may also be formed by activated granulocytes by a membrane-bound enzyme, nicotinamide adenine dinucleotide phosphate (NADPH) oxidase. Thus, tissue infiltration by neutrophils, which occurs during both ischemia-reperfusion (I/R) injury as well as systemic inflammatory disturbances, such as sepsis, increases superoxide generation.

Superoxide anion is a relatively weak free radical, but may be converted to the more potent redox species hydrogen peroxide and hydroxyl radical, in the presence of intracellular free iron, via the Fenton reaction. Normally, free iron concentrations are insufficient to support Fenton chemistry, but under conditions of severe acidosis, as occur in shock, sufficient iron is liberated to promote oxidant formation from superoxide anion. Recently, the importance of Fenton chemistry in shock has been questioned and other sources of toxic oxidant species have been proposed. Superoxide may combine, for example, with nitrogen-centered free radicals, such as nitric oxide (NO), to form the highly potent oxidant species peroxynitrite [41]. Peroxynitrite has a broad range of molecular targets, as evidenced by its effects on lipid peroxidation, protein modification [31, 42], mitochondrial respiration [43], and glutathione depletion [44]. In fact, many of the deleterious actions ascribed to NO are now recognized to be, in fact, a consequence of peroxynitrite formation. Peroxynitrite is a highly unstable species in aqueous solution at physiologic pH, and is rapidly protonated to the labile acid. Peroxynitrous acid breaks down to form a reactive oxidant, thought to be either hydroxyl radical or a vibrationally unstable intermediate with hydroxyl radical like activity.

Exposure of intact cells and tissues to exogenous or endogenously generated oxidants, such as hydrogen peroxide, hydroxyl radical, and peroxynitrite, produces abundant DNA strand breaks [1, 19, 45, 46]. Exogenous and endogenously generated peroxynitrite causes DNA strand breaks *in vitro* in multiple cell types, including vascular smooth muscle, endothelium, macrophages, and myocardium [1, 2, 19, 21, 46]. Oxidative DNA damage has also been observed *in vivo*, as evidenced by the urinary excretion of the repair product 8-oxo-7,8-dihydro-2′deoxyguanosine following mesenteric I/R injury [47]. The formation of peroxynitrite has been shown to play a critical role in the development of lipid peroxidation after lung ischemia [48], epithelial hyperpermeability in immunostimulated intestinal epithelial cells [49], and tissue damage after hepatic [50], splanchnic [46], myocardial [46, 51], and renal I/R injury [52].

High local levels of NO have also been proposed to induce DNA damage, as a consequence of NO-mediated inhibition of ribonucleotide reductase [53] or other DNA repair enzymes [14, 54]. The relative importance of free radicals versus oxidants in shock-induced DNA strand breakage is a continuing matter of dispute, and has major implications for novel therapeutic approaches to the management of circulatory shock. The salutary effects of anti-oxidants on DNA strand breakage suggest that the final common trigger of DNA breaks is probably an oxidant species; this does not, however, exclude a critical role for free radicals in the generation of oxidant species, either via the Fenton reaction or the formation of peroxynitrite.

In addition to the effects of free radical and oxidant injury on PARS activation, cytokines have been implicated in post-transcriptional regulation of PARS activity. Interferon-gamma (IFN-γ), released in shock states by activated T lymphocytes and natural killer cells, upregulates PARS activity in cultured macrophages but has no effect on the transcriptional regulation of PARS nor on the steady-state expression of PARS mRNA [55]. IFN-γ has been shown to dose-dependently trigger DNA strand breakage, suggesting that its induction of PARS activity may be mediated indirectly via an allosteric effect on PARS. The mechanism by which IFN-γ triggers DNA injury is unknown; it is possible that IFN-γ induces DNA strand breakage via an induction of cytotoxic free radicals or oxidants, but this remains to be explored.

Pathologic Roles of PARS

Energetic Depletion

PARS activation induces the immediate formation of poly(ADP-ribose), arising from the catalytic cleavage of NAD. Poly(ADP-ribose) is rapidly degraded, with a half-live in the range of minutes to several hours [28]. At low levels of DNA strand breakage, the duration of PARS activation and the consumption of NAD are trivial. At higher levels of DNA damage, however, PARS activation is persistent and NAD consumption may rapidly progress to near total depletion, with drastic alterations in cellular metabolism [1, 29, 33, 46, 56]. A futile cycle of polymeric synthesis and degradation rapidly ensues, assuring the consumption of the enzymatic substrate NAD [33, 46]. Because NAD plays a pivotal role in glycolysis, the tricarboxylic acid (TCA) cycle, and electron transport, PARS-mediated consumption of NAD impairs cellular oxidative phosphorylation and ATP formation [33]. In particular, the blockade of electron transport prevents reducing equivalents from interacting with molecular O_2. As a consequence, cellular respiration is inhibited even in the presence of O_2 concentrations exceeding the Vmax for cytochrome aa3. The result is intracellular energetic exhaustion, manifested by a low energy charge and inadequate high energy phosphates to maintain cellular homeostasis [46].

Evidence for this cellular "suicide" mechanism, first proposed by Berger [33], has been obtained in a variety of cell types exposed to exogenous sources of oxidant stress [46, 57, 58]. PARS activation in vitro is involved in xanthine oxidase-mediated ATP depletion [59], O_2 radical and NO mediated toxicity [14, 60], hydrogen peroxide induced damage [57], and in xanthine oxidase or peroxynitrite-induced mitochondrial dysfunction [61, 62]. Activation of PARS and the consequent reduction of intracellular energetics have also been observed following endogenous exposure to peroxynitrite in immunostimulated cells [19]. In cultured macrophages, for example, LPS stimulation simultaneously upregulates NO production by the inducible NO synthase (iNOS) and superoxide production by NADPH oxidase, resulting in in situ peroxynitrite formation, DNA strand breakage, and PARS activation [19]. Inhibition of iNOS activity or scavenging of superoxide prevents peroxynitrite formation, as judged by the formation of nitrotyrosine, a "footprint" of nitrosative stress [63]. Inhibition of PARS activity has no effect on peroxynitrite or DNA strand break formation but blocks the loss of cellular energetics [45]. Thus, endogenous levels of oxidant formation are sufficient *in vitro* to activate PARS and induce energetic failure.

The importance of the peroxynitrite-induced PARS pathway to cellular energetic failure, relative to the independent effects of the peroxynitrite precursor NO, is a matter of current debate [64]. It is clear that NO *per se* is highly toxic to aconitase, a critical enzyme in the TCA cycle, depending upon the ambient conditions of pH and O_2 tension (PO_2) [65]. Under conditions of relative hypoxia or mild acidosis which are characteristic of shock, NO toxicity to aconitase is greatly potentiated [65]. Moreover, under anoxic conditions in which peroxynitrite is not formed, exogenous NO potently inactivates aconitase [65]. NO has also been associated with the inactivation of other sulfhydryl containing enzymes, including the electron transport chain proteins NADH-ubiquinone-oxidoreductase and succinate-ubiquinone oxidoreductase [66–69]. As would be expected from the inhibition of these enzymes, exposure of cells to NO donors reduces ATP and cellular respiration, but has little effect on NAD [56]. None of the energetic changes induced by NO donors are reversed by PARS inhibitors, demonstrating that NO is independently capable of producing cellular energetic failure by a PARS-independent mechanism [56].

In contrast to the PARS-independent cytotoxicity of NO, peroxynitrite exposure of intestinal epithelial cells, macrophages, smooth muscle cells, and endothelial cells results in the depletion of both NAD and ATP, effects which are reversed by PARS inhibition [1, 2, 70]. These data suggest that there are two parallel mechanisms of energetic depletion induced by free radicals and oxidants [56]. NO inhibits the activity of enzymes in glycolysis and oxidative phosphorylation via the inactivation of sulfur-containing catalytic centers [65–69]. Peroxynitrite, and other oxidants, in contrast, inhibit intracellular energetics via the induction of DNA strand breaks and the activation of PARS [1]. At very high levels of oxidant exposure, however, PARS inhibition becomes ineffective [21], suggesting that overwhelming oxidant stress triggers multiple pathways of injury, in addition to PARS activation. The existence of PARS-dependent and PARS-independent pathways of cellular injury has been confirmed in murine islet cells in which the PARS gene has been disrupted [60]. Mutant cells are protected from moderate levels of reactive O_2 species (ROS), but are susceptible to higher levels of oxidant stress, indicating the presence of an alternative pathway of cell death which does not require PARS activation and NAD depletion [60].

Regulation of gene expression

In vivo inhibition of PARS activity has been shown to have a salutary effect on inflammatory injury in a variety of experimental models [2, 3, 15, 17, 20–22, 25, 71]. Many of these benefits have been related to the blockade of energetic depletion in conditions associated with oxidant-induced DNA strand breakage [3]. Interestingly, PARS inhibition also has potent effects on the recruitment of effector cells into the inflammatory focus, which would not be predicted from its actions on cellular energy charge. For example, PARS inhibition virtually eliminates neutrophil infiltration in experimental models of endotoxicosis, carageenan-induced pleurisy, and splanchnic ischemia-reperfusion injury [3, 16, 71]. This action has also been reproduced in PARS knockout animals [15], implying that PARS activity in some way modulates the expression of pro-inflammatory signaling molecules, such as chemokines or intercellular adhesion receptors.

Because cell surface adhesion molecules are a prime determinant of granulocytic adhesion and trans-endothelial migration of activated neutrophils from the blood stream into injured tissue, we examined the effect of PARS on the expression of intercellular adhesion molecule (ICAM)-1. Under constitutive conditions, ICAM-1 is constitutively expressed on the endothelial cell surface at low levels. During inflammation, ICAM-1 expression is upregulated in the vascular wall and may also be expressed in parenchymal cells. Using a strain of mice in which the PARS gene has been specifically disrupted, we have observed a total suppression of inflammatory-induced upregulation of ICAM-1 expression in an experimental model of colitis. Similar findings were obtained in colitic rats treated with a PARS inhibitor. These findings are supported by *in vitro* observations that PARS inhibition blocks ICAM-1 expression in immunostimulated endothelial cells [72]. We have also determined in cultured intestinal epithelial cells that PARS inhibitors suppress interleukin(IL)-1β mediated induction of C3, an early component of the complement pathway which generates C5a, a potent chemotaxin (unpublished data). Taken together, these data from studies of cultured cells and experimental *in vivo* models suggest that PARS plays a critical role in signal transduction of pro-inflammatory signals.

The mechanism by which PARS regulates the expression of pro-inflammatory genes, such as ICAM-1 and C3, may be related to its effect on the induction of the transcription factor AP-1, a heterodimer composed of varying combinations of the *c-fos* and *jun* families. AP-1 binding to the 5′ flanking regions of human ICAM-1, C3, and *c-fos* is required for their full transcriptional activation [72]. Inhibition of PARS activity in cultured cells potently blocks oxidant-induced *c-fos* mRNA expression and AP-1 activation [10]. Since the *c-fos* promoter itself has an AP-1 consensus site [10], *c-fos* activation may induce a self-amplifying cycle of gene activation. Of interest, *c-fos* activation by superoxide anion induces a poly ADP-ribosylation of *c-fos* itself [10]. Whether this post-translational modification of *c-fos* is required for AP-1 activation has not been explored. Although the role of PARS activation in *c-fos* expression has not yet been demonstrated *in vivo*, the fact that PARS regulates a critical transcription factor involved in the recruitment of neutrophils to an inflammatory focus suggests that PARS may contribute to a positive-feedback loop in shock.

Several studies have reported that high doses of certain PARS inhibitors block the IL-1β mediated iNOS expression in rodent pancreatic beta islet cells [73]. The PARS inhibitor 5-iodo-6-amino-1,2-benzopyrone (INH2BP) has also been associated with a reduction in the endotoxin-induced expression of tumor necrosis factor (TNF)-α, IL-6, iNOS, and cyclooxygenase-2 *in vitro* in murine macrophages and *in vivo* in rats [18]. Simultaneously, INH2BP increased expression of the anti-inflammatory cytokine IL-10 [18]. The inhibitory effect of the INH2B in this system could not be accounted for by an effect on the nuclear translocation of nuclear factor-kappa B (NF-κB), a pro-inflammatory transcription factor implicated in the transcriptional regulation of many shock-induced genes. Interestingly, the lipopolysaccharide(LPS)-mediated induction of mitogen activated protein (MAP) kinase activity in RAW cells was entirely prevented by pre-treatment with a variety of PARS inhibitors, suggesting that PARS activity may be required for MAP kinase activation [18]. Since MAP kinase occupies a critical role in the transduction of multiple intracellular inflammatory cascades, it is conceivable that many of the anti-inflammatory effects of PARS inhibition may be accounted for at this level.

In assessing the role of PARS activation on iNOS expression, it is important to distinguish the effects of micromolar doses of INH2BP from suprapharmacologic doses of nicotinamide [73]. The latter studies have observed iNOS inhibition by PARS inhibitors at concentrations in the range of 20–50 mM, a level which is also associated with generalized inhibition of RNA and protein synthesis. Since nicotinamide is a relatively weak PARS inhibitor, it is not possible to determine whether its inhibition of iNOS expression is a PARS-dependent phenomenon or reflects a broad cytotoxic effect on the cell. 3-aminobenzamide, which is a somewhat more potent PARS inhibitor than nicotinamide, does not inhibit iNOS-derived NO production in endotoxic rats [21] in contrast to the results described above for INH2BP [73]. This discrepancy may just reflect the log-fold difference in potency between 3-aminobenzamide and INH2BP. Definitive resolution of this issue should be provided in the near future by study of endotoxic PARS knockout mice.

Development of a Working Hypothesis Relating PARS and Circulatory Shock

The above data suggest the following working hypothesis (Fig. 1): Shock-induced cytokines stimulate free radical formation by stimulating xanthine oxidase activity and *de novo* iNOS expression and by recruiting activated neutrophils which express NADPH oxidase. Oxidants are formed from the interaction of superoxide and NO and by iron-catalyzed oxidation of superoxide. Oxidants induce AP-1 formation and generate DNA single-strand breaks. DNA strand breaks activate PARS, which in turn strongly potentiates AP-1 expression, resulting in greater expression of the AP-1 dependent genes ICAM-1 and C3. Generation of C5a (derived from C3), in combination with increased endothelial expression of ICAM-1, recruits more activated leukocytes to inflammatory foci, producing greater oxidant stress. The cycle is thus renewed as the increase in oxidant stress triggers more DNA strand breakage. The proposed cycle of inflammatory activation will be potentiated in systems where PARS-dependent MAP kinase activation also contributes to oxidant formation and granulocyte recruitment. According to the proposed scenario, which still requires careful validation but is strongly supported by multiple lines of evidence, PARS is the critical determinant of a positive-feedback cycle of inflammatory injury.

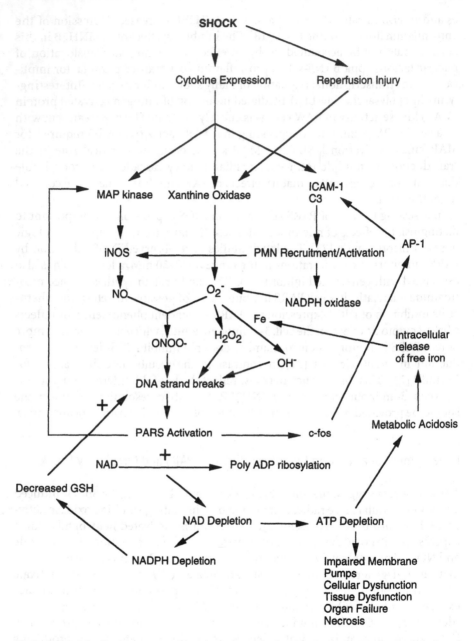

Fig. 1. Schematic diagram representing the proposed role of PARS activation in shock-induced tissue injury

The loss of NAD induced by PARS activation may accelerate this cycle by interfering with the energy-dependent reduction of oxidized glutathione, the principal intracellular anti-oxidant and the most abundant thiol found in mammalian cells [74]. NAD is the precursor for NADP, which plays a critical role in bioreductive synthetic pathways and the maintenance of reduced glutathione pools [33]. In the absence of adequate cellular levels of reduced glutathione, resulting from energetic failure or overwhelming oxidant exposure [75], further oxidant stress is unopposed, resulting in greater DNA strand breakage. Other factors contributing to ATP depletion, such as frank ischemia, would also be expected to potentiate the deleterious effect of PARS activation via their negative effect on cellular anti-oxidant capacity.

Interestingly, PARS activity appears to have a counterregulatory effect on IFN-γ induced genes. Overexpression of PARS mRNA inhibits major histocompatability complex (MHC) Class II gene expression, whereas a decrease in PARS activity, resulting from the expression of an anti-sense PARS mRNA construct, enhances MHC Class II expression [76]. The aggregate effect of PARS on IFN-γ induced gene expression *in vivo* has not been examined.

The relative balance of PARS-mediated activation of AP-1 and MAP kinase dependent genes and PARS-mediated inhibition of IFN-γ dependent genes is unknown. Based upon the available *in vivo* data, which indicate that PARS activation is strongly pro-inflammatory, it is probable that the effect on IFN-γ gene expression is not predominant. We thus favor the hypothesis that pharmacologic inhibition of PARS should have a profound effect on the course of inflammatory injury in shock. PARS stands at the crossroads of multiple intersecting pathways of inflammatory injury, creating a self-amplifying cycle of oxidant-driven damage. Experimental evidence derived from studies utilizing PARS inhibitors or murine strains with a targeted disruption of the PARS gene, as described below, in fact supports the centrality of PARS activation in the pathogenesis of shock.

Pharmacologic Inhibitors of PARS Activity

Many of the experimental data used to implicate PARS activation as a critical factor in shock have relied upon pharmacologic agents which inhibit PARS. As with all enzymatic systems, the use of pharmacologic agents to inhibit activity raises concerns of specificity. In particular, most of the commonly utilized PARS inhibitors, including 3-aminobenzamide and nicotinamide, have significant side effects [27]. These concerns have often been addressed by the parallel use of various structurally unrelated PARS inhibitors, demonstrating that the effects observed are unlikely to represent non-specific actions, but rather, are related to the specific inhibition of PARS activity. More recently, the availability of a murine strain in which the PARS gene has been genetically disrupted [77] has permitted more rigorous examination of the role of PARS in oxidant-mediated injury *in vitro* and inflammatory injury *in vivo*. Fibroblasts obtained from PARS deficient mice, for example, are resistant to moderate levels of peroxynitrite-induced injury [21]. In a model of sepsis induced by intraperitoneal administration of zymosan, PARS deficient animals have significantly reduced systemic inflammatory response *in vivo* compared to the wild-type littermate controls [15]. PARS knockout mice also have significantly reduced infarct size in a cerebrovascular occlusion model [78], similar to the neuroprotective effects of inhibiting PARS [79].

The consistent agreement between pharmacologic and gene knockout studies suggests that the inhibitors are specific.

The classic agents used to inhibit PARS activity are 3-aminobenzamide and nicotinamide. The potency of these agents is relatively poor, making them unattractive for clinical applications. The IC_{50} for 3-aminobenzamide and nicotinamide are 33 and 210 μM, respectively, and significant inhibition does not become manifest below millimolar concentrations [27]. Nonetheless, a clinical trial of nicotinamide for the treatment of diabetes mellitus has been undertaken. Several new, highly potent inhibitors have been developed, in which a carbonyl group is built in a second ring system conjugated with a six-membered aromatic ring [27]. The most potent of these are 4-Amino-1,8-naphthalimide (IC_{50} 0.18 μM), 2H-benz[c]isoquinolin-1-one[6(5H)-phenanthridinone] (IC_{50} 0.30 μM), and 1,5-dihydroxyisoquinoline (IC_{50} 0.39 μM) [27]. These agents are associated with significant *in vivo* side effects, including hypotension (personal communication: Parke-Davis Pharmaceuticals), that limit their clinical potential. More promising PARS inhibitors are under development and may become available for clinical use in the next decade [27]. In particular, a recently described agent, 5-iodo-6-amino-1,2-benzopyrone [80], has a log fold greater potency as a PARS inhibitor, relative to 3-aminobenzamide, and shows remarkable efficacy in cell-based systems and *in vivo* [18].

Nearly all PARS inhibitors examined to date, including 3-aminobenzamide and nicotinamide, act in a competitive mode at low concentrations but become mixed-type inhibitors at higher concentrations [27]. Since PARS is a multi-functional enzyme, with distinct domains related to DNA binding, substrate (NAD) binding, and poly ADP ribosylation (chain initiation, elongation, and branching), there are numerous opportunities for enzymatic inhibition; thus, multiple sites exist for a non-competitive mode of inhibition. A frequent problem with many of the novel PARS inhibitors described to date is a lack of aqueous solubility [27]. Indeed, most existing potent PARS inhibitors require solubilization in organic solvents, such as dimethylsulfoxide, which makes them less attractive for parenteral clinical application. The outstanding exception is the highly potent and water soluble PARS inhibitor 4-amino-1,8-naphthalimide (IC_{50} 18 nM) [14, 27].

The effect of *in vivo* PARS inhibition is likely to be complicated by cell-specific responses to oxidative injury and PARS activation. Whereas oxidant-induced PARS activation and energetic failure appear to be the case with most cell types, in hepatocytes inhibition of PARS is without effect on the oxidative death of the cells [81]. The apparent resistance of hepatocytes to PARS-mediated injury may be due to the high capacity of the liver to generate NAD [31]. Whether other cell types are also resistant to the effects of PARS inhibition is currently unknown. An additional factor effecting the susceptibility of cells to PARS inhibition is the state of cellular differentiation. PARS is expressed at high levels in rapidly dividing cells, such as enterocytes and keratinocytes. Terminal cellular differentiation is associated with a marked decrease in PARS activity. In the intestine, for example, nuclei from non-dividing but differentiating ring cells in the upper crypts and on the villi contain no more than 10% of the PARS activity of the lower-crypt cell nuclei [82].

The use of PARS inhibitors may be particularly appropriate in acute conditions, such as shock, where issues of toxicity related to long-term administration are less relevant. Since PARS has been implicated in numerous physiologic housekeeping functions, such as gene repair, transcription, and cell cycling, there is an obvious concern that chronic administration of PARS inhibitors may have unacceptable toxicities. Chronic *in vitro* administration of high doses of the PARS inhibitor nicotinamide, for example, reduces β-islet cell function [83]. PARS inhibition has also been associated with an increase in sister chromatid exchange [84]. The effect of long-term PARS inhibition on gene repair is concerning, with respect to the opportunity for malignant transformation. Many have argued that PARS activation is required to eliminate genetically damaged cells, thereby reducing oncogenic potential [85]. Whether PARS actually plays a critical or indispensable role in genetic repair is still open to question. In fact, PARS inhibition by 3-aminobenzamide actually facilitated rapid ligation of DNA excision-repair patches [86] and suppressed malignant transformation in cells with DNA damage induced by irradiation and chemical carcinogens [87].

Whether described toxicities are idiosyncratic effects of the particular PARS inhibitor, or an effect of PARS inhibition *per se*, is unclear. Targeted disruption of the PARS gene might be expected to provide a definitive answer to the question of potential long-term toxicity of PARS inhibition, although this approach is not functionally equivalent to pharmacologic inhibition since the lack of PARS activity is ontogenic. PARS knock-out mice appear superficially to have an unremarkable phenotype, although approximately 30% of animals spontaneously develop a dermatitis [77]. The rapid division of keratinocytes, and the corresponding high levels of PARS activity in basal cells, suggest that PARS may play an important role in cellular differentiation. Chronic inhibition of PARS activity may therefore be problematic in regenerative tissues, such as the gut and skin. Surprisingly, there have been no reports that PARS deficient animals have inadequate gene repair, given the importance of this function traditionally assigned to PARS. Assuming that PARS in fact does participate in DNA repair, the phenotype of the PARS knock out animals implies that redundant cellular mechanisms may be able to compensate for the absence of the enzyme. As with any anti-inflammatory approach, PARS inhibitors may interfere with immune clearance of pathogens. In the case of bacterial infection, this has yet to be explored. The situation is complicated with respect to the effect of PARS inhibition on viral infection, since some PARS inhibitors are virostatic and have been proposed, in fact, as antiviral therapies [88].

Pharmacologic Effects of PARS Inhibitors

Oxidant-Induced *in vitro* Injury

PARS inhibition protects cultured cells from free radical and oxidant mediated injury. Inhibition of PARS activity significantly improved survival of islet cells co-cultured with activated macrophages [89] and exposed to chemical NO donors [90]. PARS inhibitors are also protective against oxidant exposure in a wide variety of cell types, including pulmonary endothelial and epithelial cells, enterocytes, and neurons [14, 29, 31, 56, 65, 91]. Recently, we showed that exogenous exposure of cultured human enterocytes and pulmonary epithelial cells to peroxynitrite resulted in a profound depletion of NAD, followed temporarily by a reduction in ATP and loss of epithelial monolayer barrier function [56,92]. Inhibition of PARS preserved intracellular energetics and ameliorated the disruption of epithelial permeability [56]. The protective effects of PARS inhibitors on oxidant-induced reduction in cellular respiration have now been confirmed in PARS deficient fibroblasts [21].

Endotoxic Shock

Endotoxic shock is a systemic inflammatory process produced by a cascade of inflammatory mediators which trigger the widespread activation of leukocytes and the production of toxic levels of free radicals and oxidants, including peroxynitrite [93]. The primary role of oxidant production and neutrophil recruitment in shock suggests that PARS inhibitors may be particularly effective as novel therapeutics. In the past year, experimental *in vivo* evidence has demonstrated the protective effect of PARS inhibitors [2] and the PARS$^{-/-}$ genotype [15] in various models of systemic inflammation. Of signal importance, PARS inhibitors have been shown to restore mitochondrial respiration and intracellular NAD$^+$ in cells harvested from endotoxic animals [20]. This evidence supports the central hypothesis that PARS activation is a critical determinant of energetic failure in sepsis.

The loss of intracellular energetics in endotoxic shock appears to be systemic, with evidence of impaired respiration in multiple cell types [20, 21]. The pathologic manifestations of PARS-mediated energetic depletion depend to a large extent upon the physiologic role of the particular tissue in question. Our laboratory has focused on the role of oxidant-induced energetic failure in the vasculature, since hypocontractility of the vascular smooth muscle plays a major role in the development of ischemia and end-organ injury in septic shock. Using a rat model of severe endotoxic shock, we have observed that treatment with the PARS inhibitor nicotinamide one hour after administration of LPS, maintained higher blood pressure levels without affecting the level of iNOS expression [20]. In order to confirm that the improvement in blood pressure was related to changes in the vascular response, as opposed to an effect on myocardial contractility, vessels were harvested three hours after LPS administration and examined for *ex vivo* contractile responses to graded doses of norepinephrine. *In vivo* inhibition of PARS restored 50% of the endotoxin-induced loss of vascular contractility [20], confirming the existence of a PARS-dependent mechanism of vascular failure. Moreover, treatment with the more potent PARS inhibitor 3-aminobenzamide in the same model fully restored *ex vivo* vascular contractility [2].

Endotoxic shock is also associated with formation of peroxynitrite in the vascular intima [93], suggesting that oxidant-mediated injury of the endothelium might account for the loss of endothelial vasodilatory responsiveness in septic shock. In order to test whether PARS activation might contribute to the loss of endothelial function in shock, vessels harvested from endotoxic rats were pre-contracted with norepinephrine and allowed to relax in response to the NO-dependent vasodilator acetylcholine. Endotoxic shock induced a more than 60% loss in endothelial-dependent relaxation, compared to a 35% decrease in vessels taken from animals treated *in vivo* with the PARS inhibitor 3-aminobenzamide [21]. These data suggest that PARS activation may play a significant role in endothelial injury in shock. It is, thus, likely that PARS-mediated injury might also affect other critical functions of the endothelium which are deranged in sepsis, including the development of capillary leak and microvascular thrombosis.

Survival is the ultimate criterion for therapeutic success in clinically-relevant initiatives to treat circulatory shock. In order to test whether PARS inhibitors affect mortality, a lethal model of murine endotoxic shock was utilized (120 mg/kg IP) in which mortality at 42 hours is > 90%. Treatment with the PARS inhibitor 3-aminobenzamide prevented any deaths for the first 18 hours (relative to 40% survival in the untreated group). At 42 hours, 50% of the treated animals survived, confirming the dramatic protective effect of PARS inhibition [2]. A dose-dependent protective effect of the PARS inhibitor INH2BP was also observed in the same model of murine endotoxic shock; PARS inhibition prevented any mortality at 18 hours post-LPS administration and increased survival at 42 hours to 60% [18]. Studies examining the effect of endotoxin in PARS$^{-/-}$ animals are currently underway and should establish, unequivocally, the role of PARS activation in endotoxic shock.

Splanchnic Ischemia-Reperfusion Injury

Splanchnic ischemia of sufficient duration primes the intestinal epithelium for a reperfusion injury, mediated by free radical and oxidant generation by enterocytes and infiltrating leukocytes in the gut mucosa. Injury to the bowel is manifested histologically by edema and lifting of the mucosa away from the underlying basement membrane. Functional changes are noted by the loss of vectorial transport and the increase in the transepithelial passage of macromolecules from the lumen to the circulation [94]. The loss of intestinal barrier function is related to the formation of free radicals and oxidants, such as NO, superoxide, peroxynitrite, and hydroxyl radical [95], and may be ameliorated by agents which catalyze the dismutation of superoxide [96, 97] or block the formation of iNOS-derived NO [98]. Although all organs may be susceptible to reperfusion injury, the intestine is particularly vulnerable due to the large concentration of mucosal xanthine oxidase, a rate limiting enzyme of nucleic acid degradation which catalyzes the formation of O_2-derived free radicals during the early phase of reperfusion [96]. At later stages of reperfusion, neutrophils infiltrate into the mucosa and contribute to the generation of superoxide anion via a membrane NADPH oxidase [99]. In fact, strategies which prevent neutrophil infiltration significantly reduce bowel injury [100].

The emphasis on oxidant injury and neutrophil recruitment in splanchnic I/R injury suggests that PARS activation may play a critical role in mediating tissue injury. The protective effects of PARS inhibition was recently demonstrated in a rat model of splanchnic artery occlusion and reperfusion, in which the celiac and superior mesenteric arteries were clamped for 45 minutes, followed by one hour of reperfusion [3]. I/R injury resulted in a significant decrease in mean arterial blood pressure, an increase in neutrophil infiltration into the gut mucosa, as assessed by myeloperoxidase activity, and marked histologic injury to the ileum. The production of the oxidant peroxynitrite in response to IR injury was suggested by the oxidation in the plasma of dihydrorhodamine-123 to rhodamine (which reflects peroxynitrite-mediated oxidation) and by immunohistochemical evidence of nitrotyrosine formation in the mucosa. Nitrosation of tyrosine residues is a semi-quantitative measure of nitrosative stress, which includes but is not specific for peroxynitrite-induced oxidation. I/R injury also injured vascular endothelial and smooth muscle function in this model, as evidenced by the decreased contraction of isolated aortic rings to catecholamine stimulation and the diminished relaxation of vessels to the vasodilating effects of acetylcholine [3]. A functional loss of the gut mucosa was also appreciated by the increased permeability of the mucosal epithelium to the lumen to plasma flux of a fluorescein-labeled 4000 MW dextran. I/R injury induced an increase in PARS activity in intestinal epithelial cells, as measured 10 minutes after the start of reperfusion. Inhibition of PARS activity by *in vivo* administration of 3-aminobenzamide prior to reperfusion was strongly protective, reducing histologic injury and improving blood pressure, restoring *ex vivo* vascular contractility and endothelium-dependent relaxation, and limiting reperfusion-induced hyperpermeability [3]. Of considerable interest, PARS inhibition virtually eliminated the massive increase in I/R induced neutrophil infiltration. Most importantly, in the absence of PARS inhibition, none of the animals survived I/R injury, whereas all shocked animals treated with 3-aminobenzamide survived. These data provide strong support to the role of PARS activation in splanchnic I/R injury and augur well for future therapeutic opportunities utilizing PARS inhibition. Recently, we have confirmed the role of PARS in mediating mesenteric I/R injury, utilizing a gene-targeted PARS deficient murine model. PARS knock-out mice had less evidence of tissue injury than wild-type littermate controls, as judged by the levels of lipid peroxidation and had virtually no increase in neutrophil recruitment into the gut, or in remote organs such as the lung, during the reperfusion phase.

The value of PARS inhibitors in I/R injury has been recently extended to other forms of injury, unrelated to systemic shock. PARS inhibitors, for example, have been shown to limit infarct size in experimental models of middle cerebral occlusion/reperfusion [79], and skeletal and myocardial I/R injury [22, 101]. 3-aminobenzamide also attenuated the myocardial dysfunction caused by global ischemia and reperfusion in the isolated perfused lapine heart [101]. Thus, the role of PARS activation in I/R injury appears to be a unifying principle, not confined to a particular vascular distribution. It can be expected, therefore, that PARS inhibitors may be efficacious in a variety of clinical conditions typified by regional shock, including stroke and myocardial infarction.

Conclusion

The loss of end-organ respiration in shock depends upon the loss of O_2-carrying blood flow to peripheral tissues and the capacity of the cells to take up and utilize the O_2 as the final electron receptor in the process of oxidative phosphorylation. Substantial data from *in vivo* models have confirmed that the activation of PARS interferes with both perfusion and respiration in various shock states. Although the loss of respiration in shock is obviously complex, and no single mechanism can fully account for the entire derangement, it is clear that PARS activity is involved in many, if not all of the critical determinants of tissue oxygenation and utilization. The importance of PARS to this process may also derive from the fact that PARS activation creates a self-amplifying positive-feedback cycle, which if unchecked may rapidly lead to massive oxidant production and tissue injury. By its effect on neutrophil recruitment, PARS activity potentiates the formation of oxidant-induced DNA strand breaks, the very trigger which allosterically up-regulates its own activity. The potency of this mechanism of injury may also provide the clinician one day with an equally valuable therapeutic target. New PARS inhibitors are under active development. Their potential utility in multiple clinical indications, aside from shock, is sure to hasten their early arrival. Issues of toxicity, especially long-term, remain and may deter the clinical use of PARS inhibitors in the treatment of chronic disease. But, for the intensivist confronted with the emergent and acute condition of circulatory shock, PARS inhibitors may provide a remarkably potent addition to the current, rather limited, armamentarium of agents to preserve cellular respiration.

References

1. Szabó C, Zingarelli B, O'Connor M, Salzman AL (1996) DNA strand breakage, activation of poly-ADP ribosyl synthetase, and cellular energy depletion are involved in the cytotoxicity in macrophages and smooth muscle cells exposed to peroxynitrite. Proc Natl Acad Sci USA 93:1753–1758
2. Szabó C, Zingarelli B, Salzman AL (1996) Role of poly-ADP ribosyltransferase activation in the vascular contractile and energetic failure elicited by exogenous and endogenous nitric oxide and peroxynitrite. Circ Res 78:1051–1063
3. Cuzzocrea S, Zingarelli B, Constantino G, et al (1997) Beneficial effects of 3-aminobenzamide, an inhibitor of poly (ADP-ribose) synthetase in a rat model of splanchnic artery occlusion and reperfusion. Br J Pharm 121:1065–1074
4. Lautier D, Lageux J, Thibodeau J, Ménard L, Poirier GG (1993) Molecular and biochemical features of poly (ADP-ribose) metabolism. Mol Cell Biochem 122:171–193
5. Durkacz BW, Omidiji O, Gray DA, Shall S (1980) (ADP-ribose)n participates in DNA excision repair. Nature 283:593–596
6. Satoh MS, Lindahl T (1992) Role of poly(ADP-ribose) formation in DNA repair. Nature 356:356–358
7. Poirier GG, de Murcia G, Jongstra-Bilen J, Niedergang C, Mandel P (1982) Poly(ADP-ribosyl)ation of polynuclesomes causes relaxation of chromatin structure. Proc Natl Acad Sci USA 79:3423–3427
8. Ohashi Y, Ueda K, Hayaisha O, Ikai K, Niwa O (1984) Induction of murine teratocarcinoma cell differentiation by suppression of poly(ADP-ribose) synthesis. Proc Natl Acad Sci USA 81:7132–7136

9. Simbulan-Rosenthal CM, Rosenthal DS, Hilz H, et al (1996) The expression of poly(ADP-ribose) polymerase during differentiation-linked DNA replication reveals that it is a component of the multiprotein DNA replication complex. Biochemistry 35:11622–11633

10. Amstad PA, Krupitza G, Cerutti PA (1992) Mechanism of c-fos induction by active oxygen. Cancer Res 52:3952–3960

11. Berger NA, Kaichi AS, Steward PG, Klevecz RR, Forrest GL, Gross SD (1978) Synthesis of poly(adenosine diphosphate ribose) in synchronized Chinese hamster cells. Exp Cell Res 117:127–135

12. Whitacre CM, Hashimoto H, Tsia ML, Chatterjee S, Berger SJ, Berger NA (1995) Involvement of NAD-poly(ADP-ribose) metabolism in p53 regulation and its consequences. Cancer Res 55:3697–3701

13. Kun E, Kirsten E, Milo GE, Kurian P, Kumari HL (1983) Cell cycle-dependent intervention by benzamide of carcinogen-induced neoplastic transformation and in vitro poly(ADP-ribosyl)ation of nuclear proteins in human fibroblasts. Proc Natl Acad Sci USA 80:7219–7223

14. Zhang J, Dawson VL, Dawson TM, Snyder SH (1994) Nitric oxide activation of poly (ADP-ribose) synthetase in neurotoxicity. Science 263:687–689

15. Szabó C, Lim LH, Cuzzocrea S, et al (1997) Inhibition of poly (ADP-ribose) synthetase attenuates neutrophil recruitment and exerts antiinflammatory effects. J Exp Med 186:1041–1049

16. Cuzzocrea S, Zingarelli B, Gilad E, Hake P, Salzman AL, Szabó C (1998) Protective effects of 3-aminobenzamide, an inhibitor of poly (ADP-ribose) synthase in a carrageenan-induced model of local inflammation. Eur J Pharm 342:67–76

17. Szabó, Zingarelli, Salzman (1996) Peroxynitrite-mediated activation of poly-ADP ribosyl synthetase contributes to the vascular failure in shock. In: Okada K, Ogata H (eds) Shock: From molecular and cellular level to whole body. Elsevier Scientific Publishers, Amsterdam, pp 3–14

18. Szabó C, Wong H, Bauer PI, et al (1997) Regulation of components of the inflammatory response by 5-iodo-6-amino-1,2-benzopyrone, an inhibitor of poly (ADP-ribose) synthetase and pleiotropic modifier of cellular signal pathways. Int J Oncol 10:1093–1104

19. Zingarelli B, O'Connor M, Wong H, Salzman AL, Szabó C (1996) Peroxynitrite-mediated DNA strand breakage activates poly-ADP ribosyl synthetase and causes cellular energy depletion in macrophages stimulated with bacterial lipopolysaccharide. J Immunol 156:350–358

20. Zingarelli B, Salzman AL, Szabó C (1996) Protective effects of nicotinamide against nitric oxide mediated vascular failure in endotoxic shock: potential involvement of poly ADP ribosyl synthetase. Shock 5:258–264

21. Szabó C, Cuzzocrea S, Zingarelli B, O'Connor M, Salzman AL (1997) Endothelial dysfunction in endotoxic shock: importance of the activation of poly (ADP ribose) synthetase (PARS) by peroxynitrite. J Clin Invest 100:723–735

22. Zingarelli B, Cuzzocrea S, Zsengeller Z, Salzman AL, Szabó C (1997) Beneficial effect of inhibition of poly-ADP ribose synthetase activity in myocardial ischemia-reperfusion injury. Cardiovasc Res 36:205–215

23. Gilad E, Zingarelli B, Salzman AL, Szabó C (1997) Protection by inhibition of poly (ADP-ribose) synthetase against oxidant injury in cardiac myoblasts in vitro. J Mol Cell Cardiol 29:2585–2597

24. Zingarelli B, Ischiropoulos H, Salzman AL, Szabó C (1997) Amelioration by mercaptoethylguanidine of the vascular and energetic failure in haemorrhagic shock in the anesthetised rat. Eur J Pharm 338:55–65

25. Cuzzocrea S, Zingarelli B, O'Connor M, Salzman AL, Caputi AP, Szabó C (1997) Role of peroxynitrite and activation of poly (ADP-ribose) synthetase in the vascular failure induced by zymosan-activated plasma. Br J Pharm 122:493–503

26. Ikejima M, Noguchi S, Yamashita R, et al (1909) The zinc fingers of human poly(ADP-ribose) polymerase are differentially required for the recognition of DNA breaks and nicks and the consequent enzyme activation. J Biol Chem 265:21907–21913

27. Banasik M, Komura H, Shimoyama M, Ueda K (1992) Specific inhibitors of poly (ADP-ribose) synthetase and mono (ADP-ribosyl) transferase. J Biol Chem 267:1569–1575

28. Boulikas T (1992) Poly(ADP-ribose) synthesis and degradation in mammalian nuclei. Anal Biochem 203:252–258
29. Thies RL, Autor AP (1991) Reactive oxygen injury to cultured pulmonary artery endothelial cells: mediation by poly ADP-ribose polymerase activation causing NAD depletion and altered energy balance. Arch Biochem Biophys 286:353–363
30. Watson AJ, Askey JN, Benson RS (1995) Poly (adenosine diphosphate ribose) polymerase inhibition prevents necrosis induced by H_2O_2 but not apoptosis. Gastroenterology 109: 472–482
31. Kirkland JB (1991) Lipid peroxidation, protein thiol oxidation and DNA damage in hydrogen peroxide-induced injury to endothelial cells: Role of activation of poly (ADP-ribose) polymerase. Biochim Biophys Acta 1092:319–325
32. Ueda K, Hayaishi O (1985) ADP-ribosylation. Ann Rev Biochem 54:73–100
33. Berger NA (1991) Oxidant-induced cytotoxicity: a challenge for metabolic modulation. Am J Respir Cell Mol Biol 4:1–3
34. Rawling JM, Alvarez-Gonzalez R (1997) TFIIF, a basal eukaryotic transcription factor, is a substrate for poly(ADP-ribosyl)ation. Biochem J 324:249–253
35. Maruta H, Matsumura N, Tanuma S (1997) Role of (ADP-ribose)n catabolism in DNA repair. Biochem Biophys Res Commun 246:265–269
36. Yokoyama T, Kawamoto T, Mitsuuchi Y, et al (1990) Human poly(ADP-ribose) polymerase gene: cloning of the reporter region. Eur J Biochem 194:521–526
37. Suzuki H, Uchida K, Shima H, et al (1987) Molecular cloning of cDNA for human poly(ADP-ribose) polymerase and expression of its gene during HL-60 cell differentiation. Biochem Biophys Res Commun 146:403–409
38. Taniguchi T, Morisawa K, Ogawa M, Yamamoto H, Fujimoto S (1988) Decrease in the level of poly(ADP-ribose) synthetase during nerve growth factor-promoted neurite outgrowth in rat pheochromocytoma PC12 cells. Biochem Biophys Res Commun 54:1034–1040
39. Umezawa K, Akaike T, Fujii S, et al (1997) Induction of nitric oxide synthesis and xanthine oxidase and their roles in the antimicrobial mechanism against Salmonella typhimurium infection in mice. Infect Immun 65:2932–2940
40. Akaike T, Ando M, Oda T, et al (1990) Dependence on O_2^- generation by xanthine oxidase of pathogenesis of influenza virus infection in mice. J Clin Invest 85:739–745
41. Salzman AL (1995) Nitric oxide in the gut. New Horizons 3:352–364
42. Rubbo H, Radi R, Trujillo M, et al (1994) Nitric oxide regulation of superoxide and peroxynitrite-dependent lipid peroxidation. Formation of novel nitrogen-containing oxidized lipid derivates. J Biol Chem 269:26066–26075
43. Radi R, Rodriguiz M, Castro L, Telleri R (1994) Inhibition of mitochondrial electron transport by peroxynitrite. Arch Biochem Biophys 308:89–95
44. Barker JE, Bolanos JP, Land JM, Clark JB, Heales SJ (1996) Glutathione protects astrocytes from peroxynitrite-mediated mitochondrial damage: implications of neuronal/astrocytic trafficing and neurodegeneration. Dev Neurosci 18:391–396
45. Szabó C, Salzman AL (1995) Endogenous peroxynitrite is involved in the inhibition of cellular respiration in immuno-stimulated J774.2 macrophages. Biochem Biophys Res Commun 209:739–743
46. Schraufstatter IU, Hinshaw DB, Hyslop PA, Spragg RG, Cochrane CG (1986) Oxidant injury of cells: DNA strand-breaks activate polyadenosine diphosphate-ribose polymerase and lead to depletion of nicotinamide adenine dinucleotide. J Clin Invest 77:1312–1320
47. Loft S, Larsen PN, Rasmussen A, et al (1995) Oxidative DNA damage after transplantation of the liver and small intestine in pigs. Transplantation 59:16–20
48. Ischiropoulos H, al-Mehdi AB, Fisher AB (1995) Reactive species in ischemic rat lung injury: contribution of peroxynitrite. Am J Physiol 269:L158–L164
49. Unno N, Menconi M, Smith M, Fink M (1995) Nitric oxide mediates interferon gamma induced hyperpermeability in cultured human intestinal epithelial monolayers. Crit Care Med 23:1170–1176
50. Ma TT, Ischiropoulos H, Brass CA (1995) Endotoxin-stimulated nitric oxide production increases injury and reduces rat liver chemoluminescence during reperfusion. Gastroenterology 108:463–469

51. Mattheis G, Sherman MP, Buckberg GD, Hayborn DM, Young HH, Ignarro LJ (1992) Role of L-arginine-nitric oxide pathway in myocardial reoxygenation injury. Am J Physiol 162: H616-620
52. Yu L, Gengaro PE, Niederberger M, Burke TJ, Schrier RW (1994) Nitric oxide: a mediator in rat tubular hypoxia/reoxygenation injury. Proc Natl Acad Sci USA 91:1691-1695
53. Lepoivre M, Fiesch F, Coves J, Thelander L, Fontecave M (1991) Inactivation of ribonucleotide reductase by nitric oxide. Biochem Biophys Res Commun 79:442-448
54. Wink DA, Laval J (1994) The Fpg protein, a DNA repair enzyme, is inhibited by the biomediator nitric oxide in vitro and in vivo. Carcinogenesis 15:2125-2129
55. Berton G, Sorio C, Laudanna C, Menegazzi M, Carcerceri De Prati A, Suzuki H (1991) Activation of human monocyte-derived macrophages by interferon g is accompanied by increase of poly(ADP-ribose) polymerase activity. Biochim Biophys Acta 1091:101-109
56. Kennedy MS, Denenberg AG, Szabó C, Salzman AL (1998) Activation of poly-ADP ribosyl synthetase mediates cytotoxicity induced by peroxynitrite in human intestinal epithelial cells. Gastroenterology (in press)
57. Cochrane CG (1991) Mechanisms of oxidant injury of cells. Mol Aspects Med 12:137-147
58. Junod AF, Jornot L, Peterson H (1989) Differential effects of hyperoxia and hydrogen peroxide on DNA damage, polyadenosine diphosphate-ribose polymerase activity, and nicotinamide adenine dinucleotide and adenosine triphosphate contents in cultured endothelial cells and fibroblasts. J Cell Physiol 140:177-185
59. Aalto TK, Raivio KO (1993) Nucleotide depletion due to reactive oxygen metabolites in endothelial cells: effect of antioxidants and 3-aminobenzamide. Pediatr Res 34:572-576
60. Heller B, Wang ZQ, Wagner J, et al (1995) Inactivation of the poly (ADP-ribose) polymerase gene affects oxygen radical and nitric oxide toxicity in islet cells. J Biol Chem 270: 11 176-11 180
61. Bulkart V, Koike T, Brenner HH, Kolb H (1992) Oxygen radicals generated by the enzyme xanthine oxidase lyse rat pancreatic islet cells in vitro. Diabetologia 35:1028-1034
62. Szabó C, Day BJ, Salzman AL (1996) Evaluation of the relative contribution of nitric oxide and peroxynitrite to the suppression of mitochondrial respiration in immunostimulated macrophages, using a novel mesoporphyrin superoxide dismutase analog and peroxynitrite scanvenger. FEBS Lett 381:82-86
63. Singer II, Kawka DW, Scott S, et al (1996) Expression of inducible nitric oxide synthase and nitrotyrosine in colonic epithelium in inflammatory bowel disease. Gastroenterology 111: 871-885
64. Szabó, Salzman (1996) The physiology and pathophysiology of nitric oxide in the lung. In: Wilmott R (ed) The pediatric lung. Birkhauser Publishing Ltd, Basel, pp 279-310
65. Gardner PR, Constantino G, Szabó C, Salzman AL (1997) Nitric oxide sensitivity of the aconitases. J Biol Chem 272:25 071-25 076
66. Drapier J-C, Hibbs JB (1994) Differentiation of murine macrophages to express nonspecific cytotoxicity in L-arginine-dependent inhibition of mitochondrial iron-sulfur enzymes in the macrophage effector cells. J Immunol 14:2829-2838
67. Stadler J, Curran RD, Ochoa JB, et al (1994) Effect of endogenous nitric oxide on mitochondrial respiration of rat hepatocytes in vitro and in vivo. Arch Surg 126:186-191
68. Kurose I, Kato S, Ishii H, et al (1993) Nitric oxide mediates lipopolysaccharide-induced alteration of mitochondrial function in cultured hepatocytes and isolated perfused liver. Hepatology 18:380-388
69. Welsh N, Eizirik DL, Bendtzen K, Sandler S (1991) Interleukin-1b-induced nitric oxide production in isolated rat pancreatic islets requires gene transcription and may lead to inhibition of the Krebs cycle enzyme aconitase. Endocrinology 129:3167-3173
70. Szabó C, Ferrer-Sueta G, Zingarelli B, Southan GJ, Salzman AL, Radi R (1997) Mercaptoethylguanidine and related guanidine nitric oxide synthase inhibitors react with peroxynitrite and protect against peroxynitrite-induced oxidative damage. J Biol Chem 272: 9030-9036
71. Szabó C, Zingarelli B, Cuzzocrea S, Salzman AL (1997) Poly (ADP-ribose) synthetase modulates expression of P-selectin and ICAM-1 in myocardial ischemia-reperfusion injury. Jap J Pharmacol 75:101P (Abst)

72. Roebuck KA, Rahman A, Lakshminarayanan V, Janakidevi K, Malik AB (1995) H_2O_2 and tumor necrosis factor-alpha activate intercellular adhesion molecule 1 (ICAM-1) gene transcription through distinct cis-regulatory elements within the ICAM-1 promoter. J Biol Chem 270:18966–18974

73. Akabane A, Kato I, Takasawa S, et al (1995) Nicotinamide inhibits IRF-1 mRNA induction and prevents IL-1 beta-induced nitric oxide synthase expression in pancreatic beta cells. Biochem Biophys Res Commun 215:524–530

74. Martensson J, Jain A, Meister A (1990) Glutathione is required for intestinal function. Proc Natl Acad Sci USA 87:1715–1719

75. Schoenberg MH, Beger HG (1990) Oxygen radicals in intestinal ischemia and reperfusion. Chem Biol Inter 76:141–161

76. Qu Z, Fujimoto S, Taniguchi T (1994) Enhancement of interferon-g-induced major histocompatability complex class II gene expression by expressing an antisense RNA of poly-(ADP-ribose) synthetase. J Biol Chem 269:5543–5547

77. Wang ZQ, Auer B, Sting L, et al (1995) Mice lacking ADPRT and poly (ADP-ribosylation) develop normally but are susceptible to skin disease. Genes Dev 9:510–520

78. Eliasson MJL, Sampei K, Mandir AS, et al (1997) Poly(ADP-ribose)polymerase gene disruption renders mice resistant to cerebral ischemia. Nature Med 3:1089–1095

79. Takahashi K, Greenberg JH, Jackson P, Maclin K, Zhang J (1997) Neuroprotective effects of inhibiting poly(ADP-ribose) synthetase on focal cerebral ischemia in rats. J Cereb Blood Flow Metab 17:1137–1142

80. Bauer PI, Kirsten E, Young LJT, et al (1996) Modification of growth related enzymatic pathways and apparent loss of tumorigenicity of a ras-transformed bovine endothelial cell line by treatment with 5-iodo-6-amino-1,2-benzopyrone. Int J Oncol 8:239–252

81. Yamamoto K, Tsukidate K, Farber JL (1993) Differing effects of the inhibition of poly(ADP-ribose) polymerase on the course of exudative cell injury in hepatocytes and fibroblasts. Biochem Pharmacol 46:483–491

82. Porteous JW, Furneaux HM, Pearson CK, Lake CM, Morrison A (1979) Poly (adenosine diphosphate ribose) synthetase activity in nuclei of dividing and of non-dividing but differentiating intestinal epithelial cells. Biochem J 180:455–463

83. Reddy S, Salari-Lak N, Sandler S (1995) Long-term effects of nicotinamide-induced inhibition of poly(adenosine diphosphate-ribose) polymerase activity in rat pancreatic islets exposed to interleukin-1 beta. Endocrinology 136:1907–1912

84. Oikawa A, Tohda H, Kanai M, Miwa M, Sugimura T (1980) Inhibitors of poly(adenosine diphosphate ribose) polymerase induce sister chromatid exchanges. Biochem Biophys Res Commun 97:1311–1316

85. Nagele A (1995) Poly(ADP-ribosyl)ation as a fail-safe, transcription-independent, suicide mechanism in acutely DNA-damaged cells: a hypothesis. Radiat Environ Biophys 34:251–254

86. Cleaver JE, Park SD (1986) Enhanced ligation of repair sites under conditions of inhibition of poly(ADP-ribose) synthesis by 3-aminobenzamide. Mutat Res 173:287–290

87. Borek C, Morgan WF, Ong A, Cleaver JE (1984) Inhibition of malignant transformation in vitro by inhibitors of poly(ADP-ribose) synthesis. Proc Natl Acad Sci USA 81:243–247

88. Vladimirov VG, Krasiltnikov II, Volgarev AP, Platonov VG (1991) An experimental study of ADP-ribosylation inhibitors as anti-influenza agents. Vopr Virusol 36:293–295

89. Burkart V, Kolb H (1993) Protection of islet cells from inflammatory cell death in vitro. Clin Exp Immunol 93:273–278

90. Radons J, Heller B, Bürkle A, et al (1994) Nitric oxide toxicity in islet cells involves poly-(ADP-ribose) polymerase activation and concomitant NAD^+ depletion. Biochem Biophys Res Commun 199:1270–1277

91. Kallmann B, Burkhart V, Kröncke KD, Kolb-Bachofen V, Kolb H (1992) Toxicity of chemically generated nitric oxide towards pancreatic islet cells can be prevented by nicotinamide. Life Sciences 51:671–678

92. Szabó C, Saunders C, O'Connor M, Salzman AL (1996) Peroxynitrite causes energy depletion and increases permeability via activation of poly-ADP ribosyl synthetase in pulmonary epithelial cells. Am J Respir Mol Biol 60:105–109

93. Szabó C, Salzman AL, Ischiropoulos H (1995) Endotoxin triggers the expression of an inducible isoform of nitric oxide synthase and the formation of peroxynitrite in the rat aorta in vivo. FEBS Lett 363:235–238
94. Salzman AL, Wollert PS, Wang H, et al (1993) Intraluminal oxygenation ameliorates ischemia/reperfusion-induced gut mucosal hyperpermeability in pigs. Circ Shock 40:37–46
95. Granger DN, Rutili G, McCord JM (1981) Superoxide radicals in feline intestinal ischemia. Gastroenterology 81:22–23
96. Granger DN, Hollwarth ME, Parks DA (1986) Ischemia-reperfusion injury: role of oxygen-derived free radicals. Acta Physiol Scand 548:47–63
97. Kurose I, Wolf R, Grisham MB, Granger DN (1994) Modulation of ischemia/reperfusion-induced microvascular dysfunction by nitric oxide. Circ Res 74:376–382
98. Unno N, Wang H, Menconi MJ, et al (1997) Inhibition of inducible nitric oxide synthase ameliorates endotoxin-induced gut mucosal barrier dysfunction in rats. Gastroenterology 113:1246–1257
99. Grisham MB, Hernandez LA, Granger DN (1986) Xanthine oxidase and neutrophil infiltration in intestinal ischemia. Am J Physiol 251:G567–G574
100. Kubes P, Hunter J, Granger DN (1992) Ischemia/reperfusion-induced feline intestinal dysfunction: importance of granulocyte recruitment. Gastroenterology 103:807–812
101. Thiemermann C, Bowes J, Myint FP, Vane JR (1997) Inhibition of the activity of poly(ADP ribose) synthase reduces ischemia-reperfusion injury in the heart and skeletal muscle. Proc Natl Acad Sci USA 94:679–683

Cellular Responses to Hypoxia: Possible Relevance to Multiple Organ Failure in Critical Illness?

P. T. Schumacker and N. S. Chandel

Introduction

Clinically, tissue hypoxia can be defined as a condition arising when some cells do not receive sufficient oxygen (O_2) to meet their metabolic needs. Critically ill patients are constantly at risk of sustaining hypoxic tissue injury as a result of lung gas exchange failure, tissue hypoperfusion, or dysfunction of the microcirculatory system responsible for regulating O_2 delivery (DO_2) in accordance with local oxygen demands. Accordingly, much attention in critical care is focused on assessing the adequacy of tissue DO_2 and on maintaining adequate levels of O_2 delivery in patients with organ system failure.

Studies of isolated cells have shown that O_2 uptake (VO_2) does not become limited by O_2 availability until the local O_2 tension (PO_2) falls to nearly anoxic levels. When the extracellular PO_2 is decreased to values of less than ~ 5 torr, the gradient for O_2 diffusion between the cell membrane and the mitochondria becomes insufficient to support mitochondrial respiration, which becomes limited by the extracellular PO_2 [1]. Many studies have examined the sequence of events that occur when the DO_2 to tissues is halted during ischemia, both at the cellular level and at the level of intact tissues. Of course, an important difference between ischemia and anoxia is the accumulation of lactate, carbon dioxide (CO_2), potassium (K^+) and other tissue metabolic products in the former, which may modify the response to the anoxia that develops. The physiological mechanisms of ischemic tissue injury have been studied extensively, and many excellent reviews are available [2]. The purpose of this chapter is rather to focus on recent laboratory investigation that has examined the cellular responses to more moderate degrees of hypoxia. Emerging new evidence suggests that many cells can detect and respond to changes in PO_2 within the physiological range, defined as PO_2 values between 5 and 50 torr. We refer to this as cellular hypoxia, although it is important to note that cells have more than enough O_2 to sustain metabolic activity in this range. Moreover, many cells in intact tissues normally function in this PO_2 range, so it is probably incorrect to think of it as pathophysiologic. Nevertheless, a better understanding of how cells detect and respond to hypoxia may yield insight into the mechanisms of cell injury that develop during anoxia or ischemia, which may be useful in developing strategies to protect cells from the consequences of these events. Recent laboratory studies are beginning to reveal that cells can both detect and respond to moderate hypoxia by adjusting their energy utilization, gene expression, and other cell processes. These responses may help to protect both the cells themselves and the organism as a whole if faced with more severe or prolonged O_2 deprivation.

Attempting to draw conclusions about organ function in critically ill patients based on studies of cultured cells is naive at best, and potentially dangerous at its worst. Nevertheless, it is interesting to speculate about the possible relationship between the events in hypoxic tissue and those seen in studies of different types of cells under controlled O_2 conditions. Undoubtedly, a clear understanding of how cells in intact tissues behave during moderate hypoxia will have to await more careful studies in the future.

Background

Production of ATP via Aerobic and Anaerobic Sources

Biochemically, cells use O_2 in a variety of different reactions. However, the most critical of these involves the generation of adenosine triphosphate (ATP) during aerobic respiration. Most of the ATP used by the cell is produced by mitochondrial electron transfer-linked phosphorylation, which accounts for more than 90% of the O_2 utilized by the cell. All mammalian cells have the ability to generate ATP in the absence of O_2, through the process of substrate-level phosphorylation. However, it is well known that this process yields only 2 moles of ATP per mole of glucose consumed, as opposed to 38 moles when oxidized fully via glycolysis followed by mitochondrial respiration. Moreover, because approximately 18 times as much glucose is used to generate ATP anaerobically as is used for aerobic respiration, few cells have sufficient carbohydrate stores to sustain anaerobic glycolysis for prolonged periods without becoming depleted of this valuable substrate. Although it might seem that normal rates of ATP generation could be maintained for a short time by anaerobic glycolysis, few cells normally express sufficient levels of glycolytic enzymes required to achieve glycolytic fluxes that could supply ATP at rates needed to sustain normal resting metabolic activities. At best, substrate level phosphorylation can supply only a fraction of the ATP that cells require to sustain normal resting activities. Consequently, when aerobic respiration is limited by a lack of O_2, the rate of ATP utilization by the cell must decrease. Finally, it is well known that anaerobic metabolism of glucose yields two molecules of lactate, which contributes to the generation of a metabolic acidosis. In many cells this acidosis inhibits glycolytic flux by inhibiting the activity of certain glycolytic enzymes, further limiting the ability of cells to generate ATP in the absence of O_2.

Mitochondrial Function

Normally, the rate of electron transport (and thus the rate of O_2 uptake) is tightly coupled to the rate of ATP utilization by the cell. Mitochondria produce ATP by oxidizing substrates and transferring the reducing equivalents through a series of carriers with successively increasing affinities for electrons [3, 4]. At several of these steps, sufficient free energy is released to drive ion pumps that expel protons from the inner mitochondrial matrix. The last of these steps involves cytochrome aa_3, also known as cytochrome c oxidase, the terminal enzyme of the mitochondrial electron transport system [5]. This enzyme binds O_2 with high affinity and transfers four electrons, eventually generating water. Cytochrome aa_3 represents the last of three electron transport sites where proton pumping occurs, thus contributing to the generation of an electrochemical gradient for H^+ across the inner mitochondrial membrane [6]. Proton pumping also occurs at the nicotinamide adenine dinucleotide (NADH) dehydrogenase and at the b-c_1 complex. The resulting electrochemical potential ($\Delta\psi$) is comprised of a pH gradient (ΔpH, typically about 1 pH unit) and a voltage gradient (ΔV, typically about 140 mV). Another enzyme complex in the inner membrane called the F_0F_1-ATP synthase uses the free energy stored in that electrochemical gradient to generate ATP from adenosine diphosphate (ADP) + inorganic phosphate (Pi). Analogous to a turbine, the ATP synthase allows protons to move down their electrochemical gradient, entering the mitochondrial matrix and tending to dissipate the potential. The free energy released in this process is used to drive the synthase, generating ATP in the process.

Many factors can influence the rate of mitochondrial electron transport and O_2 consumption in a cell, but the most important regulator in many cell types is the availability of ADP + Pi [7]. As ATP is utilized for cellular processes, ADP + Pi returned to the mitochondria provide substrates for the ATP synthase. When ATP utilization by the cell decreases, the decrease in return of ADP + Pi to the mitochondria limits the activity of the ATP synthase [3]. When the ATP synthase activity decreases, the mitochondrial transmembrane potential ($\Delta\psi$) tends to increase. This tends to reduce electron transport because the greater electrochemical gradient across the inner mitochondrial membrane tends to hinder proton pumping, which is linked to electron transport. Other factors, including availability of substrates and the mitochondrial ionized calcium concentration can also influence mitochondrial respiration. Finally, some of the mitochondrial $\Delta\psi$ is used to pump substrates or ions into the mitochondrial matrix. For example, Ca^{2+} pumps in the inner mitochondrial membrane rely on the electrochemical gradient to sequester Ca^{2+} ions from the cytosol. This can be shown experimentally by incubating intact isolated mitochondria in buffered solutions containing high Ca^{2+} concentrations. Those mitochondria virtually abolish their synthesis of ATP, diverting most of their $\Delta\psi$ to Ca^{2+} pumping. However, under normal conditions in intact cells there is little doubt that the availability of ADP and Pi represent major elements regulating the rate of mitochondrial respiration [6]. Because this is determined by the rate of ATP utilization, cell respiration is tightly coupled to the rate of ATP utilization.

The high binding affinity of cytochrome aa_3 for O_2, allows mitochondria to sustain normal levels of respiration (and ATP synthesis) until the availability of O_2 falls to very low levels. Based on measurements with the purified enzyme [8], VO_2 should not decrease until mitochondrial PO_2 falls below 1 torr. Indeed, studies of respiration in intact cells and in isolated mitochondria have shown this to be the case. If O_2 does fall to respiration-limiting levels, the rate of electron transport becomes limited by the availability of O_2 and cellular respiration decreases. In that situation the mitochondrial potential is liable to decrease because the rate of proton extrusion decreases [9, 10]. Dissipation of the mitochondrial potential is dangerous because it may lead to the opening of the mitochondrial permeability transition (MPT) pore [11], which leads to the release of calcium ions from mitochondria to the cytosol, mitochondrial swelling, and ultimately can lead to cell death. To delay this event, some cells are capable of sustaining mitochondrial potential by using ATP to drive the ATP synthase in reverse. Obviously, mitochondrial ATP synthase cannot function in both directions at the same time. Therefore, the cell must either be generating by using the potential, or maintaining the potential at the expense of glycolysis-derived ATP. Because the ability of the cell to generate ATP anaerobically is limited, cells can only protect mitochondrial potential for a short time by this mechanism.

One can look at the mitochondrial potential as representing a balance between the rate of electron transport and the rate of ATP synthesis [12]. Factors that increase electron transport tend to augment the potential by augmenting proton extrusion, while factors such as ATP synthesis tend to dissipate the potential by allowing the entry of protons down their electrochemical gradient. The relationship between the rate of electron transport and the rate of ATP synthesis is reflected in the coupling ratio for the mitochondria. Mitochondrial uncoupling agents often act as protonophores in the inner mitochondrial membrane, allowing protons to leak into the mitochondria and thereby shunting them past the ATP synthase. Consequently, electron transport proceeds and respiration occurs, but ATP generation can be abolished if the electrochemical gradient is sufficiently dissipated.

Mitochondrial PO_2

When given excess metabolic substrates, respiration by isolated mitochondria has been shown to remain independent of PO_2 until the PO_2 falls below 1–2 torr [13, 14]. Presumably, the lower critical O_2 concentration for isolated mitochondrial, as opposed to intact cell respiration relates to the diffusion resistance offered by the cell membrane and cytosol [15]. When these are removed in preparing mitochondrial suspensions, the PO_2 at cytochrome oxidase remains closer to the PO_2 in the solution. Indeed, when cytochrome oxidase is isolated from mitochondria and studied in solution, critical PO_2 values of less than 1 torr are frequently seen.

While some investigators have argued that mitochondria typically function at PO_2 values in the range of 1–2 torr, this is not normally the case. The following analysis should demonstrate why mitochondrial PO_2 is normally within a few torr of the extracellular PO_2 (Fig. 1). Consider a suspension of isolated cells in a stirred solution where the PO_2 is maintained at a constant level, say, 100 torr. If the mitochondrial PO_2 were 1 torr, then the O_2 flux into the cell (VO_2) would be

Fig. 1. Schematic diagram illustrating O_2 transport from the cell membrane to the mitochondrion. Diffusive O_2 transport (VO_2) occurs because a small PO_2 difference exists between the extracellular space and the mitochondrion (ΔPO_2). Above a critically low extracellular PO_2, changes in the extracellular PO_2 are matched by identical changes in mitochondrial PO_2

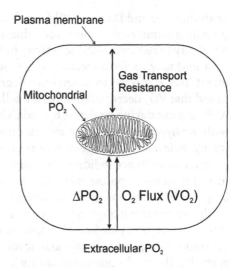

determined as the ratio of the driving gradient for O_2 diffusion (the difference between extracellular PO_2 and mitochondrial PO_2, or 99 torr in this example) and the diffusive transport resistance between the cell surface and the mitochondria. If the extracellular PO_2 were then reduced to 50 torr and mitochondrial PO_2 remained at 1 torr, the VO_2 of the cell would have to decrease because the driving gradient for diffusion would decrease ($50 - 1 = 49$ torr) while the diffusive transport resistance would not change. Yet in experiments where cell VO_2 has been measured as the extracellular PO_2 decreases, it has been shown that cellular VO_2 remains constant until the PO_2 reaches a value in the range of 3–7 torr. Assuming that the resistance to diffusion between the cell surface and the mitochondria does not change as a function of O_2 concentration, the observation that VO_2 is independent of PO_2 above ~ 5 torr would mean that the difference between mitochondrial and extracellular PO_2 must remain constant as the extracellular PO_2 fluctuates, above the critical PO_2 of 5 torr. In other words, mitochondrial PO_2 must remain within a few torr of extracellular PO_2 under physiologic conditions.

Down-regulation of Cellular Metabolism During Moderate Hypoxia

Intact Tissues

Many previous studies have evaluated the relationship between DO_2 and VO_2 in intact tissues. These studies have shown that VO_2 remains constant as the DO_2 is reduced, until a critical DO_2 is reached [16]. An assumption of those studies is that O_2 demand remains constant as the DO_2 changes. However, there is evidence that some tissues may have the ability to reduce metabolic activity in states where the DO_2 is reduced, possibly resulting in a correction in the DO_2 to VO_2 ratio. In intact porcine myocardium, Arai et al. [17] and Pantley et al. [18] found evidence of metabolic suppression when epicardial blood flow was reduced by 50%. In other studies, Lee and Downey [19] found evidence of metabolic suppression in iso-prenaline-stimulated canine myocardium during partial reduction of blood flow. An ability to reduce metabolic activity in the face of decreasing DO_2 (hypoxic adaptation) may confer protection in the face of more severe hypoxic challenge. In intact liver subjected to progressive decreases in blood flow, Dishart et al. [20] found that VO_2 decreased before ATP fell, which was suggestive of a decrease in ATP demand during moderate hypoxia. Collectively, these findings are consistent with the hypothesis that mammalian cells may decrease metabolic demand during hypoxia, although the evidence is indirect.

Stronger evidence indicates that some lower vertebrate species have an ability to dramatically suppress metabolic activity, thereby allowing them to survive long exposures to anoxic environments [21]. For example, the Western painted turtle can survive being kept under near anoxic conditions for many weeks at a time [22]. Hepatocytes from that species can maintain normal cellular ATP concentrations despite being kept anoxic for more than 24 hrs. Recent evidence suggests that these cells possess an ability to significantly suppress protein synthesis [23], membrane ion channel conductivity [24, 25] and ATP demand during extreme hypoxia [26]. This allows cells to maintain ATP levels via anaerobic glycolysis, which is adequate by virtue of the low rate of ATP utilization. Not surprisingly, these cells die rapidly under anoxic conditions if 2-deoxyglucose is administered to block glycolytic activity. Clearly, mammalian cells are not capable of surviving days or weeks of anoxia because they do not possess mechanisms that allow them to virtually abolish ATP demand. However, increasing evidence suggests that many species do have an ability to partially suppress ATP demand when the DO_2 is reduced, and can activate this response when the level of hypoxia is relatively moderate.

Isolated Cells

Recent studies have begun to identify cellular mechanisms in higher organisms that allow cells to reduce their O_2 demands in states where DO_2 is moderately, but not critically reduced [27]. Classical studies dating from the 1920's have shown that cellular VO_2 remains independent of O_2 concentration until the cellular PO_2 falls below a critical value in the range of 4–7 torr [1, 28, 29]. However, a common feature among many of those studies was the short duration of hypoxia, which may have prevented the development of an adaptive response in the cells.

Using primary cultures of hepatocytes in suspension, we examined the effects of more prolonged, moderate hypoxia on cellular O_2 demand [27, 30]. Cells were seeded at low density (10^7 cells/250 ml media) into spinner flasks equipped with polarographic O_2 electrodes allowing measurement of the PO_2 in the solution. O_2 was supplied by gassing the head space above the liquid. As shown in Figure 2, cells maintained under normoxic conditions ($PO_2 > 100$ torr) showed no significant change in O_2 uptake over 14 hrs. When the PO_2 was then lowered to ~20 torr, O_2 uptake decreased by approximately 50% within several hours, without any loss of cell viability. These reduced respiratory rates were maintained for the

Fig. 2. Effects of prolonged moderate hypoxia on O_2 consumption by rat hepatocytes in suspension culture. Cells in the normoxic flask were kept at $PO_2 \sim 120$ torr throughout; whereas PO_2 was reduced from 120 to ~ 20 torr in the hypoxic flask at t = 14 hrs, and returned to 120 torr at t = 38 hrs. O_2 uptake was measured at the study PO_2 in aliquots obtained anaerobically from the flask. (From [27] with permission)

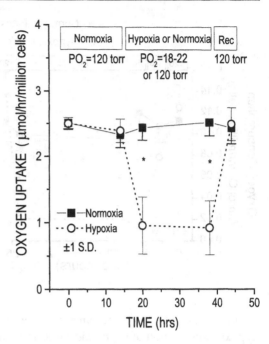

duration of hypoxia. When the PO_2 of the hypoxic flask was restored to the level of the control flask, cellular VO_2 returned to baseline levels within a few minutes. Both the normoxic and the hypoxic cells released lactate into the media, although hypoxic cell release was slightly greater than from normoxic controls. However, the calculated rate of ATP utilization (based on aerobic plus anaerobic sources) revealed that ATP utilization had decreased by $\sim 50\%$ in the hypoxic group. Thus, these findings reveal a true decrease in the demand for ATP, rather than a shift from aerobic to anaerobic sources. Collectively, these results indicate that hepatocytes can undergo reversible decreases in respiration during hypoxia that are non-lethal and reversible after the PO_2 is restored.

Is this response only seen in mammalian hepatocytes? The answer to this question appears to be no. Figure 3 shows the effect of a similar level of hypoxia on the respiratory rates of embryonic chick cardiomyocytes studied in suspension culture [31]. When the PO_2 of the media was decreased, these cardiomyocytes underwent a reversible decrease in respiration, which was evident within 10 minutes. This state of inhibition was maintained for the duration of hypoxia, and was rapidly reversible when normoxic conditions were restored. As with the hepatocytes, these responses occurred at PO_2 values well above "critical PO_2" values where O_2 availability begins to limit respiration.

Cultured cardiomyocytes grown on glass cover slips exhibit spontaneous contractions after 2–3 days in culture, and can be used to study the utilization of ATP for contraction. Contracting cells can be placed in a flow-through chamber, permitting the study of contraction under controlled O_2 conditions. Figure 4 shows the effect of prolonged moderate hypoxia on spontaneous contraction in these cells [32]. Consistent with their decrease in VO_2, contractile motion (calculated as

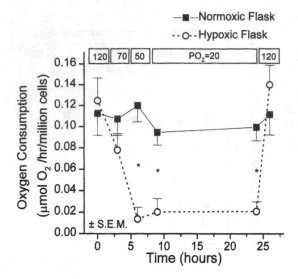

Fig. 3. Effects of prolonged moderate hypoxia on O_2 consumption by embryonic chick cardiomyocytes in suspension culture. Cells in the normoxic flask were kept at PO_2 ~ 120 torr throughout; whereas PO_2 was reduced from 120 to 70, 50 and 20 torr in the hypoxic flask, and returned to 120 torr at $t = 24$ hrs. O_2 uptake was measured at the study PO_2 in aliquots obtained anaerobically from the flask. (From [31] with permission)

the product of rate × contraction amplitude) was decreased in these cells during hypoxia. Restoration of normoxic conditions was associated with a slow but progressive return of contractile motion, without loss of cell viability. Combined with the hepatocyte data, these studies suggest that many diverse cell types have the ability to reduce ATP demand during moderate hypoxia, resulting in a decrease in O_2 demand by the cells. ATP production appears to remain well-matched to ATP demand, which is consistent with the conclusion that this is an adaptive, rather than a pathophysiologic response.

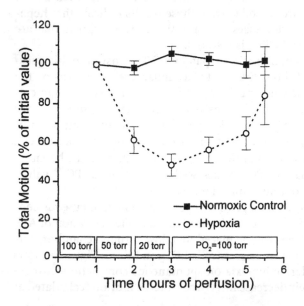

Fig. 4. Effects of moderate hypoxia on spontaneous contractile motion of cultured embryonic chick cardiomyocytes on glass cover slips. Cell motion was quantified as the product of rate and magnitude of deflection. Hypoxia ($PO_2 = 50$ or 20 torr) produced reversible suppression of contractile motion that recovered after normoxia was restored ($PO_2 = $ 100 torr). (Data from [32])

Cellular Oxygen Sensing During Hypoxia

How do Mitochondria Sense Hypoxia?

The cellular responses described above were seen at moderate levels of hypoxia, where the cell PO_2 was significantly higher than the critical level needed to support normal levels of respiration. Indeed, hepatocytes exposed to moderate levels of hypoxia continued to function at normal levels of VO_2 for 2–3 hours, indicating that lack of O_2 was not the cause of the decrease in respiration. Moreover, the use of isolated cells in stirred suspensions or of monolayers superfused with media under controlled O_2 conditions precludes the possibility that significant gradients in O_2 could have existed between the cells and the perfusate. Therefore, these responses to hypoxia imply the existence of a cellular O_2 sensor capable of detecting the changes in PO_2 and activating the cellular response (e.g., a decrease in ATP utilization).

Many putative mechanisms of cellular O_2 sensing have been identified in vertebrate species, but experimental studies linking these potential mechanisms to the functional responses in cells are incomplete. An increasing body of data suggests that mitochondria may act as the O_2 sensor mediating the decrease in respiration seen during moderate hypoxia. For years, mitochondria have been listed among the potential sites of O_2 sensing [33], based on the fact that they are responsible for the majority of the O_2 consumed by the cell. Moreover, they contain the O_2-binding enzyme cytochrome aa_3, which functions as the terminal respiratory complex in the electron transport chain. However, the binding affinity of cytochrome aa_3 for O_2 is high, such that the rate of electron transport does not begin to become limited by O_2 availability until the PO_2 falls to less than 1 torr. If the electron transport system is not affected until the cell is virtually anoxic, how could this system functionally detect changes in O_2 within the physiological range of PO_2? This perplexing question has led many investigators to dismiss mitochondria as a potential site of O_2 sensing.

More recent evidence has begun to re-examine the possibility that mitochondria may function as cellular O_2 sensors. To understand how this could occur, it is necessary to consider several studies of mitochondrial function during hypoxia. As described above, the rate of electron transport (and thus the rate of VO_2) is tightly coupled to the rate of ATP utilization by the cell [34]. In most cells, respiration under resting conditions is less than 20% of the maximal rate; therefore, cytochrome aa_3 functions at a fraction of its maximal capacity (Vmax). Experimentally, it is possible to study the maximal capacity of cytochrome aa_3 by measuring the respiration rate of the cell when the compound TMPD (N,N,N′,N′-tetramethyl-p-phenylenediamine, a non-enzymatic reductant for cytochrome c) is used to supply electrons directly to cytochrome c. Recall that cytochrome c is the electron carrier protein that supplies electrons to cytochrome aa_3. Under basal conditions less than 20% of the pool of cytochrome c is reduced. Consequently, a cytochrome c molecule that binds to cytochrome aa_3 has only a 20% chance of being reduced, and therefore able to transfer an electron. The reducing agent TMPD can enter the cell and donate electrons directly to cytochrome c. At sufficiently high concentrations, TMPD can fully reduce the pool of cytochrome c. In that case, an electron can be transferred every time cytochrome c binds to aa_3 and the respiratory rate of the cell increases to a maximal rate. Under those conditions, the respiratory rate of the cell increases by 5–7 fold and reflects the Vmax of cytochrome oxidase. In this assay, a mitochondrial uncoupling agent such as FCCP normally would also be administered to dissipate the mitochondrial potential, to allow a maximal rate of respiration to be attained. Also, ascorbate is added to keep the TMPD in a reduced state. Otherwise, progressive oxidation of TMPD would occur.

According to classical mitochondrial studies, the maximal rate of cytochrome aa_3 activity should remain independent of PO_2 until a very low O_2 concentration is reached. However, respiration by cultured cardiomyocytes incubated with TMPD was found to be PO_2-dependent below an O_2 tension of ~50 torr (Fig. 5) [31]. These results suggest that the Vmax of cytochrome oxidase is O_2-dependent in these cells at PO_2 values within the physiologic range. To test this possibility more explicitly, Chandel et al. [8] studied the activity of isolated bovine heart cytochrome aa_3 in buffered solutions. The enzyme was incubated in stirred solutions at 25 °C at different PO_2 values for 4 hrs. Aliquots were then transferred to a respirometer where the activity (Vmax) of the oxidase was studied under different PO_2 conditions by adding excess substrate and measuring the rate of O_2 consumption. As expected, cytochrome aa_3 assayed at PO_2 values > 50 torr exhibited a normal Vmax, regardless of the incubation PO_2. However, the Vmax of cytochrome aa_3 measured at PO_2 values < 40 torr was decreased by ~50% in enzyme that had been incubated at PO_2 levels of < 40 torr for 2–4 hrs. Collectively, these studies show that the Vmax of the oxidase decreases reversibly when the mitochondria have been exposed to physiological hypoxia. While many different cell types from different organisms show a similar response, it now appears that some cell types require a longer exposure to low PO_2, while other cell types exhibit a decreased Vmax within minutes after exposure to hypoxia. For example, hepatocytes began to decrease VO_2 after 2–3 hrs of hypoxia, whereas cultured cardiomyocytes decreased respiration much more quickly. In all cells studied to date, increasing the extracellular PO_2 to > 50 torr is associated with a rapid and complete restoration of Vmax.

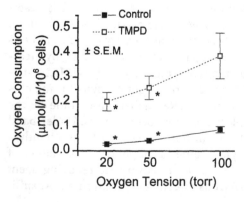

Fig. 5. Comparison of basal respiration (Control) and cytochrome oxidase maximal activity (TMPD respiration) in embryonic cardiomyocytes. TMPD respiration decreases as a function of PO_2 at 50 and 20 torr, indicating the Vmax of the oxidase becomes PO_2-dependent during moderate hypoxia. This characteristic allows mitochondria to function as O_2 sensors. (From [31] with permission)

How do changes in the Vmax of cytochrome oxidase allow the mitochondria to function as O_2 sensors? As stated above, respiration normally operates at a fraction of the maximum capacity of the cell. Therefore, a 50% decrease in the Vmax of the oxidase does not limit or reduce basal respiration. However, to maintain its normal rate of VO_2 in the face of a decrease in Vmax of cytochrome aa_3, the redox state of the electron carriers upstream from the oxidase must shift to a more reduced state. Indeed, the concentration of NAD(P)H was found to increase in hepatocytes after 2–3 hrs at $PO_2 = 20$ torr [27, 32]. This change in mitochondrial redox may then initiate an intracellular signaling cascade culminating in the partial inhibition of cellular metabolic processes requiring ATP. A partial inhibition of ATP utilization would reduce ATP utilization and thereby reduce cellular respiration by limiting the supply of ADP to the mitochondria. In this respect, the mitochondria would function as regulators of cell metabolic activity in response to hypoxia.

What Signals do Mitochondria Generate During Hypoxia?

Newly reported evidence suggests that mitochondria increase their generation of reactive oxygen species (ROS) during moderate hypoxia. While it may seem paradoxical that ROS production should increase when the PO_2 at the mitochondria is decreased, it is important to remember that ROS production is a function of mitochondrial redox as well as the availability of O_2. For many years it has been known that mitochondria can generate superoxide anions by transfer of single electrons from ubisemiquinone to O_2 [35]. Subsequent dismutation of superoxide by superoxide dismutase (SOD) leads to the generation of hydrogen peroxide (H_2O_2) in cells. Factors that increase mitochondrial reduction (e.g., the mitochondrial inhibitor antimycin A), tend to prolong the lifetime of ubisemiquinone, thereby augmenting the production of superoxide. By contrast, inhibitors that block electron flow contributing to the formation of ubisemiquinone (e.g., the compound rotenone) tend to attenuate ROS formation. In experimental studies where mitochondrial redox was increased during simulated ischemia, ROS production was dramatically increased despite PO_2 values in the range of 2–4 torr [36]. If hypoxia decreases the Vmax of cytochrome oxidase, then ROI signaling should increase during hypoxia due to the increase in mitochondrial redox that would occur.

To test this hypothesis, Duranteau et al. [37] measured ROS formation in cultured cardiomyocytes using the dye 2,7-dichlorofluorescin diacetate (DCFH-DA). This non-fluorescent dye enters the cells, where the acetate groups are cleaved by cytosolic esterases. This traps the reduced, nonfluorescent compound (DCFH) in the cell. Intracellular ROS, especially peroxides, can oxidize DCFH, forming the fluorescent compound 2,7-dichlorofluorescein (DCF) which can be measured. Quantitative fluorescence microscopy can thereby be used to assess ROS generation.

Figure 6 shows a plot of DCF fluorescence in cardiomyocytes when the extracellular PO_2 was decreased from ~ 107 torr to different levels of hypoxia. Within

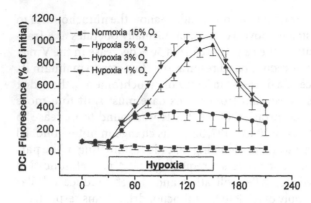

Fig. 6. Effects of moderate hypoxia on DCFH fluorescence in contracting cardiomyocytes. Baseline normoxic measurements were made during 15% O_2; hypoxia was initiated at t = 30 min and normoxia was restored at t = 150 min. Progressive increases in DCFH signals are indicative of increased ROS generation, probably hydrogen peroxide. (From [37] with permission)

< 30 min, significant increases in ROS generation were detected, which decreased when the PO_2 was subsequently returned to $PO_2 > 100$ torr. Other experiments showed that these changes in DCFH oxidation could be attenuated by administering the mitochondrial inhibitors rotenone and TTFA, indicating that these ROS originated from the mitochondrial electron transport chain. Moreover, a PO_2-dependence of ROS generation was noted, with progressively greater ROS signals observed as the O_2 was reduced from 5% O_2 to 1% O_2. The paradoxical increase in ROS generation at lower PO_2 appears to be due to the change in cytochrome aa_3 redox state as a consequence of its change in Vmax during hypoxia. In this manner, cytochrome oxidase appears to function as an O_2 sensor, which signals a reduction in PO_2 via changes in mitochondrial redox and subsequent ROS generation.

Are the ROS Generated During Hypoxia Involved in the Cellular Response to Hypoxia?

If increases in ROS generated during hypoxia participate in the intracellular signaling responsible for the down-regulation of energy demand, then it should be possible to alter the functional response of the cell to hypoxia by intervening in the ROS signaling pathway. In studies recently published [32], addition of the thiol-reducing agent 2-mercaptopropionyl glycine, completely abolished the decrease in contractile motion seen during hypoxia (2% O_2) in cardiomyocytes. Presumably this agent enhances the scavenging of H_2O_2 by maintaining the cellular pool of reduced glutathione, a substrate needed by glutathione peroxidase. This finding suggests that H_2O_2 is involved in the signaling sequence linking the O_2 sensor (mitochondria) with the functional response (contraction). Similarly, addition of exogenous H_2O_2 during normoxia mimicked the effect of hypoxia by eliciting a progressive decrease in contractile motion, which was fully reversible after its washout [32]. Indeed, the time course of inhibition and recovery were very similar.

In summary, increasing evidence suggests that mitochondria may function as cellular O_2 sensors responsive to changes in PO_2 within the physiological range.

It is conceivable that cytochrome oxidase may mediate this transduction process by adjusting its activity in response to lowered PO_2, eliciting an increase in mitochondrial reduction which results in an increase in ROS generation. Although high levels of ROS generated by mitochondria may potentially damage the cell via oxidation of lipids, proteins and desoxyribonucleic acid (DNA), these low levels of ROS appear to function as signaling elements linking the O_2 sensor to the functional response. Future studies will be required to determine whether this transduction process is involved in other cellular responses to hypoxia. For example, it is possible that a similar process may be involved in the activation of gene transcription responsible for vascular endothelial growth factor (VEGF) which promotes the development of new blood vessels in hypoxic tissues, activation of the expression of glycolytic enzymes which would augment glycolytic capacity, or expression of erythropoietin which stimulates the formation and maturation of red blood cells. More work will be required to fully establish the significance of mitochondria as O_2 sensors in normal tissues and in pathophysiologic states.

Possible Relevance to Organ System Failure

In a simplistic sense it is possible to classify cellular ATP utilization into two categories; those functions necessary for survival of the cell, and those functions that contribute to the function provided by the intact tissue. Examples of the former might include the maintenance of electrochemical gradients, repair of oxidant damage, and replacement or repair of effete enzymes. Without these essential functions, cell survival would be immediately threatened. Although a deterioration of organ system functions such as contraction, maintenance of endothelial or epithelial barrier function, or secretion of neurotransmitters, hormones or signaling substances would eventually threaten the survival of the organism, these functions are not essential for the individual cells contributing to the overall function. An ability of cells to selectively inhibit non-essential functions when hypoxia threatens to limit ATP production might be protective, and could allow the cells to survive a more extended or more severe decrease in O_2 availability.

In critically ill patients, organ system failure often involves a partial inhibition of ATP-dependent processes related to cell function, rather than a failure due to massive loss of cell viability. Of course it is possible that some apoptosis may occur in organ failure, but the ability to recover organ function in those patients surviving organ failure suggests that the problem represents an impairment of integrated cell function rather than viability. It is interesting to speculate that a relationship may exist between the suppression of cellular function seen during hypoxia in laboratory studies and the failure of cells in intact tissues during organ system failure. Inflammatory mediators or cell hypoxia in malperfused tissues may contribute to the suppression of tissue function, through activation of signaling pathways describe above. However, further work is required to test this possibility.

Conclusion

Although classical studies have shown that cells maintain normal rates of respiration during brief periods of hypoxia until critically low O_2 concentrations are reached, more recent data indicates that cells have the ability to suppress ATP demand and mitochondrial respiration during more prolonged periods of moderate hypoxia. The data suggest that cells detect physiological levels of hypoxia via an O_2 sensing mechanism that involves mitochondria. Alterations in mitochondrial redox during hypoxia result in the generation of ROS by mitochondria, which appear to activate subsequent signal transduction steps resulting in the inhibition of ATP demand. This response can be inhibited by agents that augment the scavenging of H_2O_2 during hypoxia, or mimicked during normoxia by administering agents that augment ROS production in cells. The resulting inhibition of cell function and metabolic demand appears limited to non-essential cell functions related to organ system function. The possible activation and involvement of such a mechanism during organ system failure is interesting, but will require further work to establish.

References

1. Jones DP, Kennedy FG (1982) Intracellular oxygen supply during hypoxia. Am J Physiol 243: C247–C253
2. Granger DN, Korthuis RJ (1995) Physiologic mechanisms of postischemic tissue injury. Annu Rev Physiol 57:311–332
3. Brown GC (1992) Control of respiration and ATP synthesis in mammalian mitochondria and cells. Biochem J 284:1–13
4. Balaban RS (1990) Regulation of oxidative phosphorylation in the mammalian cell. Am J Physiol 258:C377–C389
5. Cooper CE (1990) The steady-state kinetics of cytochrome c oxidation by cytochrome oxidase. Biochim Biophys Act 1017:187–203
6. Jones DP, Shan X, Park Y (1992) Coordinated multisite regulation of cellular energy metabolism. Annu Rev Nutr 12:327–343
7. Kadenbach B, Barth J, Akgun R, Freund R, Linder D, Possekel S (1995) Regulation of mitochondrial energy generation in health and disease. Biochim Biophys Act 1271:103–109
8. Chandel NS, Budinger GRS, Schumacker PT (1996) Molecular oxygen modulates cytochrome c oxidase function. J Biol Chem 271:18672–18677
9. Andersson BS, Aw TY, Jones DP (1987) Mitochondrial transmembrane potential and pH gradient during anoxia. Am J Physiol 252:C349–C355
10. Aw TY, Andersson BS, Jones DP (1987) Mitochondrial transmembrane ion distribution during anoxia. J Appl Physiol 252:C356–C361
11. Griffiths EJ, Halestrap AP (1995) Mitochondrial non-specific pores remain closed during cardiac ischaemia, but open upon reperfusion. Biochem J 307:93–98
12. DiLisa F, Blank PS, Colonna R, Gambassi G, Silverman HS, Stern MD, Hansford RG (1995) Mitochondrial membrane potential in single living adult rat cardiac myocytes exposed to anoxia or metabolic inhibition. J Physiol 486:1–13
13. Rumsey WL, Schlosser C, Nuutinen EM, Robiolio M, Wilson DF (1990) Cellular energetics and the oxygen dependence of respiration in cardiac myocytes isolated from adult rat. J Biol Chem 265:15392–15399
14. Wilson DF, Erecinska M, Drown C, Silver IA (1979) The oxygen dependence of cellular energy metabolism. Arch Biochem Biophys 195:485–493

15. Jones DP, Mason HS (1978) Gradients of oxygen concentration in hepatocytes. J Biol Chem 253:4874-4880
16. Schumacker PT, Cain SM (1987) The concept of a critical oxygen delivery. Intensive Care Med 13:223-229
17. Arai AE, Pantely GA, Anselone CG, Bristow J, Bristow JD (1991) Active downregulation of myocardial energy requirements during prolonged moderate ischemia in swine. Circ Res 69:1458-1469
18. Pantley GA, Malone SA, Rhen WS, Anselone CG, Arai A, Bristow J, Bristow JD (1990) Regeneration of myocardial phosphocreatine in pigs despite continued moderate ischemia. Circ Res 67:1481-1493
19. Lee S-C, Downey HF (1993) Downregulation of oxygen demand in isoprenaline stimulated canine myocardium. Cardiovasc Res 27:1542-1550
20. Dishart MK, Schlichtig R, Tonnessen TI, Rozenfield RA, Simplaceanu E, Williams D, Gayowski TJP (1998) Mitochondrial redox state as a potential detector of liver dysoxia in vivo. J Appl Physiol 84:791-797
21. Buck LT, Land SC, Hochachka PW (1993) Anoxia-tolerant hepatocytes: model system for study of reversible metabolic suppression. Am J Physiol 265:R49-R56
22. Ultsch GR, Jackson DC (1982) Long-term submergence at 3°C of the turtle Chrysemys picta bellii, in normoxic and severely hypoxic water. i. Survival, gas exchange and acid-base status. J Exp Biol 96:11-28
23. Land SC, Buck LT, Hochachka PW (1993) Response of protein synthesis to anoxia and recovery in anoxia-tolerant hepatocytes. Am J Physiol 265:R41-R48
24. Perez-Pinzon MA, Rosenthal M, Sick TJ, Lutz PL, Pablo J, Mash D (1992) Downregulation of sodium channels during anoxia: a putative survival strategy of turtle brain. Am J Physiol 262:R712-R715
25. Perez-Pinzon MA, Chan CY, Rosenthal M, Sick T (1992) Membrane and synaptic activity during anoxia in the isolated turtle cerebellum. Am J Physiol 263:R1057-R1063
26. Buck LT, Hochachka PW, Schon A, Gnaiger E (1993) Microcalorimetric measurement of reversible metabolic suppression induced by anoxia in isolated hepatocytes. Am J Physiol 265:R1014-R1019
27. Schumacker PT, Chandel N, Agusti AGN (1993) Oxygen conformance of cellular respiration in hepatocytes. Am J Physiol 265:L395-L402
28. Warburg O, Kubowitz F (1929) Atmung bei sehr kleinen Sauerstoffdrucken. Biochem Z 214:5-18
29. Wilson DF, Rumsey WL, Green TJ, Vanderkooi JM (1988) The oxygen dependence of mitochondrial oxidative phosphorylation measured by a new optical method for measuring oxygen concentration. J Biol Chem 263:2712-2718
30. Chandel NS, Budinger GRS, Choe SH, Schumacker PT (1997) Cellular respiration during hypoxia: Role of cytochrome oxidase as the oxygen sensor in hepatocytes. J Biol Chem 272:111-112
31. Budinger GRS, Chandel N, Shao ZH, Li CQ, Melmed A, Becker LB, Schumacker PT (1996) Cellular energy utilization and supply during hypoxia in embryonic cardiac myocytes. Am J Physiol 14:L37-L53
32. Budinger GRS, Duranteau J, Chandel NS, Schumacker PT (1998) Hibernation during hypoxia in cardiomyocytes: role of mitochondria as the oxygen sensor. J Biol Chem 273:3320-3326
33. Bunn HF, Poyton RO (1996) Oxygen sensing and molecular adaptation to hypoxia. Physiol Rev 76:839-885
34. Kadenbach B (1986) Regulation of respiration and ATP synthesis in higher organisms: Hypothesis. J Bioenerg Biomembr 18:39-54
35. Turrens JF, Alexandre A, Lehninger AL (1985) Ubisemiquinone is the electron donor for superoxide formation by complex III of heart mitochondria. Arch Biochem Biophys 237:408-414
36. Vanden Hoek TL, Shao Z, Li C, Schumacker PT, Becker LB (1997) Mitochondrial electron transport can become a significant source of oxidative injury in cardiomyocytes. J Mol Cell Cardiol 29:2441-2450
37. Duranteau J, Chandel NS, Kulisz A, Shao Z, Schumacker PT (1998) Intracellular signaling by reactive oxygen species during hypoxia in cardiomyocytes. J Biol Chem 273:11619-11624

The Mitochondrial Permeability Transition

A. P. Halestrap

Introduction

Under normal physiological conditions, the mitochondrial inner membrane is impermeable to all but a few selected metabolites and ions. The relative impermeability of the mitochondrial inner membrane is essential for the maintenance of the membrane potential and pH gradient that drive adenosine triphosphate (ATP) synthesis during oxidative phosphorylation. If this permeability barrier is disrupted, mitochondria become uncoupled and the proton-translocating ATPase actively hydrolyzes, rather than synthesises, ATP. Were this to occur in a cell, ATP concentrations could not be maintained even by glycolysis. Unless the pore could close again, the cell would be destined to die, since ATP is required to maintain the integrity of the cell. Eventually, the permeability barrier of the plasma membrane would be compromised through phospholipase A_2 action, and leakage of cell contents, and disruption of ion gradients would then ensure cell death. Such a non-specific increase in the permeability of the inner mitochondrial membrane can occur when the mitochondrial matrix calcium concentration ($[Ca^{2+}]$) is greatly increased, especially when this is accompanied by oxidative stress, adenine nucleotide depletion and mitochondrial depolarization. This phenomenon, known as the mitochondrial permeability transition (MPT), is associated with the opening of a non-specific pore in the mitochondrial inner membrane, which transports any molecule of < 1500 Daltons [1–4]. The conditions required to induce the MPT are exactly those found in tissues subjected to reperfusion after a period of ischemia (reperfusion injury) or in cells exposed to a variety of chemical insults that cause oxidative stress. Indeed there is increasing evidence that the MPT may be critical in the transition from reversible to irreversible cell injury and necrosis. Furthermore, the MPT has now been implicated as the "central executioner" in apoptosis. This chapter will provide a brief review of what is known about the molecular mechanism of the MPT and its regulation, and then summarize the evidence for its critical role in reperfusion injury and other insults leading to necrotic and apoptotic cell death, including the action of cytokines implicated in multiple organ failure (MOF).

The Molecular Mechanism of the MPT

Early data showed that the MPT allows all solutes < 1500 Daltons to enter the mitochondrial matrix and is reversed immediately by chelation of calcium (Ca^{2+}) with EGTA. These data implied the presence of a Ca^{2+}-dependent, non-specific channel in the inner mitochondrial membrane, but for many years it was argued that activation of mitochondrial phospholipase A_2 leading to a non-specific increase in the permeability of the inner membrane phospholipid bilayer was responsible [5]. However, when it was demonstrated that the MPT can be specifically and totally inhibited by sub-micromolar concentrations of the immunosuppressive drug cyclosporin A (CsA) without any effect on phospholipase A_2 activity, this view became untenable [6–8]. The immunosuppressive action of CsA is mediated by a complex between cytosolic cyclophilin (CyP-A) and CsA that inhibits calcineurin, a Ca-sensitive protein phosphatase [9]. The known action of CsA as an immunosuppressive agent suggested to us that effects of CsA on the MPT might also involve a member of the CyP family within the matrix [8] and subsequent studies have confirmed this, leading to the proposed mechanism of MPT shown in Figure 1. Our model proposes that a non-specific channel is formed by a conformational change of the adenine nucleotide translocase (ANT), an integral inner mitochondrial membrane protein whose normal function is to catalyze the transport of ATP out of the mitochondrial matrix in exchange for adenosine diphosphate (ADP) [10]. Calcium is required to trigger this conformational change, the process being facilitated by another matrix protein,

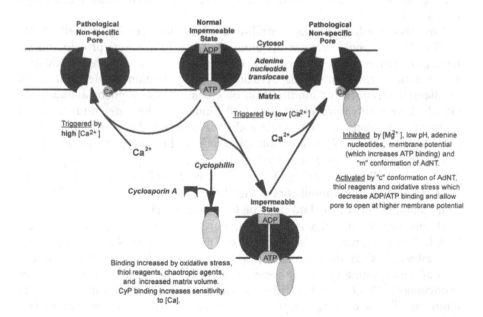

Fig. 1. Proposed model for the mechanism of action of the mitochondrial permeability transition

cyclophilin-D (CyP-D), that has peptidyl-prolyl cis-trans isomerase (PPIase) activity. Evidence for this model and the mechanisms by which factors known to regulate the MPT may act are presented below.

The Role of Mitochondrial CyP in the Mitochondrial Permeability Transition

The mitochondrial matrix contains PPIase activity that is inhibited by CsA and its analogs with $K_{0.5}$ values very similar to those for inhibition of the MPT [8, 11–13]. Furthermore, the number of binding sites required for 100% inhibition of the MPT corresponds to the concentration of PPIase within the matrix (about 50 pmol per mg protein) [8, 11]. We were able to purify and N-terminal sequence the CsA-sensitive mitochondrial PPIase and so confirm that it was a member of the cyclophylin (CyP) family, most probably identical to the product of the human CyP-3 gene [14]. This is a nuclear encoded protein with a mitochondrial targeting pre-sequence that is cleaved after translocation of the protein into the matrix. It is now more usually termed CyP-D [9]. We have cloned and sequenced the cDNA for rat mitochondrial CyP (Accession number U68544). With the exception of the extreme N-terminal residue, the sequence corresponds exactly to the N-terminus sequence of the purified protein [15]. This confirms that the matrix PPIase in rat mitochondria is indeed the equivalent of human CyP-3 (CyP-D). Northern blots demonstrate that mRNA for CyP-D is present in rat muscle, heart, liver, kidney and brain and is of identical size (1.5 kb) in all tissues. This finding makes it unlikely that there are differently spliced tissue-specific isoforms [15].

Our model predicts that those conditions which enhance the sensitivity of the MPT to $[Ca^{2+}]$ would increase the binding of CyP to its target protein and we have provided evidence to show that this notion is indeed correct. Oxidative stress induced with t-butyl hydroperoxide (TBH), glutathione depletion induced by diamide treatment or modification of vicinal thiols by phenylarsine oxide (PheArs) were all shown to increase CyP binding to the inner mitochondrial membrane, concomitant with their ability to increase the sensitivity of pore opening to Ca^{2+} [16, 17]. Mild chaotropic agents and increases in matrix volume were also able to increase both CyP binding and MPT opening in response to Ca^{2+} [17]. In all cases, binding of CyP was almost totally prevented by CsA. In contrast, several other modulators of the MPT such as matrix $[Ca^{2+}]$, [ADP], pH or membrane potential had no effect on CyP binding [18].

Despite the evidence described above, there is now a body of data to suggest that CyP binding may not be essential for the opening of the MPT pore, but may rather sensitize the process to $[Ca^{2+}]$. Thus at high matrix $[Ca^{2+}]$ inhibition of pore opening by CsA is overcome in both heart mitochondria and liver mitochondria [12, 16–18]. Yet under the same conditions, CsA is able to prevent almost totally the binding of CyP-D to the inner mitochondrial membrane [16, 18].

The Role of Adenine Nucleotide Translocase in the Mitochondrial Permeability Transition

The first evidence for an involvement of adenine nucleotide translocase (ANT) in pore opening was the observation that any reagent such as carboxyatractyloside (CAT) that stabilized the "c" conformation of ANT, stimulated the MPT, whilst any reagent such as bongkrekic acid (BKA) that stabilized the "m" conformation of ANT, inhibited the MPT [8, 18, 19]. Furthermore, matrix ADP is an important modulator of pore opening that acts by decreasing the sensitivity of the calcium trigger site to $[Ca^{2+}]$. There are two ADP binding sites with K_i values of about 1 and 25 µM. The high affinity site is blocked by the inhibitor CAT, and therefore is thought to be associated with ANT [18, 20]. We have tested the ability of a range of nucleotides to inhibit the MPT, and found that only ATP and deoxy-ADP inhibit, with $K_{0.5}$ values 500 and 20 times greater than ADP, respectively. Inhibition of the MPT by these compounds correlates with their affinity for the matrix binding site of ANT [18]. Adenine nucleotide binding is antagonized by oxidative stress induced by TBH or diamide and also by thiol reagents, such as PheArs, which is known to be a powerful activator of the MPT [18]. PheArs has the greatest effect of the reagents tested, raising the $K_{0.5}$ for ADP inhibition of the MPT to >500 µM; this effect is accompanied by covalent modification of ANT [18].

Bernardi and colleagues [21–24] have provided strong evidence that the MPT is voltage-regulated, being activated as the membrane potential becomes less negative. We have suggested that the membrane potential is sensed by the ANT itself through an effect on adenine nucleotide binding. This idea is plausible, since ANT is an electrogenic carrier, transporting ATP^{4-} in exchange for ADP^{3-} with a mechanism that may well involve a potential driven conformational change that alters the affinity of the adenine nucleotides on either side of the membrane [10]. In support of this hypothesis, we have demonstrated that in mitochondria depleted of adenine nucleotides by pyrophosphate treatment, not only is the MPT much more sensitive to $[Ca^{2+}]$, but it is also no longer voltage sensitive [12, 18]. Oxidative stress shifts the voltage dependence of the MPT, allowing the pore to open at more negative potentials. Two distinct thiol groups have been implicated in this effect, one sensitive to oxidation of glutathione, for example by TBH or diamide, and the other responding to the redox state of matrix NAD(P) [23, 25, 26]. ANT is known to have three cysteine residues that show differential reactivity to various thiol reagents in a conformation-dependent manner. These cysteine residues may represent the thiol groups that regulate both CyP-D binding and the inhibitory effects of ADP and membrane potential on the MPT [18].

A role for ANT in the MPT is now generally accepted [1–3], but there has been debate as to whether this protein may itself form the pore or is just a regulatory component. Although it has been reported that the purified and reconstituted ANT can form Ca^{2+}-dependent channels resembling the MPT pore [27] direct evidence for an interaction of CyP-D with ANT is still lacking. Attempts at chemical cross-linking of CyP-D to ANT have so far met without success. As an alternative approach we have now overexpressed CyP-D as a glutathione-S-transferase fusion protein and are using this reagent, immobilized on sepharose-glutathione, to investigate ANT binding directly.

Other Possible Components of the MPT Pore

It has been suggested that the outer membrane porin and benzodiazepine receptor may be involved in the MPT, since these components have been reported to copurify with ANT as a complex under some conditions [2, 28, 29]. Although this proposal is attractive especially in light of the recent suggestion that the MPT is involved in the release of cytochrome c during apoptosis (see below), evidence for it is lacking. First, ligands of the mitochondrial benzodiazepine receptor are without effect on the MPT [18]. Second, the MPT can be observed in mitoplasts from which the outer membrane has been largely removed by digitonin treatment and exhibits identical properties to the MPT in normal mitochondria (unpublished data). However, it does seem likely that there may be a Ca^{2+} binding protein that provides the Ca^{2+} trigger site for the MPT, since neither CyP-D nor ANT have obvious Ca^{2+} binding motifs.

The Locus of Action of Different Modulators of the MPT

Table 1 summarizes how ANT provides a common locus for the action of the different modulators of the MPT. Binding of matrix adenine nucleotides to ANT inhibits pore formation by decreasing the affinity of the trigger site for $[Ca^{2+}]$. Adenine nucleotide binding is antagonized by the "c" conformation of the carrier,

Table 1. Proposed sites of action of known modulators of the mitochondrial permeability transition

Effect via change in cyclophilin-D binding[a]	Effect via change in nucleotide binding[a]	Direct effect on Ca^{2+} binding
Activatory		
Thiol reagents (e.g., diamide PheArs)	Thiol reagents (e.g., diamide PheArs)	High pH
Oxidative stress (e.g., TBH)	Oxidative stress (e.g., TBH)	
Increased matrix volume	"C" conformation of ANT	
Chaotropic agents		
Inhibitory		
CsA	Membrane potential	Low pH
	Membrane surface charge (e.g., trifluoperazine)	Mg^{2+}
	"M" conformation of ANT	

[a] Note that both CyP binding and ADP binding exert their effects through changes in the sensitivity of the MPT to $[Ca^{2+}]$

membrane depolarization and thiol reagents that attack a specific thiol group on ANT, perhaps Cys^{159} [18]. These perturbations all sensitize the MPT to $[Ca^{2+}]$. In contrast, the "m" conformation and increased membrane potential enhance nucleotide binding and inhibit the pore. These effectors are all without effect on CyP-D recruitment to the membrane. Chaotropic agents and increased matrix volume sensitize the MPT to $[Ca^{2+}]$ by increasing CyP-D binding, an effect that thiol reagents and oxidative stress also induce, perhaps through modification of the Cys^{56} of ANT [18]. Increased CyP-D binding facilitates the transition of ANT into its open channel state. Low pH and Mg^{2+} are thought to compete directly with Ca^{2+} at the trigger site. Trifluoperazine is a potent inhibitor of the MPT under energized but not de-energized conditions [18]. This agent was originally thought to act indirectly through inhibition of phospholipase A_2, preventing the accumulation of free fatty acids which stimulate the MPT, probably through interaction with ANT. However, inhibition occurs even without changes in free fatty acid accumulation and is now thought to be mediated by an effect on surface membrane charge that changes the voltage sensitivity of the MPT [30]

The Role of the Mitochondrial Permeability Transition in Reperfusion Injury of the Heart and Other Tissues

It is well established that when ischemic tissues are reperfused, the damage caused during anoxia is further exacerbated. This phenomenon is known as reperfusion injury and the mechanisms involved have been widely studied [2, 4, 31–34] and are summarized below. During the ischemic phase, cells endeavor, unsuccessfully, to maintain their ATP levels through glycolysis. This process leads to an accumulation of lactic acid and hence a decrease in intracellular pH (pH_i). The Na^+/H^+ antiporter seeks to correct this, loading the cell with Na^+ which requires the Na^+/K^+ ATPase to drive it out. If there is insufficient ATP to allow this, the Na^+ accumulates and also prevents Ca^{2+} from being pumped of out of the cell on the Na^+/Ca^{2+} antiporter; the process may actually be reversed and allow additional Ca^{2+} entry. During ischemia, Ca^{2+} may also enter the mitochondria by reversal of the Na^+/Ca^{2+} antiporter, but upon reperfusion, Ca^{2+} is rapidly taken up into the mitochondria by means of the uniporter. The sudden influx of oxygen (O_2) into a hypoxic cell induces the formation of O_2 free radicals through an interaction of O_2 with ubisemiquinone which is formed by respiratory chain inhibition during hypoxia. Additional O_2 free radicals are produced through the operation of xanthine oxidase. This enzyme is activated during hypoxia and is presented with high concentrations of xanthine produced by the purine degradation that occurs during hypoxia. The combination of oxidative stress and high $[Ca^{2+}]$ provides the ideal conditions for the MPT, especially in the presence of elevated cellular phosphate concentrations and depleted adenine nucleotide levels, both of which occur during ischemia. Furthermore, during the reperfusion phase, the pH_i rapidly returns to pre-ischemic values through the operation of the Na^+/H^+ antiporter, lactic acid efflux on the monocarboxylate transporter (MCT) and bicarbonate dependent mechanisms [35]. Thus, the inhibitory effect

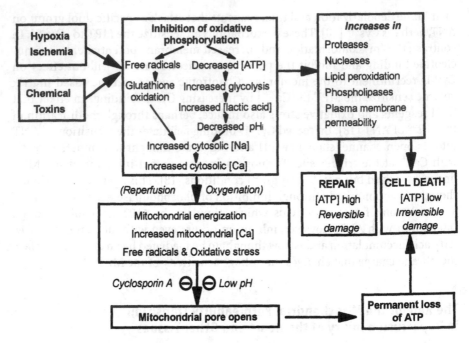

Fig. 2. Scheme summarizing the involvement of the MPT in necrotic cell death

of low pH on the MPT [36] is removed, allowing the other stimulators of the process to exert their full effect. The sequence of events described above is summarized in Figure 2 and suggests that the MPT may be central in determining whether a cell lives or dies. Indeed morphological studies confirm mitochondria become swollen and amorphous under such conditions [2, 32].

Direct Measurement of Pore Opening During Reperfusion of the Ischemic Heart

In order to establish directly that the MPT occurs in intact tissues under pathologic conditions it is necessary to measure mitochondrial pore opening *in situ*. In isolated hepatocytes subjected to oxidative stress, measurements of pore opening have been achieved using laser scanning confocal microscopy with the intracellular green fluorescent dye, calcein, in combination with the mitochondrial membrane potential sensitive red fluorescent dye tetramethylrhodamine (TMRM) [37]. Calcein only enters the mitochondria when the MPT pore opens, whilst TMRM leaves the mitochondria under these conditions. This technique has been used to show that mitochondria undergo the MPT during necrotic cell death induced by oxidative stress [37]. CsA, especially in the presence of trifluoperazine, inhibits the MPT and protects cells from death. CsA also protects isolated heart cells from irreversible injury during re-oxygenation following anoxia [38], and in these cells there is a correlation between mitochondrial $[Ca^{2+}]$ content and subsequent cell death [39].

These techniques for measuring MPT cannot easily be applied to the perfused heart and we have devised an alternative procedure that relies on the impermeability of the inner mitochondrial membrane to 2-deoxyglucose-6-phosphate [12]. Hearts are perfused in the Langendorff recirculating mode with [^{3}H]-2-deoxyglucose [DOG] which enters the heart on the glucose carrier and is then phosphorylated to DOG-6-phosphate. This compound is not further metabolized and is trapped within the cell. DOC-6-phosphate would not be expected to enter mitochondria unless the pore opens. After washing out extracellular [^{3}H]-DOG, hearts are subjected to various periods of ischemia and reperfusion, and then mitochondria prepared rapidly and assayed for [^{3}H]-DOG and citrate synthase (an indicator of mitochondrial recovery). From the [^{3}H]-DOG content of the mitochondria and a small sample of total heart homogenate, an estimation of pore opening is possible. Mitochondria prepared immediately after the ischemic period show no increase in DOG content, but those prepared following a period of reperfusion show a significant increase [12]. Pore opening is maximal after 5 min of reperfusion [34] and this time point corresponds to the period when the intracellular pH returns to pre-ischemic values [35]. Thus, our data suggest that a profound opening of the mitochondrial pore occurs only during the reperfusion phase, consistent with the predictions made above. It has been argued that pore opening is not a primary cause of cell injury, but rather a secondary phenomenon that occurs following other critical damage to the myocyte, such as breakdown of the plasma membrane permeability barrier [40]. However, if the latter were to occur, DOG would be lost from the cell before it could enter the mitochondria and thus no increase in mitochondrial DOG would be measured.

Reversal of The MPT in Hearts That Recover During Reperfusion

Recovery of heart function during reperfusion can be measured using pressure transducers to monitor heart rate, left ventricular developed pressure (LVDP), end diastolic pressure (EDP) and aortic pressure. In addition, adenine nucleotide concentrations can be determined in hearts freeze-clamped after the ischemic period or after reperfusion [41]. Reperfusion after short periods of ischemia leads to total recovery of LVDP and the ATP/ADP ratio [41], yet using the DOG technique, we have demonstrated that even under these conditions mitochondria undergo MPT [12, 34, 41]. This finding suggests that the opening of the mitochondrial pores must be transient, such that rapid resealing allows total recovery of mitochondrial function and heart performance. Unfortunately, when the MPT reverses, closure of the mitochondrial pores means that DOG remains trapped inside the mitochondria and the reversal is not detected. Detection requires a modification of the DOG technique, in which hearts are loaded with [^{3}H]-DOG during reperfusion once maximum recovery of the heart had been established (post-loading). If reversal of the MPT occurs during reperfusion, mitochondrial DOG entrapment following post-loading should be less than when DOG is present at the start of reperfusion (pre-loading). Experimental observations confirm this prediction. After 40 min of ischemia post-loading gives about 50% less mitochondrial DOG entrapment than is observed with preloading (unpublished observations). Thus, if the insult caused by ischemia/reperfusion is not too great, mitochondria can undergo a transient permeability transition, followed by closure of the pores and entrapment of DOG. The closure is presumably brought about by a decrease in matrix $[Ca^{2+}]$ that occurs as Ca^{2+} is lost from the mitochondria during the MPT. However, closure will only occur if enough "healthy" mitochondria are remaining in the cell to accumulate the released calcium and provide sufficient ATP to maintain ionic homeostasis in the cell. The balance between the number of "closed" and "open" mitochondria within any cell will be critical in determining whether a cell lives or dies. If there are too many "open" mitochondria, they will release more Ca^{2+} and hydrolyze more ATP than the "closed" mitochondria can accommodate. In contrast, if there are sufficient "closed" mitochondria to meet the cell's ATP requirements and to accumulate released Ca^{2+} without undergoing the MPT themselves, the "open" mitochondria will close again and the cell will recover.

Inhibitors of the MPT Protect Cells from Injury Caused by Oxidative Stress and Ischemia/Reperfusion

Cyclosporin: If the MPT is a critical factor in the development of reperfusion injury, CsA would be expected to provide some protection from damage. This prediction has been borne out in isolated cardiac myocytes subjected to reoxygenation following a period of hypoxia [38], in hepatocytes during chemical anoxia and oxidative stress [37, 42] and in perfused hearts subjected to isothermic global ischemia followed by reperfusion [12, 34, 41]. In the latter case, we demonstrated that hearts treated with 0.2 µM CsA showed a greater recovery of LVDP, tissue ATP/ADP ratios and functional mitochondria, whilst AMP levels and EDP (an indicator of contracture due to low ATP/ADP and elevated $[Ca^{2+}]$), were lower. No protective effect of CsA was observed on the loss of total adenine nucleotides that occurs as a result of purine degradation during hypoxia. Nor was protection from inhibition of respiratory chain function (State 3 substrate oxidation) observed [12, 34]. Inhibition of State 3 oxidation is probably caused by O_2 free radicals, formed during ischemia and reperfusion, directly modifying components of the respiratory chain [12, 33, 34, 41]. Our observations are consistent with CsA exerting its effects by preventing the MPT, which is down-stream of changes in total adenine nucleotides and free radicals. Furthermore, we have demonstrated that only analogs of CsA that block the MPT in isolated mitochondria are able to offer protection to the reperfused heart [12, 34]. The protective effect of CsA was highly concentration dependent, showing an optimal response at 0.2 µM and declining at higher concentrations [41]. A similar concentration dependence has been observed for CsA-protection of isolated cardiac myocytes subjected to reoxygenation following a period of hypoxia [38].

Antioxidants and calcium antagonists: There is extensive literature showing that antioxidants and free radical scavengers can protect the ischemic/reperfused heart from irreversible damage [2, 33, 41, 43]. Whilst there may be many processes within the cardiac myocyte that are possible targets for the action of these reagents, prevention of the MPT is clearly one of them. There is also strong evidence that mitochondrial overload accompanies reperfusion injury, and preventing this with calcium antagonists or ruthenium red, an inhibitor of mitochondrial calcium uptake, also provides protection [2, 4, 33, 34, 42]. Once again, these observations are consistent with a critical role for the MPT in reperfusion injury, but they cannot be taken as proof of such a role [38].

Low pH$_i$: There is extensive literature demonstrating that low pH (< 7.0) can protect a variety of cells, including cardiac myocytes and hepatocytes, from oxidative stress, re-oxygenation following anoxia or reperfusion following ischemia [2, 33, 44]. These effects can be brought about by using low extracellular pH or by addition of specific inhibitors of the Na$^+$/H$^+$ antiporter such as amiloride. A low pH$_i$ may have several means of exerting a protective effect on the cell, but the profound inhibition of the MPT at pH < 7.0 [36] suggests that prevention of the MPT pore may be an important one. Support for this view comes from the observation that during reperfusion of the heart the MPT pore opens over the same period of time as the pH$_i$ is restored from less than 6.5 to pre-ischemic values (> 7.0) [34, 35].

Pyruvate: It is well documented that pyruvate can protect hearts against ischemia/reperfusion and anoxia/re-oxygenation injury [45, 46]. The protective effects of pyruvate have been attributed to beneficial metabolic alterations and to protection from free radical production, since pyruvate acts as a free radical scavenger [45, 46]. However, an additional effect of pyruvate might be through inhibition of the MPT. The free radical scavenging effects of pyruvate would contribute to this protection. In addition, as a good respiratory substrate, pyruvate would generate a high mitochondrial NADH/NAD$^+$ ratio, preventing oxidation of protein thiol groups critical for modulation of the MPT voltage sensor, and also a high membrane potential which would act in concert to inhibit MPT (see above). Furthermore, pyruvate enters heart cells with a proton by means of the MCT [47]. This pyruvate entry leads to a decrease in pH$_i$ directly, but in addition pyruvate competes with lactate for transport by the MCT [47] which may lead to a greater intracellular accumulation of lactic acid and further lowering of pH$_i$. Such an effect would inhibit the MPT still further. We have demonstrated that the drop in perfusate pH of pyruvate-treated hearts on reperfusion is considerably greater than for control hearts, suggesting that pH$_i$ is significantly lower at the end of ischemia and during the reperfusion phase (unpublished observations). There is also direct evidence from nuclear magnetic resonance (NMR) studies that pyruvate causes a decrease in pH$_i$ in a low-flow model of ischemia [48]. We have used the DOG technique to confirm that the protective effect of 10 mM pyruvate (present both before and during ischemia, and during reperfusion) is accompanied by a reduction of mitochondrial pore opening during the initial stages of reperfusion and more extensive closure during later stages (unpublished observations). Indeed, in the presence of pyruvate, hearts recover 100% of their LVDP after 40 min ischemia, compared to only about 50% in the absence of pyruvate, and this is associated with DOG entrapment returning to pre-ischemic values as opposed to a 50% decrease in DOG entrapment in controls. These data are the first direct evidence that mitochondrial pore opening can reverse when hearts damaged by reperfusion recover.

Propofol: Propofol is an anesthetic agent that is frequently used during cardiac surgery and in post-operative sedation [49]. There are reports that propofol can act as a free radical scavenger [50, 51] and also that at concentrations higher than used clinically, it may inhibit the MPT in isolated mitochondria [52]. One study [53] has suggested that propofol can attenuate the effects of hydrogen peroxide induced oxidative stress in the perfused heart. We have studied the effects of propofol on recovery of hearts from ischemia (unpublished data). When added 10 min prior to ischemia and during reperfusion at 2 μg/ml, a concentration similar to that employed clinically, significant protection of hearts was observed. Thus, recovery of LVDP after 30min ischemia (means ± S.E.M.) increased from $36 \pm 8\%$ (n = 10) in control hearts to $70 \pm 11\%$ (n = 8; p < 0.05) in propofol-treated hearts. This was accompanied by a 25% decrease in mitochondrial DOG entrapment. When added to isolated heart mitochondria at the same concentration, no inhibition of the MPT was observed. Thus, the protective effect of propofol may not be through a direct effect on the MPT, but through other mechanisms such as its free radical scavenging properties causing a decrease in oxidative stress or reported inhibitory effects on Ca^{2+} channels [54, 55] leading to a reduction in Ca^{2+} overload. Nevertheless, propofol provides another example of a reagent whose protection of the heart from reperfusion injury is accompanied by a decrease in mitochondrial pore opening *in vivo*.

The Mitochondrial Permeability Transition and Apoptosis

There is recent evidence that the MPT may act as the "central executioner" of cells subjected to a range of insults, such as oxidative stress, growth factor removal or exposure to cytokines. Indeed, the mitochondria may not only determine whether cells live or die, but also whether death occurs by apoptosis or necrosis [56]. Thus, in some cells, changes in mitochondrial membrane potential ($\Delta\varphi$) occur early in apoptosis and can be inhibited by CsA, which also inhibits apoptosis. Furthermore, mitochondria are required to induce apoptosis in a cell free system and appear to do this by release of an apoptosis inducing factor which is most probably cytochrome c [57–59]. The anti-apoptotic gene product, bcl-2, is associated with the mitochondrial outer membrane and has been reported to inhibit the MPT and prevent release of cytochrome c and consequent caspase activation [58, 59].

Attractive though this hypothesis may be, there are cell types that demonstrate apoptosis without early changes in $\Delta\varphi$ or inhibition by CsA [57–60]. Nor does

CsA protect cell types from all apoptotic stimuli and may even induce apoptosis under some circumstances [60-62]. However, it is likely that cells experiencing only a modest insult may undergo a transient opening of the MPT pore which then closes again, enabling ion gradients and ATP production to be re-established. Under such conditions, sufficient swelling of the outer membrane may occur to release cytochrome c and set in motion the apoptotic cascade that causes an organized, non-inflammatory cell death by apoptosis. The controlled nature of apoptosis requires that tissue ATP content is maintained, and where this is not the case, cell death becomes necrotic [63]. Such a situation occurs when a cell experiences a sufficient insult to cause MPT pore opening that is both extensive and prolonged. Not only is cytochrome c released, but mitochondria remain uncoupled and therefore unable to generate the ATP required for maintaining cellular ionic homeostasis and repairing tissue damage. Under these conditions, damage continues unabated, leading ultimately to rupture of the plasma membrane and cell death. This uncontrolled necrotic form of cell death is inflammatory and further exacerbated as neutrophil invasion leads to yet more damage. Thus, the decision between apoptosis and necrosis may rest on the extent of the MPT, and can account for the observation that apoptosis and necrosis both occur in the reperfused heart, with the least damaged areas showing a preponderance of apoptosis over necrosis. A diagram summarizing how the MPT may act as the decisiom maker between apoptosis and necrosis is given in Figure 3.

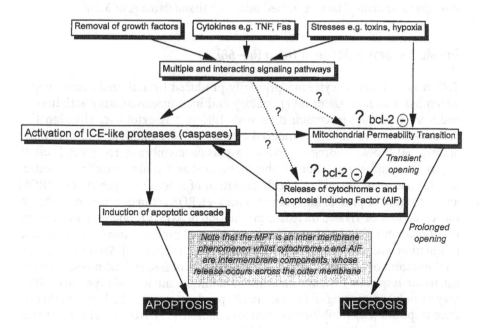

Fig. 3. Scheme illustrating how the MPT may be involved in deciding whether a cell dies by necrosis or apoptosis

The Role of the Membrane Permeability Transition in Multiple Organ Failure

MOF is a major complication of traumatic or septic shock [64, 65], but its causes are not fully understood. It appears to be the result of a massive inflammatory response, with the lungs, kidneys and liver being the organs most susceptible to damage. Although supplied with adequate O_2, they behave as is if they are hypoxic, suggesting that mitochondrial function may be impaired. During acute shock, blood flow to the intestine becomes severely restricted and subsequent restoration of blood flow leads to "reperfusion injury" which, by comparison with the heart, may well involve the MPT. This damage to the intestine may have a direct effect to breakdown the permeability barrier of the gut lumen, allowing bacteria or bacterial endotoxins to infiltrate submucosal tissues. These toxins, or the damaged gut itself, may activate immune cells in tissues and organs that are "downstream" of the mucosa (e.g. Kupffer cells in the liver, macrophages in the lamina propria of the gut) which in turn release various inflammatory mediators such as tumor necrosis factor (TNF-α) and interleukins (IL-1 and IL-6). The initial release of these factors may be sufficient to cause tissue damage alone, or they may prime the immune system which is subsequently activated massively by a further insult (the "second hit" hypothesis). The second insult may be continuing infection, anesthesia or an episode of hypertension. Following the second hit, activated neutrophils and macrophages invade tissues, release cytokines such as TNF-α and cause rapid and often irreversible damage. Whatever the initial process, TNF-α, alone or in combination with interferon γ (IFN-γ), IL-1 and IL-6, are thought to be critical factors in mediating the tissue damage of MOF.

The Mechanisms of Action of TNF-α [66–68]

TNF-α is a pleitropic cytokine, primarily produced by activated macrophages, which has a wide range of inflammatory and immunomodulatory activities. In addition, especially in combination with IFN-γ, it is cytotoxic. The signaling pathways involved in TNF-α-induced cytotoxicity are multiple, and may differ among cell types. Binding of TNF-α to plasma membrane receptors leads to G-protein-coupled activation of phospholipases and sphingomyelinases, extracellular release of arachidonic acid, formation of reactive oxygen species (ROS) and activation of protein kinases and proteases. ROS are major players in the cytotoxic actions of TNF-α. Increased production of ROS is thought to occur as the result of an inhibition of the respiratory chain, and probably involves free radical production within the mitochondrial complex III [67, 69, 70]. Secondary effects on the respiratory chain may also occur as a result of free radical-mediated damage to the respiratory chain complexes. In addition, nitric oxide synthase (NOS) may be induced, causing an increase in NO production [71] which can further reduce respiration by inhibiting cytochrome oxidase [72]. NO may also react with oxygen free radicals to produce the highly reactive peroxynitrite, which can induce additional damage to the cell [73]. Since the MPT is greatly sensitized to

$[Ca^{2+}]$ by oxidative stress it is likely that cell death induced by TNF-α, be it apoptotic or necrotic, involves the MPT [74].

Conclusion

The MPT converts the mitochondrion from an organelle that, through its production of ATP, sustains the cell in its normal function, to an instrument of death. Although the exact details of its mechanism remain elusive, there is strong evidence that the MPT involves a Ca^{2+}-mediated conformational change in ANT that converts it into a non-specific pore (Fig. 1). CyP is required to enable this conformational change and the process is further sensitized to $[Ca^{2+}]$ by oxidative stress whereas decreasing pH_i below 7.0 greatly desensitizes the MPT to $[Ca^{2+}]$. Knowledge about the mechanisms responsible for the MPT can be used to protect tissues from damage caused by stresses such as reperfusion injury and chemical insult to cells (Fig. 2). Thus CsA, free radical scavengers, and procedures to decrease pH_i can all offer protection to cells under conditions of stress.

Acknowledgements. This work was supported by project grants from the Medical Research Council and the British Heart Foundation.

References

1. Bernardi P, Broekemeier KM, Pfeiffer DR (1994) Recent progress on regulation of the mitochondrial permeability transition pore; A cyclosporin-sensitive pore in the inner mitochondrial membrane. J Bioenerg Biomemb 26:509–517
2. Halestrap AP (1994) Interactions between oxidative stress and calcium overload on mitochondrial function. In: Darley-Usmar V, Schapira AHV (eds) Mitochondria: DNA, proteins and disease. Portland Press Ltd, London, pp 113–142
3. Zoratti M, Szabo I (1995) The mitochondrial permeability transition. Biochim Biophys Acta 1241:139–176.
4. Crompton M (1990) The role of Ca^{2+} in the function and dysfunction of heart mitochondria. In: Langer GA (ed) Calcium and the heart. Raven Press Ltd, New York, pp 167–198
5. Gunter TE, Pfeiffer DR (1990) Mechanisms by which mitochondria transport calcium. Am J Physiol 258:C755–C786
6. Crompton M, Ellinger H, Costi A (1988) Inhibition by cyclosporin A of a Ca^{2+}-dependent pore in heart mitochondria activated by inorganic phosphate and oxidative stress. Biochem J 255:357–360
7. Broekemeier KM, Dempsey ME, Pfeiffer DR (1989) Cyclosporin-A is a potent inhibitor of the inner membrane permeability transition in liver mitochondria. J Biol Chem 264:7826–7830
8. Halestrap AP, Davidson AM (1990) Inhibition of Ca^{2+}-induced large amplitude swelling of liver and heart mitochondria by cyclosporin A is probably caused by the inhibitor binding to mitochondrial matrix peptidyl-prolyl cis-trans isomerase and preventing it interacting with the adenine nucleotide translocase. Biochem J 268:153–160
9. Galat A (1993) Peptidylproline cis-trans-isomerases – Immunophilins. Eur J Biochem 216:689–707
10. Klingenberg M (1980) The ADP-ATP Translocation in mitochondria, a membrane potential controlled transport. J Membr Biol 56:97–105

11. Griffiths EJ, Halestrap AP (1991) Further evidence that cyclosporin-a protects mitochondria from calcium overload by inhibiting a matrix peptidyl-prolyl cis-trans isomerase – implications for the immunosuppressive and toxic effects of cyclosporin. Biochem J 274:611–614

12. Griffiths EJ, Halestrap AP (1995) Mitochondrial non-specific pores remain closed during cardiac ischaemia, but open upon reperfusion. Biochem J 307:93–98

13. Nicolli A, Basso E, Petronilli V, Wenger RM, Bernardi P (1996) Interactions of cyclophilin with the mitochondrial inner membrane and regulation of the permeability transition pore, a cyclosporin A-sensitive channel. J Biol Chem 271:2185–2192

14. Connern CP, Halestrap AP (1992) Purification and N-terminal sequencing of peptidyl-prolyl cis-trans-isomerase from rat liver mitochondrial matrix reveals the existence of a distinct mitochondrial cyclophilin. Biochem J 284:381–385

15. Woodfield KY, Price NT, Halestrap AP (1997) cDNA cloning of rat mitochondrial cyclophilin. Biochim Biophys Acta 1351:27–30

16. Connern CP, Halestrap AP (1994) Recruitment of mitochondrial cyclophilin to the mitochondrial inner membrane under conditions of oxidative stress that enhance the opening of a calcium-sensitive non-specific channel. Biochem J 302:321–324

17. Connern CP, Halestrap AP (1996) Chaotropic agents and increased matrix volume enhance binding of mitochondrial cyclophilin to the inner mitochondrial membrane and sensitize the mitochondrial permeability transition to [Ca^{2+}]. Biochemistry 35:8175–8180

18. Halestrap AP, Woodfield KY, Connern CP (1997) Oxidative stress, thiol reagents, and membrane potential modulate the mitochondrial permeability transition by affecting nucleotide binding to the adenine nucleotide translocase. J Biol Chem 272:3346–3354

19. LeQuoc K, LeQuoc D (1988) Involvement of the ADP/ATP carrier in calcium-induced perturbations of the mitochondrial inner membrane permeability: importance of the orientation of the nucleotide binding site. Arch Biochem Biophys 265:249–257

20. Novgorodov SA, Gudz TI, Milgrom YM, Brierley GP (1992) The permeability transition in heart mitochondria is regulated synergistically by ADP and cyclosporin-A. J Biol Chem 267:16274–16282

21. Bernardi P (1992) Modulation of the mitochondrial cyclosporin-A-sensitive permeability transition pore by the proton electrochemical gradient – evidence that the pore can be opened by membrane depolarization. J Biol Chem 267:8834–8839

22. Petronilli V, Cola C, Bernardi P (1993) Modulation of the mitochondrial cyclosporin A-sensitive permeability transition pore 2. The minimal requirements for pore induction underscore a key role for transmembrane electrical potential, matrix pH, and matrix Ca^{2+}. J Biol Chem 268:1011–1016

23. Petronilli V, Costantini P, Scorrano L, Colonna R, Passamonti S, Bernardi P (1994) The voltage sensor of the mitochondrial permeability transition pore is tuned by the oxidation-reduction state of vicinal thiols – Increase of the gating potential by oxidants and its reversal by reducing agents. J Biol Chem 269:16638–16642

24. Scorrano L, Petronilli V, Bernardi P (1997) On the voltage dependence of the mitochondrial permeability transition pore – A critical appraisal. J Biol Chem 272:12295–12299

25. Costantini P, Chernyak BV, Petronilli V, Bernardi P (1996) Modulation of the mitochondrial permeability transition pore by pyridine nucleotides and dithiol oxidation at two separate sites. J Biol Chem 271:6746–6751

26. Chernyak BV, Bernardi P (1996) The mitochondrial permeability transition pore is modulated by oxidative agents through both pyridine nucleotides and glutathione at two separate sites. Eur J Biochem 238:623–630

27. Brustovetsky N, Klingenberg M (1996) Mitochondrial ADP/ATP carrier can be reversibly converted into a large channel by Ca^{2+}. Biochemistry 35:8483–8488

28. McEnery MW, Snowman AM, Trifiletti RR, Snyder SH (1992) Isolation of the mitochondrial benzodiazepine receptor – Association with the voltage-dependent anion channel and the adenine nucleotide carrier. Proc Natl Acad Sci USA 89:3170–3174

29. Beutner G, Ruck A, Riede B, Welte W, Brdiczka D (1996) Complexes between kinases, mitochondrial porin and adenylate translocator in rat brain resemble the permeability transition pore. FEBS Lett 396:189–195

30. Broekemeier KM, Pfeiffer DR (1995) Inhibition of the mitochondrial permeability transition by cyclosporin a during long time frame experiments: Relationship between pore opening and the activity of mitochondrial phospholipases. Biochemistry 34:16440–16449
31. Lemasters JJ, Thurman RG (1995) The many facets of reperfusion injury. Gastroenterology 108:1317–1320
32. Reimer KA, Jennings RB (1992) Myocardial ischemia, hypoxia and infarction. In: Fozzard HA, Jennings RB, Huber E, Katz AM, Morgan HE (eds) The heart and cardovascular system, 2nd edn. Raven Press Ltd, New York, pp 1875–1973
33. Halestrap AP, Griffiths EJ, Connern CP (1993) Mitochondrial calcium handling and oxidative stress. Biochem Soc Trans 21:353–358
34. Halestrap AP, Connern CP, Griffiths EJ, Kerr PM (1997) Cyclosporin A binding to mitochondrial cyclophilin inhibits the permeability transition pore and protects hearts from ischaemia/reperfusion injury. Mol Cell Biochem 174:167–172
35. Vandenberg JI, Metcalfe JC, Grace AA (1993) Mechanisms of intracellular pH recovery following global ischaemia in the perfused heart. Circ Res 72:993–1003
36. Halestrap AP (1991) Calcium-dependent opening of a non-specific pore in the mitochondrial inner membrane is inhibited at pH values below 7 – Implications for the protective effect of low pH against chemical and hypoxic cell damage. Biochem J 278:715–719
37. Nieminen AL, Saylor AK, Tesfai SA, Herman B, Lemasters JJ (1995) Contribution of the mitochondrial permeability transition to lethal injury after exposure of hepatocytes to t-butylhydroperoxide. Biochem J 307:99–106
38. Nazareth W, Yafei N, Crompton M (1991) Inhibition of anoxia-induced injury in heart myocytes by cyclosporin-A. J Mol Cell Cardiol 23:1351–1354
39. Miyata H, Lakatta EG, Stern MD, Silverman HS (1992) Relation of mitochondrial and cytosolic free calcium to cardiac myocyte recovery after exposure to anoxia. Circ Res 71:605–613
40. Piper HM, Noll T, Siegmund B (1994) Mitochondrial function in the oxygen depleted and reoxygenated myocardial cell. Cardiovasc Res 28:1–15
41. Griffiths EJ, Halestrap AP (1993) Protection by cyclosporin a of ischemia reperfusion-induced damage in isolated rat hearts. J Mol Cell Cardiol 25:1461–1469
42. Pastorino JG, Snyder JW, Hoek JB, Farber JL (1995) Ca^{2+} depletion prevents anoxic death of hepatocytes by inhibiting mitochondrial permeability transition. Am J Physiol 268:C676–C685
43. Reimer MA, Murry CE, Richard VJ (1989) The role of neutrophils and free radicals in the ischemic-reperfused heart: Why the confusion and controversy? J Mol Cell Cardiol 21:1225–1239
44. Bond JM, Chacon E, Herman B, Lemasters JJ (1993) Intracellular pH and Ca^{2+} homeostasis in the pH paradox of reperfusion injury to neonatal rat cardiac myocytes. Am J Physiol 265:C129–C137
45. Deboer LWV, Bekx PA, Han LH, Steinke L (1993) Pyruvate enhances recovery of rat hearts after ischemia and reperfusion by preventing free radical generation. Am J Physiol 265:H1571–H1576
46. Borle AB, Stanko RT (1996) Pyruvate reduces anoxic injury and free radical formation in perfused rat hepatocytes. Am J Physiol 270:G535–G540
47. Halestrap AP, Wang X, Poole RC, Jackson VN, Price NT (1997) Lactate transport in heart in relation to ischemia. Am J Cardiol 80A:17A–25A
48. Cross HR, Clarke K, Opie LH, Radda GK (1995) Is lactate-induced myocardial ischemic injury mediated by decreased pH or increased intracellular lactate? J Mol Cell Cardiol 27:1369–1381.
49. Bryson HM, Fulton BR, Faulds D (1995) Propofol – an update of its use in anesthesia and conscious sedation. Drugs 50:513–559
50. Green TR, Bennett SR, Nelson VM (1994) Specificity and properties of propofol as an antioxidant free radical scavenger. Toxicol Appl Pharmacol 129:163–169
51. Murphy PG, Bennett JR, Myers DS, Davies MJ, Jones JG (1993) The effect of propofol anaesthesia on free radical-induced lipid peroxidation in rat liver microsomes. Eur J Anaesth 10:261–266

52. Sztark F, Ichas F, Ouhabi R, Dabadie P, Mazat JP (1995) Effects of the anaesthetic propofol on the calcium-induced permeability transition of rat heart mitochondria: Direct pore inhibition and shift of the gating potential. FEBS Lett 368:101–104
53. Kokita N, Hara A (1996) Propofol attenuates hydrogen-peroxide induced mechanical and metabolic derangements in the isolated rat heart. Anesthesiology 84:117–127
54. Buljubasic N, Marijic J, Berczi V, Supan DF, Kampine JP, Bosnjak ZJ (1996) Differential effects of etomidate, propofol, and midazolam on calcium and potassium channel currents in canine myocardial cells. Anesthesiology 85:1092–1099
55. Li YC, Ridefelt P, Wiklund L, Bjerneroth G (1997) Propofol induces a lowering of free cytosolic calcium in myocardial cells. Acta Anaesthesiol Scand 41:633–638
56. Susin SA, Zamzami N, Castedo M, et al (1997) The central executioner of apoptosis: Multiple connections between protease activation and mitochondria in Fas/APO-1/CD95- and ceramide-induced apoptosis. J Exp Med 186:25–37
57. Liu X, Kim CN, Yang J, Jemmerson R, Wang X (1996) Induction of apoptotic program in cell-free extracts: Requirement for dATP and cytochrome c. Cell 86:147–157
58. Kluck RM, Bossy-Wetzel E, Green DR, Newmeyer DD (1997) The release of cytochrome c from mitochondria: A primary site for Bcl-2 regulation of apoptosis. Science 275:1132–1136
59. Yang J, Liu XS, Bhalla K, et al (1997) Prevention of apoptosis by Bcl-2: Release of cytochrome c from mitochondria blocked. Science 275:1129–1132
60. Garland JM, Halestrap A (1997) Energy metabolism during apoptosis. Bcl-2 promotes survival in hematopoietic cells induced to apoptose by growth factor withdrawal by stabilizing a form of metabolic arrest. J Biol Chem 272:4680–4688
61. Gottschalk AR, Boise LH, Thompson CB, Quintans J (1994) Identification of immunosuppressant-induced apoptosis in a murine B-cell line and its prevention by bcl-x but not bcl-2. Proc Natl Acad Sci USA 91:7350–7354
62. McDonald JW, Goldberg MP, Gwag BJ, Chi SI, Choi DW (1996) Cyclosporin induces neuronal apoptosis and selective oligodendrocyte death in cortical cultures. Ann Neurol 40:750–758
63. Leist M, Nicotera P (1997) The shape of cell death. Biochem Biophys Res Commun 236:1–9
64. Aranow JS, Fink MP (1996) Determinants of intestinal barrier failure in critical illness. Br J Anaesth 77:71–81
65. Biffl WL, Moore EM (1996) Splanchnic ischaemia/reperfusion and multiple organ failure. Br J Anaesth 77:59–70
66. Vilcek J, Lee TH (1991) Tumor necrosis factor. New insights into the molecular basis of its actions. J Biol Chem 266:7313–7316
67. Goossens V, Grooten J, Devos K, Fiers W (1995) Direct evidence for tumor necrosis factor-induced mitochondrial reactive oxygen intermediates and their involvement in cytotoxicity. Proc Natl Acad Sci USA 92:8115–8119
68. Wallach D, Boldin M, Varfolomeev E, Beyaert R, Vandenabeele P, Fiers W (1997) Cell death induction by receptors of the TNF family: Towards a molecular understanding. FEBS Lett 410:96–106
69. Schulze-Osthoff K, Bakker AC, Vanhaesebroeck B, Beyaert R, Jacob WA, Fiers W (1992) Cytotoxic activity of tumor necrosis factor is mediated by early damage of mitochondrial functions – Evidence for the involvement of mitochondrial radical generation. J Biol Chem 267:5317–5323
70. Hennet T, Richter C, Peterhans E (1993) Tumour necrosis factor-alpha induces superoxide anion generation in mitochondria of L929 cells. Biochem J 289:587–592
71. Horton RA, Ceppi ED, Knowles RG, Titheradge MA (1994) Inhibition of hepatic-gluconeogenesis by nitric oxide: A comparison with endotoxic shock. Biochem J 299:735–739
72. Brown GC (1995) Nitric oxide regulates mitochondrial respiration and cell functions by inhibiting cytochrome oxidase. FEBS Lett 369:136–139
73. Packer MA, Murphy MP (1995) Peroxynitrite formed by simultaneous nitric oxide and superoxide generation causes cyclosporin-A-sensitive mitochondrial calcium efflux and depolarisation. Eur J Biochem 234:231–239
74. Pastorino JG, Simbula G, Yamamoto K, Glascott PA, Rothman RJ, Farber JL (1996) The cytotoxicity of tumor necrosis factor depends on induction of the mitochondrial permeability transition. J Biol Chem 271:29792–29798

Measuring Tissue Oxygenation

The Available Clinical Tools –
Oxygen-Derived Variables, Lactate, and pHi

J. L. Vincent

Introduction

Tissue hypoxia, as the result of an abnormal relationship between oxygen supply (DO_2) and O_2 demand, is a major factor in the development and propagation of multiple organ failure. As physicians, particularly in the field of intensive care, the prevention of hypoxia and the maintenance adequate tissue perfusion are thus essential aims of therapy. Increasing DO_2 may improve survival in certain groups of patients but applying this technique to reach pre-defined values of DO_2 in all patients is not effective and could even be harmful [1, 2]. The return of the arterial pressure, and even cardiac output (CO) and DO_2, to "normal", is not a sufficient indicator of oxygenation, and other methods of assessing the adequacy of tissue oxygenation are required to complement full clinical and hemodynamic evaluation, and assist in identifying the "at risk" patient. In this chapter we will discuss the rationale, advantages, and limitations of currently available techniques for assessing tissue oxygenation.

Oxygen-Derived Variables

Oxygen Supply, Uptake and Extraction

The measurement of O_2-derived variables provides information about the amount of O_2 transported, used and extracted by the body, but gives no detail about hypoxia. DO_2 represents the amount of O_2 delivered to the peripheral tissues per minute:

$$DO_2 = CI \cdot CaO_2 \cdot 10 \qquad (1)$$

where CI represents the cardiac index and CaO_2 the arterial O_2 content.

$$CaO_2 = (Hb \cdot 1.39 \cdot SaO_2) + 0.0031 \cdot PaO_2 \qquad (2)$$

where Hb represents the hemoglobin level, SaO_2 the arterial O_2 saturation and PaO_2 the arterial O_2 tension. The amount of O_2 dissolved is relatively small and can effectively be ignored (except in the presence of severe anemia) so that equation 1 becomes:

$$DO_2 = CI \cdot Hb \cdot SaO_2 \cdot 13.9 \tag{3}$$

A fall in hemoglobin or SaO_2 will not necessarily result in a fall in DO_2 as CI can increase to compensate, but a fall in CI will result in a fall in DO_2 as Hb and SaO_2 cannot compensate acutely.

O_2 uptake (VO_2) represents the sum of all oxidative metabolic reactions in the body and can be determined indirectly from the Fick equation. In simplified form:

$$VO_2 = CI \cdot 13.9 \cdot Hb \cdot (SaO_2 - SvO_2) \tag{4}$$

where SvO_2 represents the venous O_2 saturation. The use of the thermodilution technique to measure CI is, however, unreliable in the presence of intracardiac shunt, severe tricuspid regurgitation or very low CO, potentially rendering the calculation of VO_2 inaccurate. This calculation also fails to take into account pulmonary VO_2 which can be important in patients with acute lung injury (ALI).

Alternatively, VO_2 can be measured directly by the use of metabolic carts and the analysis of expired gases using the equation:

$$VO_2 = (VI \cdot FiO_2) - (VE \cdot FeO_2) \tag{5}$$

where VI and VE are the volumes of the inspired and expired gases respectively, and FiO_2 and FeO_2 are the inspired and expired O_2 fractions respectively. The technique is cumbersome and requires endotracheal intubation for accurate measurement of expired gases. Inaccuracies may also result from the presence of gas leaks and the interference of other inhaled gases such as anesthetic agents.

The ratio of VO_2 to DO_2 represents the O_2 extraction ratio (O_2ER), and from equations 3 and 4, one can see that it can be easily calculated from arterial blood gas analysis without VO_2 and DO_2 calculations. It is also independent of the Hb in level:

$$O_2ER = VO_2/DO_2 = (SaO_2 - SvO_2)/SaO_2 \tag{6}$$

Many experimental studies have shown that as DO_2 falls, O_2ER increases enabling VO_2 to be maintained [3–9]. However, a point is reached (DO_2crit) below which the increase in O_2ER can no longer compensate for the fall in DO_2 and VO_2 falls, becoming DO_2 dependent. At this point blood lactate levels rise indicating inadequate tissue oxygenation [10, 11]. The analysis of the relationship between VO_2 and DO_2 could thus be used to assess the presence of adequate oxygenation. However, measurement of VO_2 and DO_2 involves complex calculations and cumbersome equipment if metabolic carts are used. Also, the analysis of the relationship between these two parameters could be subject to mathematical coupling of data as several variables (CI, Hb, SaO_2) are used to calculate both DO_2 and VO_2, when VO_2 is measured indirectly.

The straight-line relationship between CI and O_2ER [12] is a simpler alternative that can provide useful information in complex patients. An increase in VO_2 can be achieved by either an increase in CI, an increase in O_2ER or an increase in

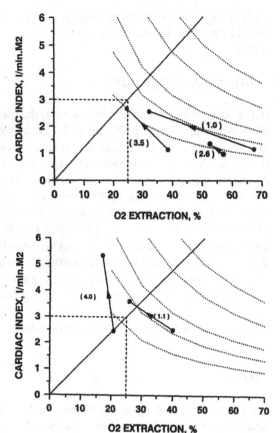

Fig. 1. Examples of the relationship between cardiac index and oxygen extraction before and during the administration of 5 mcg/kg/min of dobutamine in 5 critically ill patients, 3 with heart failure (*top panel*) and 2 with sepsis (*bottom panel*). The lactate level of each patient is shown in parentheses. VO_2/DO_2 dependency can be seen in the three patients with high lactate levels. From [12] with permission.

both. During exercise [13-15], the increase is obtained by similar increases in these two parameters. In critically ill patients, the increase in VO_2 caused by activity such as chest physiotherapy, is also caused by similar increases in CI and O_2ER [16]. To enable interpretation of this relationship, a line of reference is thus drawn through the normal values of 3 l/min/m² for CI and 25% for the O_2ER. Curvilinear lines are added to the diagram to indicate various levels of VO_2. VO_2/DO_2 dependency can be recognized by briefly increasing the DO_2 by, for example, using a small dose (5 mcg/kg/min) of dobutamine [17]. In the presence of VO_2/DO_2 independency, sequential data points will move parallel to the VO_2 isopleths. However, when VO_2/DO_2 dependency, and hence inadequate oxygenation, is present, the data points will move across VO_2 isopleths (Fig. 1). This diagram can, thus, be used to identify tissue hypoxia, and by plotting sequential values can assess the effectiveness of treatment.

SvO_2

SvO_2 can be easily measured at the bedside using a pulmonary artery catheter, either intermittently by withdrawing mixed venous blood samples, or continuously using modified catheters equipped with fiberoptic fibers. It can be influenced by SaO_2 and a more complex factor involving VO_2, CI and the Hb concentration.

$$SvO_2 = SaO_2 - VO_2/(CI \cdot Hb) \tag{7}$$

In the absence of anemia and hypoxemia, the measurement of SvO_2 thus reflects the relationship between VO_2 and CI, and hence the relationship between VO_2 and DO_2. This set of conditions occurs rarely however, and SvO_2 interpretation is thus dependent on the concomitant assessment of other parameters including CI. A reduction in SvO_2 represents an imbalance between VO_2 and DO_2 but in itself does not indicate which factor has altered. It may also be influenced by conditions affecting tissue O_2 extraction such as sepsis and acute respiratory distress syndrome (ARDS). A low SvO_2 may be a global indicator of inadequate oxygenation and of prognostic value but should not be considered in isolation as a healthy individual can have a low SvO_2 during exercise, and a low SvO_2 may be normal in a cardiac-compromised patient. Indeed therapies aimed at raising SvO_2 to normal or supranormal levels in critically patients have not been shown to improve survival [1]. The measurement of SvO_2 each time CI is assessed will enable the most reliable interpretation of these two parameters.

Lactate

Lactate is produced by many tissues, including erythrocytes, skeletal muscle and skin, as the endproduct of glycolysis. A total of 15–20 mEq/kg/day are released and a normal blood level is about 1 mEq/l. Lactate is formed from pyruvate in the cytosol in a reversible reaction catalyzed by lactate dehydrogenase (LDH).

$$\text{Pyruvate} + \text{NADH} + \text{H}^+ \leftrightarrow \text{Lactate} + \text{NAD} \tag{8}$$

The equilibrium of the reaction normally maintains a lactate/pyruvate ratio of about $10:1$. Pyruvate can be metabolized via pyruvate dehydrogenase (PDH) to acetyl-coA, which is then oxidized to carbon dioxide and water, in an irreversible reaction. Alternatively it can be transaminated with glutamate to form alanine and α-ketoglutarate. Lactate production will increase when the rate of pyruvate formation in the cytosol exceeds its utilization in the mitochondria. This may occur during strenuous exercise with a rapid rise in the metabolic rate, or in cases of reduced pyruvate dehydrogenase (PDH) activity. In conditions of adequate O_2 supply, the nicotinamide adenine dinucleotide (NADH) is used to produce adenosine triphosphate (ATP), regenerating NAD^+. However, during hypoxia, this reaction is reduced, the $NADH/NAD^+$ ratio increases and, as can be seen from equation 9, lactate levels rise.

$$\text{Lactate} \leftrightarrow \text{Pyruvate} \cdot \text{Keq} \, (\text{NADH} \cdot \text{H}^+)/\text{NAD} \tag{9}$$

As seen earlier, a fall in DO_2 causes a series of responses in an attempt to maintain a balance between ATP production and the cell's energy requirements. This is largely achieved by an increase in the amount of O_2 extracted from the blood, attained by increasing the number of perfused capillaries per unit of tissue volume. With further decreases in DO_2, this compensatory mechanism becomes inadequate to provide the mitochondria with sufficient O_2 for continued aerobic metabolism. Anaerobic metabolism must therefore be employed to provide ATP, resulting in the increased generation of lactate. Many studies confirm that this point, where VO_2 becomes DO_2 dependent, is associated with raised blood lactate levels [17–20], and levels above 2 mEq/l are widely accepted as a marker of tissue hypoxia.

The presence of raised lactate levels in circulatory shock due to low flow states, occurs predominantly as a result of anaerobic glycolysis and thus provides a marker of inadequate oxygenation. However, in sepsis the situation is more complex and tissue hypoxia, alone, does not seem to be sufficient to account for the raised levels seen. If hypoxia is the main reason for raised lactate levels, one would expect the lactate/pyruvate ratio also to increase, but studies have shown that it may remain normal in sepsis [21]. Several studies have also found that increasing DO_2 to septic patients does not decrease lactate levels [22, 23]. Using [18F] fluoromisonidazole or levels of high energy phosphates as markers of cellular hypoxia in animal models of sepsis, various groups have been unable to demonstrate the presence of hypoxia despite raised lactate levels [21, 24–27]. Other mechanisms have been proposed to account for the raised lactate levels, including reduced PDH activity [28–30], and increased aerobic glycolysis [31–33]. Activation of inflammatory cells including leukocytes may also contribute to increased lactate production. The truth of the matter is probably that lactate production is increased due to altered cellular metabolism as a result of a combination of hypoxia and other unrelated biochemical alterations.

The user of any monitoring system must be aware of its limitations, and blood lactate levels are no exception. We have already seen that their interpretation in sepsis is not straightforward. Other possible limitations include the effects of liver failure, the "wash-out" phenomenon, and the possibility of other causes of hyperlactatemia.

Liver failure: The level of lactate in the blood is a reflection of the balance between its production and its elimination. Lactate is removed predominantly by the liver, although the kidneys and the heart also play a role, and liver failure may therefore influence lactate levels. However, patients with stable cirrhosis have normal lactate levels [34] and the effect of abnormal liver function is probably just to slow the fall of levels raised as the result of shock.

The "wash-out" phenomenon: During early hypovolemic shock, poor tissue perfusion may lead to the sequestration of lactate in regional tissues. When blood flow is restored, the wash-out of this lactate could thus cause a rise in lactate, the reverse of what one would expect with an improvement in patient condition. In an animal study this effect was found to last no longer than 8 minutes after resus-

Table 1. Some causes of raised blood lactate levels

Classically considered hypoxic (type A):
- Circulatory shock
- Severe anemia
- Severe hypoxemia
- Persistent seizures or shivering

Classically considered non-hypoxic (type B):
- Biguanide toxicity
- Alcohol intoxication
- Fructose infusion
- Extensive neoplastic disease
- Severe malnutrition
- Decompensated diabetes
- Inborn errors of metabolism

citation [35] and, while it is therefore probably not significant, the possibility stresses the need for repeated measures rather than relying on a single value.

Other causes: Causes of hyperlactatemia in the critically ill, other than shock, are uncommon but must be excluded (Table 1). The traditionally quoted Cohen and Woods classification [36] which separates causes into those associated with hypoxia and those not is now essentially obsolete as in the majority of cases the hyperlactatemia is probably due to a combination of hypoxia and non-hypoxic mechanisms. For example, neoplastic disease classified as a non-hypoxic cause of hyperlactatemia may in fact have a hypoxic cause as the reduced blood supply in the center of tumors results in hypoxia.

Lactate levels are easily and rapidly measured at the bedside using automated analyzers [37]. High lactate levels have been related to prognosis in various

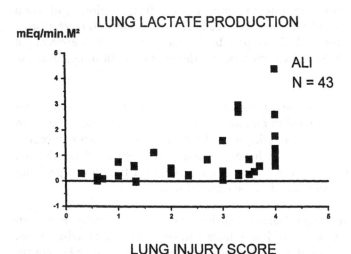

Fig. 2. Relationship between the lung lactate production and the lung injury score in patients with acute lung injury. From [44] with permission.

groups of patients [38–40] and are superior to O_2 derived variables at predicting outcome in septic patients [39,41]. The assessment of repeated values and the duration of hyperlactatemia is of more value than an isolated result [22,39,42,43]. It must be remembered that blood lactate levels represent a global marker of oxygenation and offer no information about local perfusion. The measurement of the arteriovenous difference in blood lactate across an organ may provide a means of identifying regional hypoxia although this technique is not available for routine bedside use. In a recent clinical study involving 122 patients with acute respiratory failure of various causes, De Backer et al. [44] showed that the lungs produce significantly more lactate during acute lung injury than in other causes of respiratory failure such as bronchopneumonia and cardiogenic pulmonary edema. Moreover, they observed that the amount of lactate produced was correlated to the severity of the lung disease (Fig. 2). Recent studies have shown that leukocytes may represent an important source of lactate in septic shock (unpublished observations).

Gastric intramucosal pH (pHi)

All the above methods of monitoring oxygenation provide only global measures and volunteer no information about the situation at tissue level. The gut is particularly sensitive to reductions in blood flow and the measurement of pHi has been suggested as a means of obtaining a more local indicator of hypoxia. This technique, as initially described [45], involves the insertion of a saline-filled, gas-permeable balloon into the gastric lumen. After a defined time (typically at least 30 minutes) allowing for equilibration of the saline solution with the PCO_2 of the gut lumen, a sample is withdrawn and analyzed for PCO_2 using a conventional blood gas analyzer. The pHi is then calculated using the Henderson-Hasselbalch equation:

$$pHi = 16.1 + Log_{10} (arterial [HCO_3^-] / PCO_{2tonometer} \cdot K) \tag{10}$$

where K is a time-dependent equilibration constant provided by the manufacturer which varies according to the tonometer membrane used. The technique is associated with procedural problems including variations dependent on the blood gas analyzer used, the long time interval required for equilibration and errors introduced as a result of poor saline solution manipulation. The use of gas tonometry instead of saline tonometry was therefore proposed, avoiding saline manipulation and allowing for a more rapid equilibration time. This technique has been validated *in vitro* and *in vivo* and results correlate well with those obtained from saline tonometry [46,47]. In the calculation of pHi, it is assumed that the arterial bicarbonate is identical to the intramucosal bicarbonate and thus a patient with, for example, a metabolic acidosis due to renal failure may have a low pHi without necessarily having gut hypoxia. To avoid some of the potential problems associated with the calculation of pHi, it has been suggested that the PCO_2 value itself should be used. This eliminates the need for simultaneous arterial blood sampling thus making it a more simple measure and it has been shown to have a better predictive value than pHi [43]. The PCO_2 of the gastric lumen ($PgCO_2$) is however directly influenced by the $PaCO_2$ so that it may be altered by changes in ventilatory status in the absence of any changes in regional blood flow. The use of the PCO_2 gap, the difference between $PgCO_2$ and $PaCO_2$, avoids any potential confusion in the presence of respiratory acidosis, and facilitates the correct interpretation of $PgCO_2$ values.

pHi values have been correlated with blood lactate levels and outcome, and have been shown to be of more prognostic value than O_2 derived parameters [43, 48–50]. A pHi value less than 7.35 is generally considered to indicate mucosal hypoperfusion [48, 51], and from the limited clinical data available an arterial to mucosal PCO_2 gap of greater than 8 mmHg has been suggested as an indicator of inadequate mucosal perfusion [52]. A study in children receiving extracorporeal life support found the PCO_2 gap to be a better predictor of death than hemodynamic parameters or blood lactate levels [53]. The slow equilibration times associated with the early measurements of pHi made it difficult to apply the results in the acute resuscitation situation. The automated tonometry analyzers now available make the measurement of PCO_2 a more rapid and, hence, more relevant technique [54] although it remains investigational. Only one study [55] has indicated that this form of monitoring may improve outcome and further studies are needed to confirm these results.

Conclusion

The importance of adequate tissue oxygenation in the prevention of multiple organ failure is now appreciated. We have discussed various commonly used methods of monitoring tissue oxygenation but each has its own limitations. O_2-derived variables give no information about the presence of tissue hypoxia. Blood lactate levels supply only a global indication of oxygenation status, while pHi and gastric PCO_2 provide a more regional measure. Importantly, none of the suggested measures should be used in isolation but rather as complements to a full clinical and hemodynamic assessment. The combination of blood lactate levels with pHi values has greater predictive value than either parameter alone [43], stressing the need for a holistic approach to the interpretation of patient parameters. Interpretation of individual values of any parameter should also be avoided, an evaluation of the trend in values being of greater value. Future research must focus on measures capable of identifying regional hypoxia.

References

1. Gattinoni L, Brazzi L, Pelosi P, et al (1995) A trial of goal-oriented hemodynamic therapy in critically ill patients. N Engl J Med 333:1025–1032
2. Hayes MA, Timmins AC, Yau EH, Palazzo M, Hinds CJ, Watson D (1994) Elevation of systemic oxygen delivery in the treatment of critically ill patients. N Engl J Med 330:1717–1722

3. Cain SM (1991) Physiological and pathological oxygen supply dependency. In: Gutierrez G and Vincent JL (eds) Update in intensive care and emergency medicine. Springer Verlag, Berlin, pp 114–123

4. Nelson DP, Beyer C, Samsel RW, Wood LDH, Schumacker PT (1987) Pathological supply dependence of O_2 uptake during bacteremia in dogs. J Appl Physiol 63:1487–1492

5. Bakker J, Vincent JL (1991) The oxygen supply dependency phenomenon is associated with increased blood lactate levels. J Crit Care 6:152–159

6. Zhang H, Spapen H, Benlabed M, Vincent JL (1993) Systemic oxygen extraction can be improved during repeated episodes of cardiac tamponade. J Crit Care 8:93–99

7. Zhang H, Vincent JL (1993) Oxygen extraction is altered by endotoxin during tamponade-induced stagnant hypoxia in the dog. Circ Shock 40:168–176

8. Zhang H, Vincent JL (1993) Arteriovenous differences in PCO_2 and pH are good indicators of critical hypoperfusion. Am Rev Respir Dis 148:867–871

9. Van der Linden P, Gilbert E, Paques P, Simon C, Vincent JL (1993) Influence of hematocrit on tissue O_2 extraction capabilities in anesthetized dogs during acute hemorrhage. Am J Physiol 264:H1942–H1947

10. Shibutani K, Komatsu T, Kubai K, Sarchala V, Kumar V, Bizarri DV (1983) Critical level of oxygen delivery in anesthetized man. Crit Care Med 11:640–643

11. Komatsu T, Shibutani K, Okamoto K, et al (1987) Critical level of oxygen delivery after cardiopulmonary bypass. Crit Care Med 15:194–197

12. Silance PG, Simon C, Vincent JL (1994) The relation between cardiac index and oxygen extraction in acutely ill patients. Chest 105:1190–1197

13. Weber KT, Janicki JS, McElroy PA, Reddy HK (1988) Concepts and applications of cardiopulmonary exercise testing. Chest 93:843–847

14. Astrand PO, Cuddy TE, Saltin B, Stenberg J (1964) Cardiac output during submaximal and maximal work. J Appl Physiol 19:268–274

15. Sutton JR, Reeves JT, Wagner PD, et al (1988) Operation Everest II: Oxygen transport during exercise at extreme simulated altitude. J Appl Physiol 64:1309–1321

16. Weissman C, Kemper M (1991) The oxygen uptake/oxygen delivery relationship during ICU interventions. Chest 99:430–435

17. Vincent JL, Roman A, De Backer D, Kahn RJ (1990) Oxygen uptake/supply dependency: Effects of short-term dobutamine infusion. Am Rev Respir Dis 142:2–8

18. Haupt MT, Gilbert EM, Carlson RW (1985) Fluid loading increases oxygen consumption in septic patients with lactic acidosis. Am Rev Respir Dis 131:912–916

19. Gilbert EM, Haupt MT, Mandanas RY, Huaringa AJ, Carlson RW (1986) The effect of fluid loading, blood transfusion and catecholamine infusion on oxygen delivery and consumption in patients with sepsis. Am Rev Respir Dis 134:873–878

20. Kruse JA, Haupt MT, Puri VK, Carlson RW (1990) Lactate levels as predictors of the relationship between oxygen delivery and consumption in ARDS. Chest 98:959–962

21. Tresadern JC, Threlfall CJ, Wilford K, et al (1988) Muscle adenosine 5 triphosphate and creatine phosphate concentrations in relation to nutritional status and sepsis in man. Clin Sci 75:233–242

22. Vincent JL, Dufaye P, Berre J, Leeman M, Degaute JP, Kahn RJ (1983) Serial lactate determinations during circulatory shock. Crit Care Med 11:449–451

23. Fenwick JC, Dodek PM, Ronco JJ, Phang PT, Wiggs B, Russell JA (1990) Increased concentrations of plasma lactate predict pathological dependence of oxygen consumption on oxygen delivery in patients with adult respiratory distress syndrome. J Crit Care 5:81–87

24. Hotchkiss RS, Rust RS, Dence CS, et al (1991) Evaluation of the role of cellular hypoxia in sepsis by the hypoxic marker [^{18}F] fluoromisonidazole. Am J Physiol 261:R965–R972

25. Myrvold HE, Enger E, Haljamäe H (1975) Early effect of endotoxin on tissue phosphagen levels in skelatal muscle and liver of the dog. Eur Surg Res 7:181–192

26. Chaudry IH, Wichterman KA, Baue AE (1979) Effect of sepsis on tissue adenine nucleotide levels. Surgery 85:205–211

27. Jepson MM, Cox M, Bates PC, et al (1987) Regional blood flow and skeletal muscle energy status in endotoxemic rats. Am J Physiol 253:E581–E587

28. Preiser JC, Moulart D, Vincent JL (1990) Dichloroacetate administration in the treatment of endotoxin shock. Circ Shock 30:221–228
29. Kilpatrick-Smith L, Erecinska M (1983) Cellular effects of endotoxin in vitro. I. Effect of endotoxin on mitochondrial substrate metabolism and intracellular calcium. Circ Shock 11:85–99
30. Curtis SE, Cain SM (1992) Regional and systemic oxygen delivery/uptake relations and lactate flux in hyperdynamic endotoxin treated dogs. Am Rev Respir Dis 145:348–354
31. Hotchkiss RS, Karl IE (1992) Reevaluation of the role of cellular hypoxia and bioenergetic failure in sepsis. JAMA 267:1503–1510
32. Wolfe RR, Elahi D, Spitzer JJ (1977) Glucose and lactate kinetics after endotoxin administration in dogs. Am J Physiol 232:E180–E185
33. Gore DC, Jahoor F, Hibbert JM, DeMaria EJ (1996) Lactic acidosis during sepsis is related to increased pyruvate production, not deficits in tissue oxygen availability. Ann Surg 224:97–102
34. Owen OE, Reichle FA, Mozzoli MA, et al (1981) Hepatic, gut and renal substrate flux rates in patients with hepatic cirrhosis. J Clin Invest 68:240–252
35. Leavy JA, Weil MH, Rackow EC (1988) "Lactate washout" following circulatory arrest. JAMA 260:662–664
36. Cohen RD, Woods HF (1976) Clinical and biochemical aspects of lactic acidosis. Blackwell Scientific Publications, London
37. Aduen J, Bernstein WK, Khastgir T, et al (1994) The use and clinical importance of a substrate-specific electrode for rapid determination of blood lactate concentrations. JAMA 272:1678–1685
38. Broder G, Weil MH (1964) Excess lactate: An index of reversibility of shock in human patients. Science 143:1457–1459
39. Bakker J, Gris P, Coffernils M, Kahn RJ, Vincent JL (1996) Serial blood lactate levels can predict the development of multiple organ failure following septic shock. Am J Surg 171:221–226
40. Roumen RM, Redl H, Schlag G, Sandtner W, Koller W, Goris JA (1993) Scoring systems and blood lactate concentrations in relation to the development of adult respiratory distress syndrome and multiple organ failure in severely traumatized patients. J Trauma 35:349–355
41. Bakker J, Coffernils M, Leon M, Gris P, Vincent JL (1991) Blood lactate levels are superior to oxygen derived variables in predicting outcome in human septic shock. Chest 99:956–962
42. Waxman K, Nolan LS, Shoemaker WC (1982) Sequential perioperative lactate determination: physiological and clinical implications. Crit Care Med 10:96–99
43. Friedman G, Berlot G, Kahn RJ, Vincent JL (1995) Combined measurements of blood lactate concentrations and gastric intramucosal pH in patients with severe sepsis. Crit Care Med 23:1184–1193
44. De Backer D, Creteur J, Zhang H, Norrenberg M, Vincent JL (1997) Lactate production by the lungs in acute lung injury. Am J Respir Crit Care Med 156:1099–1104
45. Fiddian-Green RG, Pittenger G, Whitehouse WM (1982) Back-diffusion of CO_2 and its influence on the intramural pH in gastric intestines of rats. J Surg Res 33:39–48
46. Creteur J, De Backer D, Vincent JL (1997) Monitoring of gastric mucosal PCO_2 by gas tonometry: In vitro and in vivo validation studies. Anesthesiology 87:504–510
47. Kolkman JJ, Zwaarekant LJ, Boshuizen L, et al (1997) In vitro evaluation of intragastric PCO_2 measurement by air tonometry. J Clin Monit 13:115–119
48. Doglio GR, Pusajo JF, Egurrola MA, et al (1991) Gastric mucosal pH as a prognostic index of mortality in critically ill patients. Crit Care Med 19:1037–1040
49. Mythen MG, Webb AR (1994) The role of gut mucosal hypoperfusion in the pathogenesis of post-operative organ dysfunction. Intensive Care Med 20:203–209
50. Ivatury RR, Simon RJ, Havriliak D, Garcia C, Greenbarg J, Stahl WM (1995) Gastric mucosal pH and oxygen delivery and oxygen consumption indices in the assessment of adequacy of resuscitation after trauma: a prospective, randomized study. J Trauma 39:128–134
51. Maynard N, Bihari D, Beale R, et al (1993) Assessment of splanchnic oxygenation by gastric tonometry in patients with acute circulatory failure. JAMA 270:1203–1210

52. Mythen M, Faehnrich j (1996) Monitoring gut perfusion. In: Rombeau JL and Takala J (eds) Gut Dysfunction in critical illness. Springer-Verlag, Berlin, pp 246–262
53. Duke T, Butt W, South M, Shann F (1997) The DCO_2 measured by gastric tonometry predicts survival in children receiving extracorporeal life support. Comparison with other hemodynamic and biochemical information. Chest 111:174–179
54. Heinonen PO, Jousela IT, Blomqvist KA, Olkkola KT, Takkunen OS (1997) Validation of air tonometric measurement of gastric regional concentrations of CO_2 in critically ill septic patients. Intensive Care Med 23:524–529
55. Gutierrez G, Palizas F, Doglio G, et al (1992) Gastric intramucosal pH as a therapeutic index of tissue oxygenation in critically ill patients. Lancet 339:195–199

Microcirculatory Flows, Microcirculatory Responsiveness, Microcirculatory and Regional (Arteriolar/Venular) O_2 Saturations

C. Ellis

Introduction

The ability to assess tissue oxygenation is essential in a wide variety of clinical settings. It is also essential in experimental studies designed to investigate the underlying causes of organ injury due to inadequate oxygen (O_2) availability. With the recognition that microvascular perfusion abnormalities may play a significant role in impaired tissue oxygenation there has been a proliferation in the past decade of experimental and clinical techniques for measuring tissue oxygenation at the microvascular level.

Some of these methodologies are refinements of existing technologies while others represent new approaches to the problem. A number of the techniques are designed to measure blood flow with the assumption that impaired blood flow will reflect a loss of O_2 delivery (DO_2) to the tissue. These techniques include laser Doppler flowmetry [1], magnetic resonance imaging (MRI) [2], microspheres [3]. Other techniques measure tissue O_2 levels, i.e., the partial pressure of O_2 (PO_2), using either surface [4] or needle O_2 electrodes [5], or O_2 levels in the vasculature as either the PO_2 in plasma with phosphorescence quenching [6] or the hemoglobin (Hb) O_2 saturation (SO_2) with near infrared spectrophotometry [7] or functional MRI (fMRI) [8]. Several approaches attempt to measure important O_2 transport parameters such as capillary transit times (combined microsphere and histology [9]) or relative changes in O_2 saturation and blood flow (combined MRI flow and fMRI [10]). At the most basic level are the intravital video microscopy (IVVM) techniques for measuring red blood cell (RBC) flow and O_2 transport in arterioles [11], venules and capillaries from direct measurements of RBC flow [12] and RBC SO_2 in these vessels [13].

Since microvascular perfusion abnormalities may be due to impaired arteriolar control of microvascular blood flow or to a loss of perfused capillaries, techniques have been developed to assess arteriolar responsiveness to a variety of stimuli [14] and to quantify changes in capillary perfusion patterns [15].

This chapter will address techniques for measuring (i) microvascular blood flow, (ii) arteriolar responsiveness to physiological or pharmaceutical stimuli, and (iii) SO_2 in arterioles, venules and capillaries and the arteriolar to venular SO_2 gradient. References to other techniques for measuring O_2 levels or O_2 transport parameters will be made where relevant to the discussion. Techniques which can be used clinically or have the potential to be used clinically will be discussed separately. Before presenting the details of the methodologies, some background information on the microvasculature and the scale of microvascular perfusion abnormalities will be presented.

Microvasculature

The term "microvasculature" refers to blood vessels that are too small to be seen without the aid of a microscope. Typically arterioles are small blood vessels on the arterial side of the capillary bed ranging in size from approximately 10 µm to 150 µm in diameter. Arterioles have smooth muscle cells and can actively alter vascular resistance. Capillaries are endothelial tubes (no smooth muscle cells) with diameters ranging from 3 to 8 µm. In some organs such as lung, mesentery and gut, capillary diameters may be substantially larger (in the range from 10–20 µm). Venules are the venous counterpart to the arteriolar vessels and their diameters tend to be larger than the corresponding arteriolar vessel. O_2 exchange between RBCs and tissue occurs in all three types of microvessels (arterioles, capillaries, venules) [16].

An example of a microvascular bed is given in Figure 1. This figure shows a composite image of the microvasculature in the extensor digitorum longus (EDL) muscle of the rat obtained using an intravital video microscopy (Leitz Metalux microscope, 10X objective, 431-nm interference filter to enhance image contrast). The overall field of view is approximately 1.6×3.0-mm. The muscle is approximately 1 mm thick and the weight of the tissue sample represented in this figure is less than 0.05 gms. The thick dark vertical line in the center of the image is the paired first order arteriole and venule (largest microvessels in a tissue are classified as 1st order, subsequent branches are 2nd, 3rd and 4th order, etc). In this tissue the 1st order arteriole is approximately 50 µm in diameter and the 1st order venule 100 µm in diameter. Second order arterioles (10 to 25 µm) branch from the 1st order arteriole (bifurcations not visible in Fig. 1) and run diagonally across the muscle fibers (oriented vertically in the image). The 2nd order arterioles branch into smaller 3rd and 4th order arterioles (terminal arterioles) that are directly connected to the capillaries. The capillary bed is made up of networks of diverging and converging capillary segments (the network of thin black lines running parallel to the muscle fibers in Fig. 1). The average distance (pathlength) across the capillary network from arteriole to venule is approximately 500 µm. The capillaries drain into collecting venules, which converge into larger 3rd and 2nd order venules (10 to 50 µm). These vessels also run diagonally across the tissue to the 1st order venule. The architecture of the microvascular bed, in this three-dimensional tissue, is not a simple ordered structure of repeating arteriolar-capillary-venular units arranged uniformly across the muscle. In some areas an arteriole tree overlaps with a venular tree without any direct vascular connections between them.

Figure 1 will be referred to throughout this chapter to help provide a perspective to the scale of the measurements that are being made by the various techniques. In making these comparisons, one should be aware that there are differ-

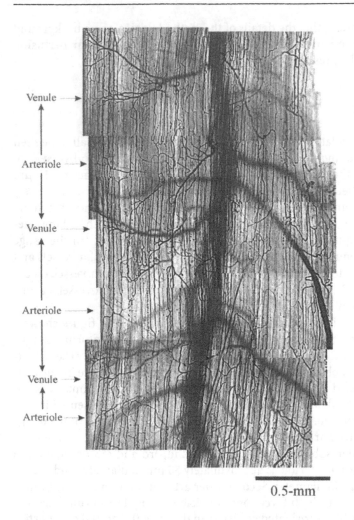

0.5-mm

Fig. 1. Composite image of the microvasculature in the extensor digitorum longus muscle of the rat obtained from video images recorded at 10 × magnification. The "Arteriole" and "Venule" labels on the left edge of the image point to the terminal ends of the arteriolar and venular trees at that location in the muscle. The arrows between the labels indicate the direction of blood flow through the capillary network that these vessels serve. Note the arteriolar-capillary-venular unit approximately 0.25 mm from the left edge of the image that overlaps the collecting venule originating at the edge of the image (second labeled venule from the top). The scale marker is 0.5 mm

ences between the microvascular bed represented in this figure and that in other organs and in other species.

In the literature there is some confusion with the use of the term microvasculature. In microsurgery, vessels 1 to 2 mm in diameter are referred to as microvessels and techniques for measuring the perfusion of these vessels are said to measure microvascular blood flow. Although these vessels are important for delivery of blood flow to the microvascular bed they should not be classified as part of the microvasculature. A number of the new medical imaging techniques (Doppler ultrasound MRI, fMRI) claim to measure microvascular perfusion or microvascular oxygenation even though the spatial resolution of these systems is not sufficient to resolve individual microvessels. The use of the term may, however, be justified since it is believed that the signal measured by these techniques originates from the microvasculature, i.e., from a population of microvessels within the sample volume [17].

Scale

Tissue oxygenation is often quantified in terms of O_2 parameters that can be derived from the entire organ, e.g. venous PO_2 or SO_2 levels, O_2 extraction ratio, average tissue PO_2 level (tPO_2), or microvascular PO_2 (mPO_2 or SO_2 (mSO_2) levels. If DO_2 to the tissue falls it is assumed that changes in these parameters will reflect the changes in tissue oxygenation. The assumption, inherent in the use of these parameters, is that impaired oxygenation will be uniform or homogeneous throughout the tissue. However, with a microvascular dysfunction, one anticipates that a maldistribution of DO_2 within the organ will have a heterogeneous effect on tissue oxygenation. In this case whole organ or mean O_2 levels will not be sufficient to describe the state of tissue oxygenation.

What data is sufficient to quantify tissue oxygenation in the presence of a maldistribution of microvascular O_2 delivery? First, one must recognize that there is significant heterogeneity of perfusion and tissue oxygenation in normal tissue. It is assumed that the observed heterogeneity reflects the microvascular regulation of DO_2 to match the local metabolic needs of the tissue. An alternative explanation is that normal healthy tissue can tolerate considerable heterogeneity of perfusion, i.e., the regulation of microvascular perfusion does not need to be that precise since diffusion exchange of O_2 between different levels of the microvasculature and the tissue ensures that all regions receive adequate DO_2 [16].

However, in disease the situation may be very different. Loss of arteriolar control of DO_2 may cause a significant maldistribution of DO_2 among arterioles. If the arteriolar dysfunction occurs at the level of 1st order arterioles then large regions of tissue (on a microvascular scale) will experience similar changes in DO_2, e.g., if DO_2 to the 1st arteriole in Figure 1 fell below the critical level for maintaining tissue oxygenation then a region larger than that represented by Figure 1 (approximately 10 mm^3 or greater) would be affected. If however, the arteriolar dysfunction occurred at the level of 2nd or 3rd order arterioles, then some regions in Figure 1 (each approximately 1 mm^3 or smaller) would be over-perfused while others would be under-perfused. Another type of microvascular dysfunction might cause an increased heterogeneity of capillary perfusion while arteriolar flow regulation remained intact. In this extreme case, the scale of impaired tissue oxygenation would be very small, i.e., less than 0.001 mm^3, the volume of tissue supplied by each capillary.

There are several challenges facing any attempt to quantify tissue oxygenation in the presence of a maldistribution of microvascular DO_2. The first is to select a technique that will have sufficient resolution to detect the abnormality. The second is to analyze and to present the data in a manner that properly represents the state of tissue oxygenation.

Microcirculatory Flow: Experimental Techniques

Techniques for measuring microvascular blood flow can be divided into invasive and non-invasive techniques. Invasive techniques include injection of microspheres, and intravital video microscopy (IVVM). Non-invasive techniques include laser Doppler flowmetry, perfusion sensitive MRI and high frequency Doppler ultrasound.

The use of labeled microspheres to measure blood flow distribution within an organ is well established. Microspheres of a diameter large enough (15 μm) to be trapped in the terminal arteriolar bed are injected into either the left atrium or the artery supplying the specific organ. The tissue is then cut into small uniform samples (from 0.1 to 2 g) and the flow within each sample calculated. The heterogeneity of perfusion can then be determined from the standard deviation (SD) of the flow measurements or as the relative dispersion (RD = SD/mean flow). Two important extensions of this technique have been developed in the past decade.

Fractal dimension: Bassingthwaighte et al. [3] have determined that the blood flow heterogeneity in a number of organs has a fractal nature. Their hypothesis was based on the observation that the relative dispersion of flow measured by microspheres increased as the spatial resolution of the measurements increased (i.e., the smaller the tissue samples the greater the value of RD). They found that the relative dispersion of flows within an organ for a given spatial resolution (sample size) could be expressed as:

$$RD(m) = RD(mref) \cdot [m/mref]1-D$$

where m is the mass of the tissue sample in grams, mref is the mass of a reference sample of arbitrary size (usually chosen to be 1 g) and D is the fractal dimension. Bassingthwaighte et al. [3] found that this relationship holds over a wide range of sample sizes indicating that the heterogeneity of microvascular blood flow follows a fractal relationship. They developed a protocol for determining the fractal dimension for each organ they analyzed. By cutting all of the samples into the smallest sample size and carefully ordering the resulting data, they were able to reconstruct the relative dispersion for a range of larger sample sizes by combining the data from adjacent pieces into larger and larger samples. Using this approach they determined that D for the myocardium was 1.2 which suggests a strong correlation between local flows (D = 1.0 indicates uniform flow; D = 1.5 indicates random flow distribution). They showed that simple fractal models of vascular networks yielded similar fractal dimensions for the computed flow distributions [18].

One would expect that the distribution of microvascular flow would be different if it were distributed based on metabolic needs rather than on the unregulated (passive) geometry of the vascular bed. Even though the degree of heterogeneity of perfusion might be the same, the distribution would be different. This would be reflected in the fractal dimension. Kleen et al. have used the approach to study myocardial blood flow heterogeneity in shock [19] and the effect of positive end-expiratory pressure perfusion patterns in the lung following lung injury [20].

Capillary transit time: The second advance in the analysis of microsphere data was the development by Allard et al. [9] of a technique for estimating capillary erythrocyte transit time. Again, the tissue is cut into small pieces and the blood flow within each is determined. The blood volume within each tissue sample is determined using chromium-51 labeled RBCs. The volume of blood associated with the capillary bed is determined from histological analysis of the proportion of capillaries to total vascular volume. The capillary erythrocyte transit time is estimated from the ratio of capillary blood volume divided by blood flow. The approach has been used to estimate regional distribution of transit times in the myocardium [9] and the small intestine [21, 22]. Walley [23] has used the distribution of capillary transit times in a simple O_2 transport model to theoretically demonstrate that heterogeneity of DO_2 impairs O_2 extraction. Walley's model was applied to data on the small intestine in endotoxemic pigs to demonstrate that increased heterogeneity of capillary transit times may account for the impaired O_2 extraction found in sepsis [21].

Allard et al. [9] made two important points about the technique which should be considered when interpreting results obtained with this approach. First, the estimate of capillary volume is based on the assumption that all vessels counted in the histological sections were perfused. In the original report myocardial blood volume showed greater heterogeneity than capillary density derived from histology, implying that there were different degrees of perfusion of the capillary bed. A change in perfused capillary density as occurs with sepsis [15] would not be detected in the estimate of capillary transit time. Second, the capillary transit time estimated from the capillary blood volume divided by the blood flow is not the same as the actual RBC transit time across the capillary bed (capillary pathlength/RBC velocity) [24–26]. Although the local blood flow is an important determinant of the red cell velocity in capillaries, capillary blood volumes estimated from histology do not reflect the distribution of capillary pathlengths from arteriole to venule. Pathlength is determined by the distance between arterioles and venules, i.e., by the architecture of the microvascular bed.

To put the capillary transit time data in perspective, the tissue sample represented by Figure 1 corresponds to less than 0.05 g. The smallest tissue samples used for estimating transit time above was 0.1 g [22] and the largest was a 1 cm length of small intestine [21]. Clearly the heterogeneity of transit times investigated in these studies correspond to heterogeneity on a much larger scale than that of the arteriolar tree or the capillary bed represented in this figure. Although microspheres are trapped in the terminal arterioles, the volume of tissue necessary to properly estimate regional flow is large relative to the scale of the microvasculature. Thus the erythrocyte capillary transit time distribution as developed by Allard et al. [9] and the fractal dimension by Bassingthwaighte et al. [3] are useful indices of the heterogeneity of regional perfusion but not directly of microvascular perfusion.

Intravital Video Microscopy

Background: Techniques for measuring microvascular blood flow using IVVM actually measure either RBC velocity or RBC supply rate and not the blood flow directly. This is an important distinction since in the microvasculature blood can no longer be considered to be a homogeneous fluid but rather a suspension of RBCs (plus white blood cells and platelets) in plasma. As the diameter of the vasculature approaches that of the size of the RBCs a number of unique rheological factors come into play that have a significant impact on microvascular perfusion.

For flow measurements, the most significant is the separation between RBCs and plasma. As blood traverses the arteriolar tree and the diameter of arterioles at each generation becomes smaller, the mean velocity of RBCs relative to the plasma becomes greater. A consequence of this phenomenon is a fall in tube hematocrit (Hct) with decreasing arteriolar diameter known as the Fahreaus effect [27]. Another consequence of the particulate nature of blood is the separation of RBCs and plasma at microvascular bifurcations [28]. As the diameter of arterioles becomes smaller there is an increase in the preferential distribution of RBCs into the vessel with the higher flow (and a preferential distribution of plasma into the vessel with the lower flow). This effect becomes more pronounced at lower Hcts [29]. Since arterioles are a branching tree structure there can be a cascade effect resulting in significant differences in Hct between arterioles. A similar phenomenon can occur in capillary networks although the mechanisms involved may be different [30].

Arteriolar measurements: Since plasma is invisible in microscope images (unless one uses a plasma marker) most techniques rely on measuring the flow of RBCs. Red cell velocities are measured based on fluctuations in light intensity obtained from the centerline of the vessel that correspond to the passage of RBCs through the vessel. The most popular techniques are based on sampling light intensity data at two locations of known separation along the vessel and determining temporal shift between the two signals (temporal correlation [11]; i.e. determining how long it takes RBCs to travel from one location to the next). In arterioles (and venules) the velocities are too high (> 1 mm/sec in the terminal arterioles) to use standard video images, so separate devices which operate at faster than video rates (30 frames/sec) have been developed.

Blood flow in arterioles and venules is estimated based on vessel diameter and an empirically derived multiplication factor of 1.6 relating centerline RBC velocity to mean blood velocity. Although Ellsworth and Pittman [31] have shown that blood flow estimated in this way does not accurately reflect arteriolar flows (due to asymmetric velocity profiles) most blood flow measurements rely on this approach.

Another approach is to measure the RBC flowrate rather than blood flowrate. In arteriolar sized vessels the velocity and Hct are too high to count the individual RBCs passing through the vessel over time. Pries et al. [32] have estimated RBC flowrate as the product of RBC velocity and the local Hct [33]. Another technique using fluorescently labeled RBCs has been developed to directly measure red cell flowrate [34]. Blood is withdrawn from the animal and labeled with a fluorescent dye. These labeled cells are then injected into the animal such that approximately 1% of the circulating RBCs are labeled. The exact numbers of labeled and unlabeled RBCs are determined using flow cytometry. The number of RBCs passing a specific point in the vessel during a measured time period are counted (for sampling statistics at least 100 labeled cells must be counted). From this data one can calculate the total number of RBCs per minute flowing through the vessel without assumptions concerning velocity profiles or plasma flowrates. However, the technique is time consuming and only vessels visible in the same field of view can be measured simultaneously.

There are few microvascular studies that have directly measured the heterogeneity of blood flow at the arteriolar level. The most extensive set of data has been compiled by Pries et. al. [32] on blood flow in the mesentery. They have measured blood flow in as many as 90 vessels in the same mesenteric microvascular bed. No data this extensive has been compiled on another microvascular bed that could be compared with the heterogeneity of perfusion estimated using fractal analysis or erythrocyte capillary transit time.

Capillary measurements: A number of techniques have been developed to measure capillary hemodynamics. Since capillaries in most organs have diameters that are less than the RBC size, RBCs must deform to enter a capillary and usually travel in single file through the vessel separated by plasma gaps. Capillary hemodynamics have been measured with similar tools to those developed for larger microvessels. Since capillary red cell velocities are much lower (mean resting velocity in skeletal muscle 0.15 mm/sec), analysis of video images is possible.

The simplest method for measuring RBC velocity is the flying spot technique developed by Tyml and Ellis [35]. The velocity of a reference spot is varied until its velocity appears to match that of the RBCs in a specific capillary. The advantage of this technique is that it can be used on video images at relatively low magnifications. Automated techniques similar to those developed for arteriolar flow have also been developed. Since capillary RBC velocity is highly variable with both zero velocities and flow reversals being common in disease models, spatial correlation techniques are better suited for capillary measurements [36].

Other parameters that are important to measure, are the number of RBCs per length of capillary (lineal density – RBC/mm; Hct can be calculated from lineal density if RBC and capillary volume are known), the number of RBCs per second passing through the capillary (supply rate – RBC/sec) and the distance between RBCs (plasma gap length, mm) [12]. As RBC velocity is not a good measure of blood flow in the microvasculature, velocity is not a good measure of RBC supply rate in capillaries since the lineal density (Hct) is highly variable among these vessels [30]. Two capillaries with the same velocity may carry very different numbers of RBCs and thus their potential for O_2 transport is very different. In capillaries with low lineal densities, the length of the plasma gap between RBCs is also very important for O_2 transport. RBCs are the primary carriers of O_2 since plasma has a very low solubility for O_2. If the plasma gap is large, O_2 in the plasma may be depleted since not enough O_2 can be transported from the RBC to the plasma to maintain the plasma PO_2 levels [37]. This effectively reduces the surface area available for O_2 diffusion from the capillary to the tissue. Thus capillaries with low lineal densities have a lower potential for O_2 transport and a lower surface area available for diffusion. Plasma gap length will play a significant role at a very low systemic Hct or in diseases that increase the heterogeneity of RBC distribution within the capillary bed. Note, the heterogeneity of these O_2 transport parameters creates a very complex situation for tissue oxygenation. Simple concepts such as capillary density and capillary transit time have less defined influences on tissue oxygenation.

We have developed a technique for measuring these parameters based on the sample of light intensities (1 pixel wide × 100 pixels long) along the axis of a capillary from video tape recordings [12]. By replaying the video tape and sampling over the time period, simultaneous data can be obtained for other capillaries in focus in the same field of view. Although computer algorithms have been developed to automatically make these measurements, we also display the data in the form of a space-time image (Fig. 2). The vertical axis of the image represents position along the capillary, and the horizontal axis the time of each sample. The dark diagonal bands are RBCs as they move through the capillary over time. The slope of a line at any location represents the velocity of that RBC at that instant. The lineal density is the number of dark bands at a specific time; the supply rate is the number of bands crossing a specific location in one second. The plasma gap length is the vertical distance between bands. The space-time image provides a rapid means of assessing the quality of the video sample and the accuracy of the computer analysis. As well, it provides a simple means of demonstrating the dynamic variability in each of these parameters over time.

Several groups have measured the spatial heterogeneity of capillary RBC velocity [38]. Tyml [39] has published data on the heterogeneity of red cell velocity

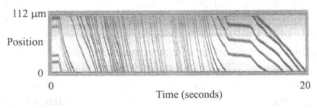

112 μm

Position

0

0   20

Time (seconds)

Fig. 2. Space-time image of red blood cell flow for 20 seconds through a 112 μm segment of a single capillary. The dark bands are the red blood cells as they traverse the sample region (from top to bottom). The light regions in between are the plasma gaps separating the red blood cells. Variation in the background light intensity along the length of the vessel can also be observed. At time zero there are four red blood cells in the sample region with zero velocity. A second later the velocity has increased and these cells rapidly leave the image. In total 55 red blood cells traverse this section of the capillary in 20 seconds with highly variable velocities (measured using the flying spot technique) in capillaries of skeletal muscle. Tyml expresses heterogeneity as the coefficient of variation (CV = SD/mean) which is the same as the relative dispersion used in the fractal analysis. He found that the heterogeneity was reduced in response to an increase in perfusion [39, 40] or a decrease in systemic Hct [41]. This data is unique because the confounding effect of temporal variations in velocity was eliminated by sampling all of the vessels in one field of view simultaneously (video tape replayed for each capillary). The region analyzed in these studies was less than 1 mm^2 with no more than two or three terminal arterioles supplying the capillaries that were analyzed. Thus the source of the heterogeneity of velocities among these capillaries originated partially from the difference in perfusion among the terminal arterioles. However, the capillary bed itself also contributed to the heterogeneity. In another study [30] on the perfusion of a capillary network supplied by a single terminal arteriole, we demonstrated that a significant amount of the heterogeneity of capillary perfusion originated within the capillary bed. The network structure of diverging and converging vessels together with the unique rheological properties of RBCs flowing through capillary bifurcations contribute to this heterogeneity. The reduction in perfusion heterogeneity among capillaries as flow increased appeared to be related to a more uniform distribution of RBCs at capillary bifurcations.

Summary: Research into fractal analysis of blood flow is significant because it provides a means for quantifying the type of flow heterogeneity that is occurring within an organ using a very simple parameter that is not dependent on the spatial resolution of the sample. Although Bassingthwaighte's original work [3] was based on microsphere data, the same analysis could be applied to flow data obtained using non-invasive techniques. The erythrocyte capillary transit time analysis is important because it attempts to quantify a maldistribution in microvascular blood flow in terms that directly apply to an O_2 transport dysfunction. The IVVM studies are significant because they demonstrate another level of heterogeneity of perfusion that cannot be quantified by the microsphere studies quoted above, i.e., the heterogeneity that originates within the capillary network itself and is not due to differences in perfusion among arterioles. Since capillaries play an important role in tissue oxygenation it is likely that changes in heterogeneity at the capillary level will play a significant role in tissue oxygenation. The heterogeneity referred to here is very different from the heterogeneity quantified using Bassingthwaighte et al.'s [3] fractal analysis or with Allard et al.'s [9] distribution of erythrocyte capillary transit times since both the scale and source of the heterogeneity is different.

Clinical Techniques

There are two techniques which can be used clinically to evaluate microvascular blood flow: laser Doppler flowmetry and perfusion sensitive MRI. Another technique in the experimental stage, high frequency Doppler ultrasound, may prove useful for clinical application in the near future.

Laser Doppler Flowmetry

Laser Doppler flowmetry measures the Doppler shift of light scattered back from red cells as they flow through the microvasculature of the sample volume of tissue independent of the orientation of the flow direction [42]. The strength of the acquired signal is a measure of the number of scattering particles and hence of the number of RBCs sampled. Thus the laser Doppler system provides a measure of the RBC "flux" or flowrate in the microcirculation. Typically the sample volume is a hemisphere 1 μm in diameter at the surface of the organ. However, the exact size of the sample volume is determined by the optical properties of the tissue and, hence, cannot be defined. The laser Doppler system cannot be calibrated nor can the output be presented in absolute terms such as mL blood/100 gm/min although several publications make this claim. However, the laser Doppler system is an excellent tool for following temporal changes in microvascular perfusion at a specific location. This system can be used to map out the spatial heterogeneity in perfusion [43] but one must be careful in interpreting these results. The light penetration depth may vary from area to area and one cannot distinguish whether the sample volume includes only capillaries, or terminal arterioles and collecting venules as well. For example, imagine moving the laser probe across the microvascular bed depicted in Figure 1. Even if capillary perfusion were relatively uniform throughout the tissue, certain regions would appear to have much higher "RBC flux" because of the concentration of arteriolar or venular vessels. The laser Doppler system is limited to making surface measurements (penetration depth approximately 1 μm).

Perfusion Sensitive MRI

Perfusion sensitive MRI has developed rapidly in the past 15 years as a non-invasive method for measuring blood flow. A variety of techniques were developed to measure flow in the macrovasculature of an organ that relied on the movement of blood relative to the stationary tissue, to generate a detectable signal. In effect, the blood itself was used as an endogenous tracer. For example, in one time-of-flight method [2], a thin slice of tissue was excited using radio-frequency pulses such that the tissue and blood would be encoded. The encoded volume associated with flowing blood would be displaced before the signal was received. By determining the spatial displacement of the volume and dividing by the time between excitation and reception, the mean velocity of the blood flow could be measured. These approaches have been refined further by allowing enough time to pass for "tagged" volumes in arteries to be displaced into the capillary bed and exchanged with the tissue. An alternate approach measures the inflow of "untagged" blood into the encoded slice. Kim and Tsekos [10] have developed a flow-sensitive alternating inversion recovery (FAIR) technique for measuring cerebral blood flow in absolute units of mL/100 gm/min. Using a 4T whole body imaging system, they reported an in-plane resolution of 0.94×0.94 mm^2 with a slice thickness of 5 mm and blood flow in absolute units. To improve temporal resolution they have extended the FAIR technique to sample multiple slices [44].

High Frequency Doppler Ultrasound

Conventional Doppler utrasound operating in the 2 to 10 Mhz frequency range can measure flow in vessels from 4 to 40 mm in diameter with velocities ranging from 10 to 100 cm/sec. This resolution is not sufficient to sample even the largest arterioles. However, high frequency Doppler ultrasound (20 to 100 MHz), does have the resolution to detect and quantify flow in individual arterioles and possibly from the capillary bed [45]. Using a high frequency (50 MHz) pulsed wave Doppler ultrasound system, Foster and colleagues [46] have reported measuring flows in arterioles as small as 20 to 35 μm. With further development this high-resolution ultrasound system will be able to map the architecture of the arteriolar bed non-invasively, while providing flow information for each vessel. However, attenuation of the high frequency ultrasound signal limits the measurement to the organ surface (penetration depth only a few millimeters).

Summary

Both the laser Doppler flowmetry system and flow sensitive MRI can sample blood flow in volumes of tissue that are smaller than that achieved with microsphere techniques. The sample volume with the laser Doppler system is smaller than for the MRI, but the measurements are limited to the surface of organs that can be exposed for study and the data cannot be presented in absolute terms. MRI can provide non-invasive flow measurements in absolute terms throughout an organ but it is a very expensive technique. Clearly, the fractal analysis of blood flow heterogeneity can be investigated using either technique. Neither system is able to measure changes in the heterogeneity of perfusion within the sample volume if the overall level of perfusion remains the same. The high frequency Doppler ultrasound system has promise for measuring flow heterogeneity on an even smaller scale, but again the measurements will be limited to the surface of an organ.

Microcirculatory Responsiveness

The responsiveness of arterioles to a variety of stimuli can be tested both *in vitro* and *in vivo*.

In Vitro

Arterioles can be isolated from a variety of organs (brain, cheek pouch, diaphragm) and cannulated with glass pipettes on the stage of a light microscope to be studied either under conditions of static pressure [47] or perfused at a known flowrate. After cannulating an arteriole, the vessel is exposed to normal physiologic pressure to ensure it develops vascular tone (i.e., constricts to approximate *in vivo* dimensions) and that there are no leaks in the system. One can then test the response of the arterioles to a variety of stimuli by measuring the change in luminal diameter at a given pressure. Repeating the measurements without an intact endothelium can be used to test the role of the vascular endothelium in the response [48]. Shear dependent phenomenon can be studied using the perfused system.

In Vivo

Similar studies can be performed on an *in vivo* microvascular preparation using an intravital microscope. A variety of preparations have been studied (pial vessels on the surface of the brain, mesentery, hamster cheek pouch, cremaster muscle, extensor digitorum longus muscle). There are two ways in which the studies have been performed. In one, the preparation is superfused with a physiological solution and the diameter of arterioles recorded. The vasoactive agent can then be added to the superfusion solution to a known concentration and the vascular response recorded [49].

A disadvantage of this approach is that the entire microvascular bed is exposed to the test substance. Changes in perfusion or pressure elsewhere in the microvascular bed may confound the response in the vessels under study.

An alternative approach, is to apply a small volume of drug at a specific site in the microvasculature [50, 51]. The microvascular preparation is covered by a layer of paraffin oil trapping a thin layer of physiological solution at the surface

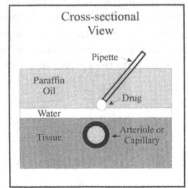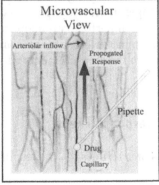

Fig. 3. The left panel shows a cross-sectional view of the application of a vasoactive drug via a micropipette to an arteriole or capillary. The pipette with a small spherical volume of drug is lowered through the paraffin oil covering the tissue until it comes in contact with the fluid layer separating the two layers. The drug rapidly disperses into the fluid layer and tissue. The right panel shows the image as seen through the intravital video microscope when the drug is applied to a specific site on a capillary. The stimulus propagates upstream to the arteriole resulting in a decrease in arteriolar diameter and a decrease in the velocity of red cells in the capillaries supplied by that arteriole

of the preparation. The drug is delivered to the site by a small pipette that is inserted through the paraffin layer over the desired site (Fig. 3). Applying the drug in this manner rather than into a superfusion solution ensures that the drug action will be mainly limited to the initial site of application. This approach has been used to demonstrate that a vasoactive drug applied locally to a capillary [52] can cause a vascular response in the supplying arteriole, i.e., a propagated response along the capillary endothelium. It has also been shown that propagated vasodilation or vasoconstriction also occurs in arterioles. The disadvantage of this approach is that the concentration of the drug at the capillary or arteriolar wall is not known. Typically the concentrations appear to be approximately 1/1000th of the concentration of the drug in the pipette.

The action of some vasoactive substances may be different whether applied to the interior (lumen) or exterior of the arteriole (e.g., ATP applied to the exterior of an arteriole causes a vasoconstriction – P2x receptor, to the interior a propagated vasodilation – P2x receptor) [53]. If this is suspected a sharpened pipette can be inserted through the wall of the arteriole and a small volume of the drug injected into the lumen.

Summary: Both the *in vitro* and *in vivo* approaches can be applied to disease models to determine whether there is an impaired vascular responsiveness at the microvascular level, and if there is, what the source of the dysfunction may be (endothelial or smooth muscle injury, excessive production of nitric oxide (NO) or the loss of the propagated response either along the capillary or arteriole). Arterioles are the main source of vascular resistance, and hence they are responsible for regulating both the magnitude and distribution of blood flow within the organ. It has been recognized for sometime that the microvascular response to changes in metabolic demand of the tissue must be integrated along the length of the arteriolar tree from capillaries to the small arterioles. An impairment of the arteriolar network's ability to regulate flow and DO_2 will have a significant impact on tissue oxygenation. If arteriolar control is lost, the passive dimensions of the microvascular bed will determine the distribution of flow. This will influence the heterogeneity of perfusion at all levels of the vascular tree.

Microcirculatory and Regional (Arteriolar/Venular) O_2 Saturation

Heterogeneity of microvascular perfusion makes the relationship between microvascular blood flow and tissue oxygenation difficult to interpret. This situation is further complicated by the diffusional exchange of O_2 across all levels of the microvascular tree and the surrounding tissue. This is best illustrated by the fall in SO_2 levels of nearly 30% as blood passes down the arteriolar tree (first discovered by Duling and Berne [54] and confirmed in a variety of tissues using a wide range of measurement techniques [16]). SO_2 at the entrance to the capillary bed ranges from 60–70%. Blood flow measurements are not sufficient to describe the oxygenation of the tissue. Changes in the heterogeneity of microvascular perfusion with disease may have unexpected effects on tissue oxygenation.

A variety of techniques have been developed to measure tissue oxygenation. Techniques have been developed for measuring SO_2 levels in arterioles and venules, and in capillaries as well as for measuring tissue or vascular PO_2 levels. A MRI technique known as functional MRI (fMRI) is sensitive to microvascular SO_2 levels. Although still an experimental tool, this approach has the potential to be used clinically. This section will deal primarily with intravital techniques for measuring SO_2 levels *in vivo*.

Spectrophotometric Analysis

Background: Hb SO_2 can be measured in the microvasculature using spectrophotometric techniques. The basic principle underlying these measurements is that light passing through a Hb solution is attenuated to a different degree depending on the wavelength of light and on degree of SO_2 of the Hb. Thus how light or dark the solution appears, its optical density (OD), can be used as a measure of the SO_2 of the Hb. There are several challenges to be overcome in applying this principle to the measurement of the SO_2 of RBCs in the microvasculature [55].

First, a change in SO_2 must cause a measurable change in the OD of the RBCs. This can be a problem in the microvasculature, since in capillaries one is attempting to measure the SO_2 of single RBCs where the pathlength of light through the cell may only be 3 to 5 µm. In arterioles and venules the pathlength may be as much as 100 to 150 µm with 20 to 30 RBCs attenuating the light at any one location. Since the amount of light absorbed by the Hb solution is also dependent on the pathlength, a wavelength of light, which is appropriate for measurement in an arteriole, will not be appropriate for a capillary. If a single cell has a measurable OD then multiple cells will appear opaque; if multiple cells have a measurable OD, a single cell will appear transparent. The solution is a careful selection of wavelengths depending on the vessel being analyzed such that there is a maximum change in OD over the range of SO_2 from 0 to 100%.

The second problem is that the pathlength through the RBCs is not known and the pathlength at any location may be quite variable from moment to moment (changes in RBC density and orientation, etc.). The solution is to make OD density measurements simultaneously at a second wavelength that is independent of the SO_2 (isosbestic wavelength). This second OD value acts as the reference OD that takes into account the pathlength (and concentration of Hb).

The third problem is light lost due to scattering from the RBCs. This is a significant problem in the larger microvessels (arterioles and venules) where the light can be scattered from multiple cells. The solution is to simultaneously sample at a third wavelength (a second isosbestic point) to account for the light lost due to scattering.

A final problem is the measurement of the light intensity incident on the RBC (needed to calculate the OD). In the mesentery where there is only a single layer of vessels this is not a problem. But in thicker tissues such as skeletal muscle, the light may have passed through multiple RBCs before reaching the vessel being sampled. This factor is a significant problem with the wavelengths used for measuring SO_2 in capillaries since it results in spatial variations in the incident light intensity. This problem can be seen in Figure 1 where there is considerable variability in the brightness of the tissue. The solution is to measure the light intensity along the length of the capillary in the absence of RBCs, i.e., as plasma gaps pass through the vessel. The bright bands between the RBCs in the space-time image (Figure 2) provide the data on the incident light intensity. For arterioles and venules this is less of a problem; the incident light intensity can be measured from the tissue beside the vessel, or by interpolating what the light intensity would be from measurements on both sides of the vessel.

SO_2 in arterioles and venules: Implementation of spectroscopy for measuring SO_2 in arterioles and venules requires simultaneous light intensity data at three wavelengths, and for capillaries simultaneous data from two wavelengths. The approach [56] with large microvessels is to sample the light intensity at one location using a fiber optic light-guide and three photodiodes, each with an appropriate interference filter (520 nm, 546 nm, 555 nm). With the fiber optic system, point measurements of SO_2 can be made at various levels of the arteriolar and venular tree.

SO_2 in capillaries: Measurement of SO_2 in capillaries has been implemented using a dual video camera system [13]. The microvascular image is split into two light-paths, passed through two separate interference filters (420 nm, 431 nm) and recorded by two separate but identical video systems. Timing information is recorded simultaneously onto both video tapes such that, during off-line analysis of the two video tapes, a computer can sample the same location along the vessel beginning at exactly the same video frame. Replaying of the video tapes permits "simultaneous" analysis of other capillaries in the field of view which are also in focus. The two video tapes are sampled and the data for each capillary is displayed in space-time images (Fig. 4). SO_2 measurements can be made at any location along the length of the vessel sampled (from 90 to 150 μm in length depending on the magnification used). Local SO_2 gradient can also be determined.

Arteriolar to venular SO_2 gradient: It is not possible to sample all microvessels in an organ or even all that are visible in a microvascular image. The challenge becomes how to design a measurement strategy that provides meaningful data on tissue oxygenation. Arteriolar data has been used to investigate the fall in SO_2 along the arteriolar tree. Capillary SO_2 data has been compiled to investigate the SO_2 levels at the arteriolar and venular ends of the capillary bed. This data has been used to determine (i) the magnitude of the fall in SO_2 levels from systemic arterial blood to the entrance of the capillary; (ii) the SO_2 levels along a length of capillary; and (iii), the arterio-venous gradient across the capillary bed. SO_2 levels at the entrance to the capillary bed (60–70% O_2 saturation) agree with measurements from arterioles [57]. RBCs in capillaries can be re-oxygenated by diffusion from nearby arterioles such that SO_2 levels may increase along the length of the capillary (i.e., the expected linear fall in SO_2 along the capillary rarely occurs) [58]. There is also evidence of considerable diffusional exchange of O_2 among

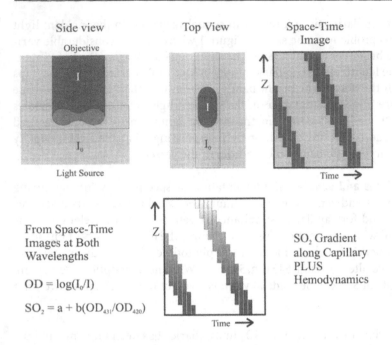

Fig. 4. This series of images demonstrates how the hemoglobin oxygen saturation (SO$_2$) of the red blood cells is calculated. Light with an incident intensity Io is absorbed by the hemoglobin as it passes through the red blood cell resulting in observed red blood cell intensity I (as illustrated in the panels labeled side and top view). The data obtained from both the 420 nm and 431 nm image are redisplayed as space-time images (panel on right) and the optical densities of the red cells at the two wavelengths are calculated (at each spatial and temporal location in the image). SO$_2$ is linearly related to the optical density ratio (OD$_{431}$/OD$_{420}$) at the two wavelengths. Color coded space-time images (bottom panel) contain information on the SO$_2$ values at any location in the capillary over time as well as the red blood cell hemodynamics

capillaries with different SO$_2$ levels or flowrates. As a consequence, the local SO$_2$ gradient in some capillaries may be greater than the a-v difference across the capillary bed.

Combining the SO$_2$ data with the hemodynamic data on RBC supply rate, the O$_2$ flow (mL O$_2$/sec) at any point along the capillary can be measured. From the a-v difference in O$_2$ flow, the amount of O$_2$ extracted (mL O$_2$/sec) from the RBCs (or gained) can be computed (Figure 5). By knowing the amount extracted and the amount delivered to the capillary one can compute the local O$_2$ extraction ratio for a single vessel. From measurement of multiple capillaries at the arteriolar end of the capillary bed one can estimate the total O$_2$ delivered (mL O$_2$/sec) to that capillary network. Similar measurements can be made at the venous end of the same network to estimate the amount of O$_2$ entering the post capillary venule, and from this compute the O$_2$ extraction ratio for this capillary network. Typically the O$_2$ extraction ratio (O$_2$ER) in a healthy animal is 15-20% across a capillary network [58].

In computing the O$_2$ER for a network of capillaries, the O$_2$ flow is used, not the SO$_2$ values, since the RBC perfusion of the capillary network is heterogeneous. To

Arteriolar end   Venular End

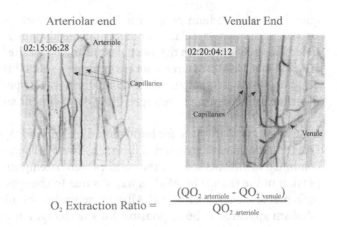

$$O_2 \text{ Extraction Ratio} = \frac{(QO_{2 \text{ artertiole}} - QO_{2 \text{ venule}})}{QO_{2 \text{ arteriole}}}$$

Fig. 5. These images illustrate how the O_2 extraction ratio across the capillary bed can be determined. SO_2 and red blood cell flow rate data are determined for capillaries at the arteriolar and venular end of the capillary bed. The O_2 extraction ratio is determined from the a–v difference in O_2 flowrate (QO_2)

estimate the mean entrance or exit SO_2 level for the capillary bed, the RBC flow weighted SO_2 levels should be used since a capillary with a high RBC supply rate will contribute more than a vessel with a low supply rate. Thus the heterogeneity of microvascular perfusion makes interpretation of SO_2 values alone, difficult.

Functional MRI: Ogawa et al. [8] were the first to demonstrate that paramagnetic deoxyHb can be used as a naturally occurring contrast agent in MRI to follow changes in microvascular oxygenation. The term applied to this method was blood oxygen level dependent contrast or BOLD. Initially it was not clear whether the signal originated from the capillary bed and small venules, or from the large veins draining the microvasculature. Menon et al. [17] provide evidence that the BOLD effect is sensitive to changes in capillary oxygenation. Using a 4T whole body system, the in-plane resolution of the fMRI system is approximately 3×3 mm^2 with a slice thickness of 5 mm. Changes in regional oxygenation in the brain have been followed in response to visual stimuli or performance of various tasks [59, 60]. Although the fMRI technique is an extremely powerful tool for the non-invasive investigation of microvascular oxygenation, the data cannot be presented in absolute units.

Summary: Although SO_2 values provide information on the O_2 levels within the microvascular bed, one cannot determine whether a change in SO_2 levels was due to a change in the magnitude of the perfusion, or a change in O_2 metabolism, or a redistribution of flow within the microvascular bed. For example, researchers are still debating whether impaired O_2 extraction in sepsis is a problem with DO_2 metabolism. The same argument holds for other techniques that determine tissue oxygenation by measuring SO_2 or PO_2 levels alone, e.g., changes in SO_2 levels measured with fMRI, tissue PO_2 measurements measured with polarographic sensors and plasma PO_2 measurements measured using phosphorescence quenching of palladium porphyrin. In the latter case, the erythrocyte – plasma separation at microvascular bifurcations means that the PO_2 levels measured will reflect the capillaries with the most plasma and hence the lowest O_2 flow rates. Although all of these measurements are extremely useful in quantifying tissue oxygenation, without simultaneous data on the vascular perfusion the situation is the same as attempting to interpret flow data without simultaneous data on O_2 levels.

Recognition of the need for both hemodynamic and O_2 data can be seen in the recent development of combined flow-sensitive MRI and fMRI techniques. In the combined MRI/fMRI studies, the authors were attempting to quantify what proportion of the change in fMRI signal was due to changes in flow versus changes in O_2 metabolism [10, 44, 61, 62]. All of these studies found that both flow and metabolism appeared to be responsible for the changes in microvascular oxygenation measured using the BOLD effect.

A final point should be considered: the scale of the O_2 measurements relative to the disturbance in microvascular oxygenation and the linearity or bias of the O_2 measurements (Fig. 6). A measurement made on a scale larger than the microvascular disturbance may not be able to detect any change in the measured parameter. It is possible that a significant redistribution of DO_2 within the microvascular bed may yield the same mean SO_2 or PO_2 level. Only significant changes that affect the entire sample volume uniformly (e.g., change in total perfusion or O_2 metabolism) are likely to be detected, and then only if O_2 metabolism is com-

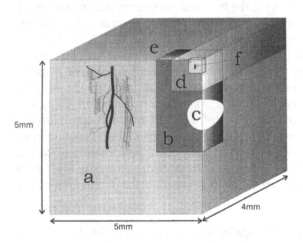

Fig. 6. This figure illustrates the scale of sample volumes associated with different measurement techniques. The line drawing in the top portion of volume "a" is a simplified version of the microvascular bed shown in Figure 1. Volume "a" is approximately the volume sampled in fMRI studies which is close to the smallest microsphere sample volumes. Volume "b" is the volume associated with the muscle shown in Figure 1. Volume "c" is the laser Doppler sample volume, and volume "d" the tissue slice sampled by the flow sensitive MRI techniques. The volume of tissue observed using intravital video microscopy (IVVM) with a 20 × objective is labeled "e" (smallest volume in top right corner of volume "a"). The short line labeled "f" in volume "e" represents analysis of a single capillary

promised. As long as the O_2 needs of the tissue are being satisfied, global measures of SO_2 and PO_2 may not be able to detect the presence of significant increases in the heterogeneity of microvascular perfusion. Walley's model [23] provides a good illustration of this when venous SO_2 levels (or whole organ O_2 extraction) are used as the measure of tissue oxygenation. This also means that interventions designed to improve tissue oxygenation by improving the distribution of DO_2 can only be detected by global measures if the tissue is supply dependent, i.e., not all of its O_2 needs are currently being met.

Conclusion

With more fundamental knowledge about the microvascular dysfunction in various diseases (and its progression over time), we will be able to make more informed choices about which methodology is appropriate for monitoring tissue oxygenation and how properly to interpret the data obtained. Techniques which combine both flow and O_2 measurements will be most useful but the resolution of these measurements relative to the scale of the microvascular O_2 transport dysfunction will be the deciding factor in selection of the appropriate methodology.

References

1. Tyml K, Ellis CG (1985) Simultaneous assessment of red cell perfusion in skeletal muscle by laser Doppler flowmetry and video microscopy. Int J Microc Clin Exp 4:397–406
2. Rutt B, Napel S (1991) Magnetic resonance techniques for blood-flow measurement and vascular imaging. Can Assoc Radiol J 42:21–30
3. Bassingthwaighte JB, King RB, Roger SA (1989) Fractal nature of regional myocardial blood flow heterogeneity. Circ Res 65:578–590
4. Sjoberg F, Gustafsson U, Lewis DH (1991) Extracellular muscle surface PO_2 and pH heterogeneity during hypovolemia and after reperfusion. Circ Shock 34:319–328
5. Buerk DG, Shonat RD, Riva CE, Cranstoun SD (1993) O_2 gradients and countercurrent exchange in the cat vitreous humor near retinal arterioles and venules. Microvasc Res 45:134–148
6. Lo LW, Jenkins WT, Vinogradov SA, Evans SM, Wilson DF (1997) Oxygen distribution in the vasculature of mouse tissue in vivo measured using a near infra red phosphor. Adv Exp Med Biol 411:577–583
7. Mancini DM, Bolinger L, Li H, Kendrick K, Chance B, Wilsor JR (1994) Validation of near-infrared spectroscopy in humans. J Appl Physiol 77:2740–2747
8. Ogawa S, Lee TM, Kay AR, Tank DW (1990) Brain magnetic resonance imaging with contrast dependent on blood oxygenation. Proc Natl Acad Sci USA 87:9868–9872
9. Allard MF, Kamimura CT, English DR, Henning SL, Wiggs BR (1993) Regional myocardial capillary erythrocyte transit time in the normal resting heart. Circ Res 72:187–193
10. Kim SG, Tsekos NV (1997) Perfusion imaging by a flow-sensitive alternating inversion recovery (FAIR) technique: application to functional brain imaging. Magn Reson Med 37:425–435
11. Duling BR, Damon DN, Donaldson SR, Pittman RN (1983) A computerized system for densitometric analysis of the microcirculation. J Appl Physiol 55:642–651
12. Ellis CG, Ellsworth ML, Pittman RN, Burgess WL (1992) Application of image analysis for evaluation of red blood cell dynamics in capillaries. Microvasc Res 44:214–225

13. Ellis CG, Ellsworth ML, Pittman RN (1990) Determination of red blood cell oxygenation in vivo by dual video densitometric image analysis. Am J Physiol 258:H1216–H1223
14. Segal SS (1991) Microvascular recruitment in hamster striated muscle: role for conducted vasodilation. Am J Physiol 261:H181–H189
15. Lam C, Tyml K, Martin C, Sibbald W (1994) Microvascular perfusion is impaired in a rat model of normotensive sepsis. J Clin Invest 94:2077–2083
16. Ellsworth ML, Ellis CG, Popel AS, Pittman RN (1994) Role of microvessels in oxygen supply to tissue. News Physiol Sci 9:119–123
17. Menon RS, Ogawa S, Hu X, Strupp JP, Anderson P, Ugurbil K (1995) BOLD based functional MRI at 4 Tesla includes a capillary bed contribution: echo-planar imaging correlates with previous optical imaging using intrinsic signals. Magn Reson Med 33:453–459
18. Van Beek JH, Roger SA, Bassingthwaighte JB (1989) Regional myocardial flow heterogeneity explained with fractal networks. Am J Physiol 257:H1670–H1680
19. Kleen M, Welte M, Lackermeier P, Habler O, Kemming G, Messmer K (1997) Myocardial blood flow heterogeneity in shock and small-volume resuscitation in pigs with coronary stenosis. J Appl Physiol 83:1832–1841
20. Kleen M, Zwissler B, Messmer K (1998) PEEP only partly restores disturbed distribution of regional pulmonary blood flow in lung injury. Am J Physiol 274:H209–H216
21. Humer MF, Phang PT, Friesen BP, Allard MF, Goddard CM, Walley KR (1996) Heterogeneity of gut capillary transit times and impaired gut oxygen extraction in endotoxemic pigs. J Appl Physiol 81:895–904
22. Connolly HV, Maginniss LA, Schumacker PT (1997) Transit time heterogeneity in canine small intestine: significance for oxygen transport. J Clin Invest 99:228–238
23. Walley KR (1996) Heterogeneity of oxygen delivery impairs oxygen extraction by peripheral tissues: theory. J Appl Physiol 81:885–894
24. Tyml K, Ellis CG, Safranyos RG, Fraser S, Groom AC (1981) Temporal and spatial distributions of red cell velocity in capillaries of resting skeletal muscle, including estimates of red cell transit times. Microvasc Res 22:14–31
25. Sarelius IH (1990) An analysis of microcirculatory flow heterogeneity using measurements of transit time. Microvasc Res 40:88–98
26. Sarelius IH (1986) Cell flow path influences transit time through striated muscle capillaries. Am J Physiol 250:H899–H907
27. Albrecht KH, Gaehtgens P, Pries A, Heuser M (1979) The Fahraeus effect in narrow capillaries (i.d. 3.3 to 11.0 micron). Microvasc Res 18:33–47
28. Pries AR, Ley K, Claassen M, Gaehtgens P (1989) Red cell distribution at microvascular bifurcations. Microvasc Res 38:81–101
29. Pries AR, Fritzsche A, Ley K, Gaehtgens P (1992) Redistribution of red blood cell flow in microcirculatory networks by hemodilution. Circ Res 70:1113–1121
30. Ellis CG, Wrigley SM, Groom AC (1994) Heterogeneity of red cell perfsuion in capillary networks supplied by a single arteriole, in resting skeletal muscle. Circ Res 75:357–368
31. Pittman RN, Ellsworth ML (1986) Estimation of red cell flow microvessels: consequences of the Baker-Wayland spatial averaging model. Microvasc Res 32:371–388
32. Pries AR, Secomb TW, Gaehtgens P, Gross JF (1990) Blood flow in microvascular networks. Experiments and simulation. Circ Res 67:826–834
33. Pries AR, Kanzow G, Gaehtgens P (1983) Microphotometric determination of hematocrit in small vessels. Am J Physiol 245:H167–H177
34. Sarelius IH, Duling BR (1982) Direct measurement of microvessel hematocrit red cell flux, velocity, and transit time. Am J Physiol 243:H1018–H1026
35. Tyml K, Ellis CG (1982) Evaluation of the flying spot technique as a television method for measuring red cell velocity in microvessels. Int J Microcirc Clin Exp 1:145–155
36. Tyml K, Sherebrin MH (1980) A method for on-line measurements of red cell velocity in microvessels using computerized frame-by-frame analysis of television images. Microvasc Res 20:1–8
37. Federspiel WJ, Popel AS (1986) A theoretical analysis of the effect of the particulate nature of blood on oxygen release in capillaries. Microvasc Res 32:164–189

38. Duling BR, Damon DH (1987) An examination of the measurement of flow heterogeneity in striated muscle. Circ Res 60:1-13
39. Tyml K (1987) Red cell perfusion in skeletal muscle at rest and after mild and severe contractions. Am J Physiol 252:H485-H493
40. Tyml K, Cheng L (1995) Heterogeneity of red blood cell velocity in skeletal muscle decreases with increased flow. Microcirculation 2:181-193
41. Tyml K, Budreau CH (1992) Effect of isovolemic hemodilution on microvascular perfusion in rat skeletal muscle during a low flow state. Int J Microcirc Clin Exp 11:133-142
42. Oberg PA (1990) Laser-Doppler flowmetry. Crit Rev Biomed Eng 18:125-163
43. Harrison DK, Abbot NC, Beck JS, McCollum PT (1993) A preliminary assessment of laser Doppler perfusion imaging in human skin using the tuberculin reaction as a model. Physiol Meas 14:241-252
44. Kim SG, Tsekos NV, Ashe J (1997) Multi-slice perfusion-based functional MRI using the FAIR technique: comparison of CBF and BOLD effects. NMR Biomed 10:191-196
45. Christopher DA, Burns PN, Armstrong J, Foster FS (1996) A high-frequency continuous-wave Doppler ultrasound system for the detection of blood flow in the microcirculation. Ultrasound Med Biol 22:1191-1203
46. Christopher DA, Burns PN, Starkoski BG, Foster FS (1997) A high-frequency pulsed-wave Doppler ultrasound system for the detection and imaging of blood flow in the microcirculation. Ultrasound Med Biol 23:997-1015
47. Dietrich HH, Kajita Y, Dacey Jr RG (1996) Local and conducted vasomotor responses in isolated rat cerebral arterioles. Am J Physiol 271:H1109-H-1116
48. Nagi MM, Ward ME (1997) Modulation of myogenic responsiveness by CO_2 in rat diaphragmatic arterioles: role of the endothelium. Am J Physiol 272:H1419-H1425
49. Jackson WF (1991) Nitric oxide does not mediate arteriolar oxygen reactivity. Microcirc Endothelium Lymphatics 7:199-215
50. Dietrich HH, Tyml K (1992) Capillary as a communicating medium in the microvasculature. Microvasc Res 43:87-99
51. Segal SS, Neild TO (1996) Conducted depolarization in arteriole networks of the guinea-pig small intestine: effect of branching of signal dissipation. J Physiol 496:229-244
52. Dietrich HH, Tyml K (1992) Microvascular flow response to localized application of norepinephrine on capillaries in rat and frog skeletal muscle. Microvasc Res 43:73-86.
53. Ellsworth ML, Forrester T, Ellis CG, Dietrich HH (1995) The erythrocyte as a regulator of vascular tone. Am J Physiol 269:H2155-H2161
54. Duling BR, Berne RM (1970) Longitudinal gradients in periarteriolar oxygen tension. A possible mechanism for the participation of oxygen in local regulation of blood flow. Circ Res 27:669-678
55. Pittman RN (1986) In vivo photometric analysis of hemoglobin. Ann Biomed Eng 14:119-137
56. Pittman RN, Duling BR (1975) A new method for the measurement of percent oxyhemoglobin. J Appl Physiol 38:315-320
57. Ellsworth ML, Popel AS, Pittmar RN (1988) Assessment and impact of heterogeneities of convective oxygen transport parameters in capillaries of striated muscle: experimental and theoreti. Microvasc Res 35:341-362
58. Ellsworth ML, Pittman RN (1990) Arterioles supply oxygen to capillaries by diffusion as well as by convection. Am J Physiol 258:H1240-H1243
59. Menon RS, Ogawa S, Strupp JP, Ugurbil K (1997) Ocular dominance in human V1 demonstrated by functional magnetic resonance imaging. J Neurophysiol 77:2780-2787
60. Ramsey NF, Kirkby BS, Van Gelderen P, et al (1996) Functional mapping of human sensorimotor cortex with 3D BOLD fMRI correlates highly with H2(15)O PET rCBF. J Cereb Blood Flow Metab 16:755-764
61. Davis TL, Kwong KK, Weisskoff RM, Rosen BR (1998) Calibrated functional MRI: Mapping the dynamics of oxidative metabolism. Pro Natl Acad Sci USA 95:1834-1839
62. Kim SG, Ugurbil K (1997) Comparison of blood oxygenation and cerebral blood flow effects in fMRI: estimation of relative oxygen consumption change. Magn Reson Med 38:59-65

Monitoring the Systemic Circulation in Sepsis with Microelectrodes

C. P. Winlove, M. Sair, and T. W. Evans

Introduction

Sepsis and septic shock cause substantial morbidity, occurring in around 1% of hospitalized patients. The associated mortality is 10–20%, amounting to an estimated 100,000 deaths per year in the USA alone [1, 2]. Thus, significant circulatory failure occurs in around 40% of patients with Gram negative bacteremia, and in those that develop septic shock the mortality is in excess of 60%. Death is usually attributable to multiple organ dysfunction syndrome (MODS) rather than refractory hypotension *per se* [3]. Despite advances in the supportive strategies used in modern intensive care, the mortality rate has remained disappointingly high, although it is possible that the incidence of sepsis and the associated syndromes is rising because of the widespread application of immunomodulating therapies in ageing Western populations. Finally, the lack of a unified definition of sepsis and its associated syndromes until recently has rendered comparison between epidemiological studies from different centers and continents at best difficult and at worst impossible.

Classification (Consensus Definitions)

Not all patients with systemic inflammatory processes have an identifiable infective cause, although the clinical endpoints are often indistinguishable. Similarly, patient outcome is not determined by the nature of the causative microorganism. In this sense, a sustained inflammatory response, frequently progressing to MODS may be triggered by an initiating (non-infective) event. Examples of conditions characterized by such a systemic inflammatory response syndrome (SIRS) include trauma, acute pancreatitis, burns or inadequate resuscitation from hemorrhagic shock. Acute lung injury (ALI) and its extreme manifestation, the acute respiratory distress syndrome (ARDS) represent the most common manifestations of end organ inflammation/failure and affect up to 30% of patients with non-pulmonary sepsis [4]. Highlighting the need for a consensus definition of sepsis and sepsis-related syndromes around which future investigations can be made, a recent conference stressed the importance of the spectrum of severity of such illnesses and conceptualized a series of overlapping clinical entities underlined by the inflammatory response [5] (Fig. 1). It was hoped that such def-

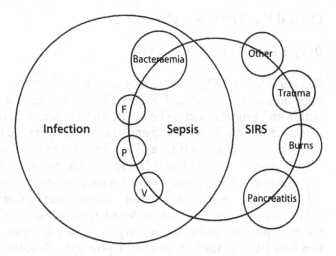

Fig. 1. The relationship between sepsis, the systemic inflammatory response syndrome (SIRS) and infection. Abbreviations: F, fungemia; P, parasitemia; V, viremia

initions (shown in Table 1) would improve detection, permit early therapeutic intervention and allow standardization of research protocols.

Table 1. Definitions of sepsis and sepsis-related syndromes (from [2] with permission)

Infection: Microbial phenomenon characterised by an inflammatory response to the presence of microorganisms or the invasion of normally sterile host tissue by those organisms.

Systemic Inflammatory Response Syndrome (SIRS): The systemic inflammatory response to a variety of severe clinical insults and manifested by two or more of the following:
- Temperature > 38 or $< 36\,°C$
- Heart rate > 90/min
- Respiratory rate > 20/min or $PaCO_2 < 4.3$kPa
- White blood cells $> 12,00$ /mm^3 or $> 10\%$ immature (band) forms

Sepsis: The systemic response to infection, manifest by two or more of the above.

Severe sepsis: Sepsis associated with organ dysfunction, hypoperfusion or hypotension. Hypoperfusion and perfusion abnormalities may include, but are not limited to, lactic acidosis, oliguria and an acute alteration in mental status.

Sepsis-induced hypotension: A systolic blood pressure of < 90 mmHg or a reduction by 40 mmHg from baseline values in the absence of other causes of hypotension e.g. hypovolemia.

Septic shock: Sepsis-induced hypotension despite adequate fluid resuscitation, in the presence of perfusion abnormalities that may include, but are not limited to, lactic acidemia, oliguria and an acute alteration in mental status. Patients who are on inotropic or vasopressor support may not be hypotensive at the time that perfusion abnormalities are measured.

Multiple organ dysfunction syndrome: Presence of altered organ function in an acutely ill patient such that homeostasis cannot be maintained without intervention.

Clinical Manifestations of Sepsis

Oxygen Delivery and Tissue Uptake

Oxygen delivery (DO_2) to the tissues must be sufficient to meet the varying metabolic demands of health and disease. Clearly, demand for O_2 varies enormously within and between vascular beds. The distribution of O_2 is dependent upon efficient alveolar-capillary gas exchange, the O_2 carrying capacity of blood, the adequacy of cardiac output (CO) and the diffusion of O_2 across the endothelium in respiring tissues (Fig. 2). Blood flow through mammalian tissues is frequently independent of arterial blood pressure across the physiological range (i.e., is auto-regulated). The mechanism of autoregulation may be due in part to a myogenic reflex, or a regulatory mechanism based upon the effects of O_2 concentration and tissue respiration on the pre-capillary arteriole [6]. Carbon dioxide (CO_2), hydrogen ions (H^+), potassium ions (K^+), prostaglandins, lactate and adenosine are possible candidates as signal species. The tissue distribution of blood is also regulated by the actions of neural and endothelial cell-derived signals on small resistance vessels and pre-capillary sphincters.

The transfer of O_2 across the endothelium and into the extracellular space is influenced by the O_2 tension gradient, capillary transit time [7] and capillary

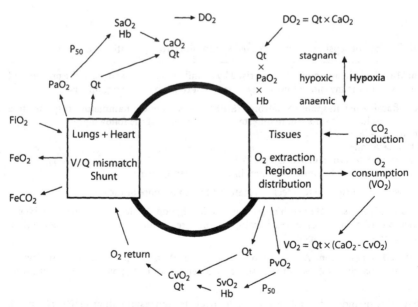

Fig. 2. Tissue oxygenation cycle from systemic to peripheral microcirculation, tissue hypoxia may result from a failure of oxygen delivery to meet tissue demand. Recent interest has moved from centrally-derived measurement (left side of circle) to the effects of sepsis on microcirculatory regulation of oxygenation (right side of circle). Abbreviations: CaO_2, arterial oxygen content; CvO_2 mixed venous oxygen content; Qt, cardiac output; Hb, hemoglobin; V/Q, ventilation-perfusion; SaO_2 arterial oxygen saturation; SvO_2 mixed venous oxygen saturation.

density [8]. In health, DO_2 exceeds oxygen consumption (VO_2) and must accommodate a three to four fold increase in demand during exercise. The body can augment tissue O_2 both by increasing CO and by extracting more arterial O_2 in response to increased requirements. Thus, the oxygen extraction ratio (O_2ER) ranges from 0.25 at rest to a peak of 0.8 during maximal exercise in conditioned individuals. In most tissues, anaerobic metabolism becomes dominant when demand begins to exceed supply, generally at O_2ER greater than 0.6, a point referred to as the anerobic threshold.

Oxygen Delivery and Uptake during Sepsis and Sepsis-Related Syndromes

The relationship between DO_2 and VO_2 in sepsis has been the subject of controversy and has been investigated extensively. DO_2 to tissues can be altered by manipulating the individual components from which it is derived; principally blood flow (CO) and arterial oxygen content. VO_2 seems to be independent of changes in DO_2 above a certain critical value (cDO_2) under physiological conditions. Decreasing DO_2 in this range results in a rise in O_2ER and increased arteriovenous oxygen difference. Below cDO_2, reductions in DO_2 lead to a fall in VO_2 in a supply-dependent fashion, irrespective of the nature of the precipitating hypoxic insult [9]. Although this biphasic relationship was described initially in animal models and anesthetized human subjects, reports of a single-phase component relationship in critically ill patients resulted in the concept of pathological supply-dependency and covert tissue O_2 debt [10–12]. Moreover, the discovery that post operative survival was better in some high risk patients who could achieve supranormal values of DO_2, VO_2 and CO following the administration of intravenous fluids and inotropic drugs subsequently lead to an assertion that so-called goal-directed therapy aimed at achieving these ends could reverse tissue hypoxia in critically ill patients and reduce mortality [13, 14]. To date evidence has actually contradicted this assertion [15, 16], even suggesting that "driving" patients with sepsis and related syndromes to achieve higher levels of DO_2 may be detrimental. Such controversies highlight the pitfalls of utilizing derived measurements in the critically care setting. Thus, it has becoming increasingly clear over the past decade that traditional "whole body" means of assessing tissue oxygenation in critically ill individuals, particularly those with sepsis and related syndromes are only crude indicators of local tissue perfusion. Moreover, assumptions made concerning the relative importance of tissue VO_2 and DO_2 based on centrally-determined observations may not be justified or valid. The increasing awareness of the importance of peripheral vascular function and regulation of regional blood flow has moved research efforts away from systemic hemodynamic indices of perfusion to the investigation of the microcirculation.

The Definition and Detection of Tissue Hypoxia
by Clinical and Physiological Methods in the Critically Ill

Tissue hypoxia may be defined as a condition in which cells display abnormal O_2 utilization leading to anaerobic metabolism. Clinical assessment may indicate specific organ dysfunction through the presence of recognized signs (mental obtundation, decreased urine output, etc.). Techniques such as magnetic resonance spectroscopy can be used to characterize metabolic changes at the cellular level, but none of these are easily applicable at the bedside. Current understanding is therefore based largely on biochemical assays such as blood lactate, which is easy to measure and can be followed sequentially to assess prognosis or the patient response to therapy. Thus, when tissue hypoxia becomes extensive it is manifest in increased serum lactate concentrations. Lactic acidosis may result from hypoxic conditions in which anaerobic production of lactate occurs globally (e.g., shock) or through focal (e.g. bowel infarction) or non-hypoxic causes (e.g., delayed clearance of lactate, accelerated aerobic glycolysis and dysfunction or pyruvate dehydrogenase). Plasma lactate has been shown to have adverse prognostic significance in critically ill patients [17]. As discussed above, the use of changes in VO_2 in response to changes in DO_2 has not proved particularly useful in determining the care of the critically ill patient. Similarly, mixed venous oxygen saturation (SvO_2), although useful in identifying cardiogenic or hypovolemic shock, is less useful in sepsis. Thus, a critical value of SvO_2 that defines inadequate DO_2 is difficult to determine. Changes in venoarterial carbon dioxide pressure gradient have also been used as a reflection of tissue hypoxia. However, it is prone to errors because $PaCO_2$ is not very different from $MvCO_2$ and its interpretation depends upon absolute values.

Gastric tonometry derives gastric intramucosal pH (pHi). The mucosal layers of the stomach are highly vulnerable to decreases in perfusion/oxygenation; and pHi, although in principle specific to the stomach, is often used to assess the global adequacy of perfusion. pHi may be a good prognostic indicator of patient outcome in the ICU in a selected subgroup but the technique is expensive, difficult to use, operator dependent and time consuming [18].

Thus, there is no gold standard for the detection of tissue hypoxia. There are no specific clinical signs and no clear cut thresholds for any single laboratory test. Global measurements of the adequacy of tissue perfusion are either cumbersome and difficult to use or inaccurate in reflecting regional blood flow. The way forward seems to require the development of new technology for the bedside measurement of regional blood flow and oxygen metabolism.

The Role of Microelectrodes in the Study of Sepsis

Methodology

The first demonstration of the electrochemical determination of O_2 concentration was over 100 years ago, but voltammetric and amperometric techniques were not used in O_2 microelectrodes *in vivo* until the 1940s. Since then time, they have been used extensively to measure the concentration of O_2 in a variety of tissues including surgical flaps, healing wounds, subcutaneous tissues, intervertebral discs, aortic wall and skeletal and cardiac muscle [19]. Microelectrodes afford a means of continuously monitoring changes in analyte concentration [19–21] and are therefore capable of measuring the physiological changes which occur in specific microcirculatory beds in sepsis and their response to therapeutic interventions. O_2 is obviously an analyte of primary importance and the amperometric assay of O_2 on noble metal, or occasionally carbon, electrodes has been employed in physiology for many years [22–23]. This methodology, using either needle electrodes which can be inserted into the tissue or surface electrodes which are attached to the organ surface, is now well established and is summarized below.

Indicators of anaerobic metabolism, such as glucose and lactate, can also be determined using microelectrodes. Most employ an enzyme, for example glucose- or lactate-oxidase, although various means of detecting the end-products of the enzyme reaction or coupling the reaction directly to the electrode exist. Some designs, notably the dialysis probe in which the electrodes and enzyme are contained in microdialysis tubing, have proved stable in tissue for long periods of time. As far as we are aware, however, none have been used in sepsis-related research.

A current focus of research in sepsis is the identification of the mediators and signal molecules which determine the tissue response. Many such species (e.g., nitric oxide, NO) are short-lived *in vivo* and microelectrodes offer a valuable means of determining their concentrations in tissue. Particular attention is now being paid to the role of NO in sepsis and various electrodes designed to detect it *in vivo* have been described, some of which are now offered commercially. Some such devices promise sufficient stability and sensitivity to enable measurements to be made in tissue, but none have been applied in clinical or experimental sepsis. The literature also contains descriptions of electrodes designed to detect other agents implicated in the pathophysiology of sepsis including superoxide, and metabolic markers such as adenosine.

The changes in the central circulation that characterize sepsis are relatively completely documented, but little is known about those of the microcirculation. Specifically, whether the latter are causative or compensatory to central circulatory changes is unclear, as are their effects on nutrient delivery and metabolite removal. Most measurements of tissue perfusion are based on the use of particulate tracers, such as radiolabeled microspheres. The measurement of flow is derived from the number of particles trapped in the microcirculatory bed. The method therefore relies on the relationship between vessel and particle radius and in conditions such as sepsis, which are associated with profound changes in vessel caliber and patency, some care is required in the interpretation of data. Moreover, in studies of tissue metabolism the key parameter is the rate of delivery of nutrients or removal of metabolites. Although under many conditions such exchange is blood-flow limited, this is not always so, particularly if processes such as transport through the interstitium or lymphatic clearance is important. Under these conditions, measurements of the exchange of a diffusible rather than a particulate indicator provides the most relevant information. Measurements of the rate of uptake or clearance of an inhaled inert gas have been employed for many years to measure whole-organ exchange [24]. With the aid of microelectrodes, these measurements can be made at the level of the microcirculation, and even combined with measurements of O_2 concentration [25–28].

Specific Methods

Electrochemical methods fall into two broad classes: potentiometry, in which the working electrode is in equilibrium with the analyte and the electrode potential gives a measure of the analyte concentration; and voltammetry/amperometry in which the electrode is driven away from its equilibrium potential and the resultant current is measured. The necessary circuitry is shown schematically in Figure 3. In brief, a redox reaction occurs at the working electrode, the rate of which can be determined from the current generated. The relationship between current and applied voltage is highly non-linear (Fig. 4). In the plateau region, the current is limited by the availability of analyte at the electrode surface and so, if diffusivity is constant, is proportional to the concentration of analyte.

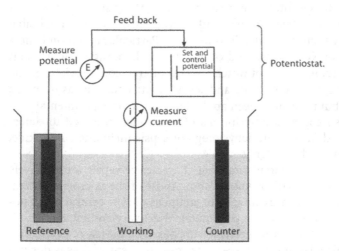

Fig. 3. A schematic illustration of the principle of amperometric assay. The working electrode is the site of a redox reaction involving the analyte of interest. The reference electrode (normally calomel or Ag/AgCl) maintains a constant reference voltage and the counter electrode provides a path of current flow to ensure that no current is drawn from the reference electrode. The circuitry maintains a constant voltage between working and reference electrodes and the resulting current is measured. These operations are normally performed by a commercial or custom made potentiostat (Note that for use in humans, electrical isolation may be required). The specificity of the assay is determined by the nature of the electrode and the applied potential. In voltammetry a time-varying potential may be applied between the electrodes, either to increase specificity (perhaps for multiple analytes) or sensitivity.

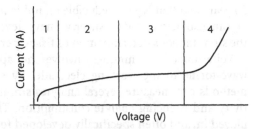

Fig. 4. A current-voltage curve for the reduction of oxygen. At low voltages the current is determined by the rate of reaction on the electrode surface. In the plateau region the current is limited by the rate of transport of anlayte to the surface, which depends on the concentration and diffusivity of the analyte and the electrode geometry. This is the domain normally chosen for amperometric measurements. The increase in current at higher voltages arises from additional electrochemical reactions (in this case, the reduction of water).

Steady state amperometry can be used to assay a range of materials, depending on the nature of the electrode and the applied potential. Its use in sepsis-related research is mainly confined to the determination of tissue oxygenation and perfusion. O_2 can be reduced at noble metals. Platinum and platinum alloys are most widely used, but gold has better electrochemical characteristics and is, in our experience, more stable in tissue. Silver (and carbon) can be useful in certain circumstances as discussed below. We generally employ electrodes 25–125 μm in diameter embedded in epoxy resin in hypodermic needles. These electrodes, and the steps necessary to prepare the electrochemical surface are described in detail elsewhere [29]. They are sufficiently robust to be inserted in a variety of tissues either in animals or humans and cause minimal tissue damage and may be sterilized by autoclave for use in humans. However, others, concerned about tissue damage have preferred to use electrodes (even multi-electrode arrays) attached to the surface of the tissue. It must be remembered, however, that the structure and metabolism of the surface may not be representative of the tissue as a whole. Using etched wires and glass insulation it is possible to make electrodes with tips only a micron or two in diameter and so, in theory, it is possible to make measurements on a cellular scale. The electrodes are, of course, extremely fragile and the small currents they generate may be difficult to measure. In addition, establishing the relationship between these highly localized measurements and whole-tissue metabolism may be problematic.

For the inert gas clearance technique of measuring tissue perfusion hydrogen is the most widely used tracer gas [30]. It can be oxidized on platinum at ~ 300 mV and the design of electrode described above is very suitable, but explosiveness limits its use in the clinical setting. Thus, the maximum concentration available in a ventilator gas mixture is 2%, which is likely to produce a current of only a few nanoamperes in tissue which, although measurable in the laboratory can pose problems in an electrically noisy clinical setting. Some authors advocate palladinization of the electrode surface to increase sensitivity, and others have attempted to generate hydrogen locally. However, we have adopted an alternative approach employing nitrous oxide (N_2O) as the tracer gas. It was established over

20 years ago that N_2O is reducible on noble metals, particularly silver [27]. Since O_2 can also be reduced on silver, we have developed a voltammetric technique for the simultaneous determination of tissue perfusion and oxygenation.

Voltammetric techniques involve the application of time-varying voltage wave-forms to the working electrode. By suitable choice of waveform, these methods can measure several analytes simultaneously, greatly increasing sensitivity and reducing analyte consumption. The methods have been widely employed in, and often specifically developed for, neurophysiology and the assay of short-lived neurotransmitters, sometimes simultaneously with O_2. They have not been extensively employed in other fields of physiology, although the availability of high speed PC-based data acquisition systems and programmable potentiostats now facilitates their implementation. We have also used voltammetry in preliminary experiments to measure changes in muscle NO in experimental sepsis.

Technical Problems

Certain artifacts arise in almost every application of microelectrodes. The first is tissue damage. In our hands, a blunt tip appears to be preferable in this respect to the more widely used cutting tip. The significance of tissue damage must be considered in relation to the size sampling region of the electrode. We have found, in most of the tissues we have studied, damage can be confined to a single layer of cells adjacent to the electrode. Therefore, if a "large"" electrode is employed, the sampling zone will extend into the surrounding, unperturbed tissue. Unless measurements are required on a cellular length scale, it therefore seems preferable to use a rather larger probe than might initially be considered, which will give a value of tissue concentration averaged over a representative volume of tissue. A second concern is the dependence of the electrode current on the diffusivity of the analyte in the tissue. The usual solution is to coat the electrochemical surface with a membrane, sufficiently impermeable to the analyte as to constitute the current-limiting resistance, thereby making the electrode current independent of diffusion in the tissue. There have been major improvements in membrane materials in recent years, in respect of both stability and tissue compatibility and materials such as Nafion can be used with some confidence. However, the third problem, that of sensor-tissue interactions is modified rather than abolished. Blood and tissue components adsorb either to a bare noble metal electrode or to a membrane. These can influence the electrode response either simply by altering the transport of the anlayte to the electrode or, in the former case, by modifying the electrochemical properties of the surface. These effects normally manifest themselves as a fall in electrode current, though with little change in the nature of the current-voltage curve, over the first few minutes following insertion into the tissue. When the electrode is removed from the tissue and placed in calibration solution, the current eventually returns to the value measured before insertion of the electrode in the tissue. We take this behavior to indicate that adsorption is rapid but desorportion is slow and the major effect is via impaired transport rather than electrochemical. Accordingly, we normally allow the electrodes to equilibrate in the tissue before beginning a series of measurements and calibrate immediately after the experiment. However, it should be noted that this interpretation cannot be proved unequivocally and some uncertainties inevitably surround the absolute values determined by the electrodes; their particular value is in the continuous recording of changes in concentration. Finally, it must be remembered that the electrode circuit involves reference and counter (in contact with the tissue) electrodes. The counter electrode is only required to provide a current path and a hypodermic needle inserted at some remote site generally suffices. The design of the reference electrode is more critical and, in our experience, is responsible for many problems of drift and instability. Ag/AgCl is generally preferred over calomel if small size or sterilization/safety in humans are considerations. Theoretically, coupling the electrode to the tissue via a salt bridge (e.g., agarose gel in saturated NaCl) to protect it from contamination and ensure an adequate supply of chloride is desirable but it is not always necessary if sufficient care is taken in the construction and positioning of the electrodes [21]. For measurements in human subjects we have found the stick-on electrodes used for electrocardiograph (EKG) recording to be satisfactory [24–30].

Experimental Studies: Animal Models of Sepsis

A number of investigators have employed the techniques described in the previous section to characterize normal tissue oxygenation in animal models and to document changes that occur under conditions of experimentally-induced sepsis. Significant interstitial tissue hypoxia has been demonstrated in endotoxemic muscle compared to sham treated animals under similar conditions. This deficit appears to be refractory to increasing inspired O_2 concentration (FiO_2) (Fig. 5). Data have also suggested that the heterogeneity of tissue oxygen tension (PtO_2), which is a characteristic of normal tissues, is reduced in endotoxemia. The basis of this is uncertain [31]. Indeed, the reason for the heterogeneity in normal tissue is also unclear although it has been identified in experiments employing both needle [32] and surface microelectrodes [33], and is therefore not attributable to artifact or electrode-induced tissue damage. Further, it is predicted by mathematical models of O_2 transport in capillary networks [8]. PtO_2 in muscle has been reported to range from 0 to 12.9 kPa with mean values varying from 2.1 to 5.8 kPa. These values may not be normally distributed and some derangement of distribution occurs between species and disease states [34]. Other studies of tissue oxygenation in sepsis have generated confusing literature, although how much variation is due to species differences and the experimental model of sepsis employed is unknown. Thus, septic pigs manifest impaired oxygenation late in the condition [36], but in rabbit muscles the impairment appears to be rapid [37]. By contrast, bladder epithelial PtO_2 appears to rise in a dose-dependent fashion following intravenous endotoxin in a resuscitated rat model [38].

Early studies therefore indicated that significant tissue hypoxia is detectable, at least in rodent endotoxemia, and is accompanied by a reduction in the normal heterogeneity of PtO_2. Moreover, attenuated tissue responsiveness to alterations

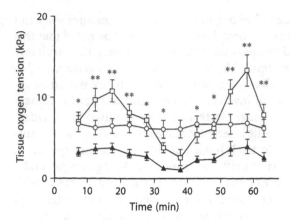

Fig. 5. Mean tissue oxygen response to changes in inspired oxygen concentration (FiO_2) in the sequence 21%, 50%, 21%, 10%, 21%, 95% in endotoxemic and control rats. Control animals (open circles) were subjected to 65 min anesthesia with either no change in FiO_2 (open circles) or the changes shown above (open squares). Endotoxemic rats (closed triangles) were also subjected to the FiO_2 changes. * denotes $p < 0.05$, ** denotes $p < 0.01$, both endotoxemic vs sham treated animals.

in PaO_2 appears to be a prominent feature of endotoxemia suggesting some impairment of tissue microvascular control.

Measurement of Tissue Perfusion

The observed reduction in the normal heterogeneity of tissue O_2 may therefore support the concept of a central cause for the measured hypoxia. Analysis of venous capillary blood O_2 content, or measurement of muscle lactate, pyruvate or acid-base balance (see above) would clearly help to clarify this issue, but the possibility remains that a significant O_2 deficit may result from locally mediated defects in flow regulation. Electrodes have been used to estimate changes in perfusion in endotoxemic animals. Normal or even increased gas delivery seems to be present, a finding inconsistent with the hypothesis of global impairment of CO and generalized diminution of tissue blood flow.

Effects of Volume Resuscitation

Volume resuscitation is a frequently advocated intervention in the management of clinical sepsis, although there are few data regarding its effects in endotoxemia-induced tissue hypoxia. In rabbit peritonitis, volume resuscitation reverses the change in muscle PtO_2 described above [37]. However, experiments in canine sepsis have suggested that this reversibility is organ specific, in that measurements of gastrointestinal mucosal PtO_2 were considerably lower than those seen in muscle, following endotoxin infusion and showed no recovery with fluid resuscitation [39]. Further work is required to establish which tissues are most at risk from hypovolemia and how much fluid replacement is required to avoid tissue hypoxia. Moreover, the nature of the replacement fluid may have important effects, increasing tissue edema due to the administration of large volumes of crystalloid potentially increasing tissue edema and aggravating the hypoxic insult.

Defects of Animals Models

How closely rodent and other models of sepsis employing a wide variety of insults resemble human sepsis is unclear. In the human, sepsis and SIRS are heterogenous conditions triggered by a wide variety of pro-inflammatory insults and manifest as a wide variety of disease severity. Experimental data are confounded by differences in patient age, co-existing disease and supportive therapy. In consequence, large numbers of patients are required to make the results of clinical trials meaningful. Endotoxemia is not synonymous with sepsis, but it represents a reproducible means of initiating an inflammatory response, despite inter and intra species variations in the response to a given dose. This is particularly apparent in the production of vasoactive mediators relevant to sepsis, such as NO. NO synthase (NOS) is expressed constitutively in the systemic and pulmonary vasculature of both rats and man, both in cultured cells and intact tissue, but although NOS induction is easily demonstrated in rodent leukocytes, evidence of induction in human inflammatory cells types has proved less forthcoming.

Studies in Humans

In healthy volunteers, low muscle PtO_2 and attenuated responses of PtO_2 to changes in blood PO_2 have been reported compared to data from normal animals. PtO_2 profiles of patients with sepsis have also been reported [40, 41] using microelectrodes which are advanced step-wise through the tissue and provided initial data suggesting that tissue hypoxia was a feature of sepsis. One study [41] contrasted muscle PtO_2 in patients with septic shock treated with norepinephrine, to normotensive critically ill controls and indicated a lower PtO_2 in the septic group (23.3 ± 22 for sepsis vs 30.6 ± 23 mm Hg for controls). Low dose dopamine infusion increased PtO_2 in healthy volunteers and critically ill patients in one study [42], an effect reversed by administration of dopamine antagonists. Dobutamine has similar effects in models of septic shock [43]. The impact of inotropic drugs on mean PtO_2 has also been reported in twenty patients with septic shock [44]. Basal PtO_2 increased during inotropic infusion in over 60% of patients studied, but no correlation was found between PtO_2 and DO_2. In other studies, skeletal muscle PtO_2 was recorded in fluid and inotrope resuscitated patients with sepsis/septic shock and compared to groups with limited infection or cardiogenic shock [45, 46]. Mean PtO_2 was considerably higher in the frankly septic patients and mean skeletal muscle PtO_2 was directly proportional to the severity of sepsis. This finding has lent some support to the concept that a primary O_2 utilisation defect exists in resuscitated sepsis, rather than a delivery problem *per se*. However, the study did not control for catecholamine administration nor for the effect of inotropic drugs. The response to ischemia was not investigated and conclusions cannot therefore be drawn regarding the O_2 extraction capabilities of muscle in septic patients.

In preliminary experiments, we have shown that changes in normal forearm perfusion and tissue oxygenation can be detected in patients with severe sepsis.

Moreover, the patients displayed a different response to transient ischemia induced by plethysmography. Under normal conditions, and following cardiopulmonary bypass, PtO_2 seems to be lower in muscle than in subcutaneous tissues. Subcutaneous PtO_2 is significantly diminished following the occlusion of forearm arterial blood flow, but rapidly returns to baseline following reperfusion. Severe sepsis is associated with increased muscle PtO_2 and significant tissue responsiveness to ischemia and reperfusion although the effects of inotropic drugs and ventilation may have influenced the results. Skin perfusion under baseline conditions was significantly greater in patients with severe sepsis and following surgery necessitating cardiopulmonary bypass compared with normal volunteers. Some impairment of regional recovery during reactive hyperemia was observed, but perfusion and oxygenation returned to baseline soon after the ischemic insult.

Conclusion

The role of tissue hypoxia and impaired cellular utilization of O_2 in the chain of events that lead inexorably to multiorgan failure in patients with septic shock is uncertain. Nevertheless, the increasing availability of computer-assisted data acquisition systems and the development of voltammetric methods to concurrently measure perfusion and oxygenation using single electrodes may mean that it is possible to simultaneously evaluate several regional vascular beds of interest in this patient population. Microelectrode techniques have to date been used mainly to measure changes in tissue oxygenation and perfusion in sepsis. Little is known of the changes in concentrations of other nutrients and metabolites. However, sensors are now available for many of these species and there appears to be no technical impediment to the immediate resolution of this important issue. Further, a key question both in research and clinical management is the involvement of species such as NO and superoxide in the development of sepsis. The electrodes which have recently been developed seem ideally suited for the assay of these short lived species in tissues. We anticipate a rapid growth of the use of microelectrodes in clinical and laboratory-based sepsis research.

Acknowledgements: Work supported by the Garfield Weston Trust and British Heart Foundation.

References

1. MacLean LD, Mulligan WG, McLean APH, Duff JH (1967) Patterns of septic shock in man – a detailed study of 56 patients. Ann Surg 166:543–562
2. Bone RC (1991) Sepsis, the sepsis syndrome, multiorgan system failure: a plea for comparable definitions. Ann Intern Med 114:332–333
3. St. John RC, Dorinsky PM (1994) Multiple organ dysfunction syndrome: pathogenesis and approach to therapy. Sem Respir Crit Care Med 15:325–333

4. Rubin DB, Wiener-Kronish JP, Murray JF (1990) Elevated von Willebrand factor antigen is an early predictor of impending acute lung injury in non-pulmonary sepsis syndrome. J Clin Invest 86:474–480
5. Bone RC. Abnormal cellular metabolism in sepsis (1992) A new interpretation [editorial comment]. JAMA 267:1518–1519
6. Berne RM (1964) Metabolic regulation of blood flow. Circ Res 15 (S1):261–268
7. Gutierrez G (1986) The rate of oxygen release and its effect on capillary O_2 tension: a mathematical analysis. Respir Physiol 63:79–96
8. Schumacker PT, Samsel RW (1989) Analysis of oxygen delivery and uptake relationships in the Kroegh tissue model. J Appl Physiol 67:1234–1244
9. Cain SM (1977) Oxygen delivery and uptake in dogs during anemic and hypoxic hypoxia. J Appl Physiol 42:228–234
10. Bihari D, Smithies M, Gimson A, Tinker J (1987) The effects of vasodilation with prostacyclin on oxygen delivery and uptake in critically ill patients. N Engl J Med 317:397–403
11. Nelson DP, Beyer C, Samsel RW, Wood LDH, Schumacker PT (1987) Pathological supply dependence of O_2 uptake during bacteraemia in dogs. J Appl Physiol 63:487–492
12. Mohsenifar Z, Jasper AC, Koerner SK (1988) Relationship between oxygen uptake and oxygen delivery in patients with pulmonary hypertension. Am Rev Respir Dis 138:69–73
13. Shoemaker WC, Appel PL, Kram HP, Waxman K, Lee T (1988) Prospective trial of supranormal values of survivors as therapeutic goals in high risk surgical patients. Chest 94:176–186
14. Yu M, Levy MM, Smith P, Takiguchi SA, Miyasaki A, Myers SA (1993) Effect of maximizing oxygen delivery on morbidity and mortality rates in critically ill patients: a prospective, randomized controlled study. Crit Care Med 21:830–838
15. Hayes MA, Timmins AC, Yau EH, Palazzo M, Hinds CJ, Watson D (1994) Elevation of systemic oxygen delivery in the treatment of critically ill patients. N Engl J Med 330:1717–1722
16. Gattinoni I, Brazzi I, Pelosi P, Iatini R, Tognoni G, Pesenti A, Fumagalli R (1995) A trial of goal-oriented hemodynamic therapy in critically ill patients. N Engl J Med 333:1025–1032
17. Bakker J, Coffernils M, Leon M, Gris P, Vincent JL (1991) Blood lactate levels are superior to oxygen-derived variables in predicting outcome in human septic shock. Chest 99:956–962
18. Gutierrez G, Ground SD (1995) Gastric tonometry: a new monitoring modality in the intensive care unit. Intensive Care Med 10:34–44
19. Whalen WJ, Spande JI (1980) A hypodermic needle PO_2 electrode. J Appl Physiol 48:186–187
20. O'Hare D, Winlove CP, Parker K (1991) Electrochemical methods for direct measurement of oxygen concentration and diffusivity in the intervertebral disc; electrochemical characterization and tissue sensor interactions. J Biomed Eng 13:304–312
21. Winlove CP, O'Hare D (1993) Electrochemical methods in physiology. Curr Topics Electrochem 2:345–362
22. Moussy F, Harrison DJ (1994) Prevention of the rapid degradation of subcutaneously implanted Ag/Ag/Cl reference electrodes using polymer coatings. Anal Chem 66:674–679
23. Clarke LC (1956) Monitor and control of blood and tissue oxygen tensions. Trans Am Soc Artif Int Organs 2:41–49
24. Corbally MC, Green HD (1990) Noninvasive measurement of regional blood flow in man. Am J Surg 160:313–321
25. Mishra SK, Haining JL (1980) Measurement of local skeletal muscle blood flow in animals by the hydrogen electrode technique. Muscle Nerve 3:285–288
26. Harrison DK, Kessler M (1989) A multiwire hydrogen electrode for *in vivo* use. Phys Med Biol 34:1397–1412
27. Albery WJ, Brooks WN, Gibson SP, Hahn CEW (1978) An electrode for PN_2O and PO_2 analysis in blood and gas. J Appl Physiol 45:637–643
28. Brooks WN, Hahn CEW, Foex P, Maynard P, Albery WJ (1980) On-line PO_2 and pN_2O analysis with an *in vivo* catheter electrode. Br J Anaesth 52:715–721
29. Hahn CEW, Brooks WN, Albery WJ, Rolfe P (1979) O_2 and N_2O analysis with a single intravascular catheter electrode. Anaesthesia 34:263–266
30. Lagerlund TD, Low PA (1994) Mathematical modeling of hydrogen clearance blood flow measurements in peripheral nerve. Comput Biol Med 24:77–89

31. Sair M, Etherington P, Curzen N, Winlove CP, Evans TW (1996) Tissue oxidation measured by microelectrode in experimental sepsis. Am J Physiol 271:H1620–H1625
32. Whalen WJ, Nair P (1970) Skeletal muscle PO_2: effect of inhaled and topically applied O_2 and CO_2. Am J Physiol 218:973–980
33. Harrison DK, Kessler M, Knauf SK (1990) Regulation of capillary blood flow and oxygen supply in skeletal muscle in dogs during hypoxaemia. J Physiol 420:431–446
34. Kessler M, Hoper J, Harrison DK, et al (1984) Tissue O_2 supply under normal and pathological conditions. Adv Exp Med Biol 169:69–80
35. Kopp KH, Sinagowitz E, Muller H (1984) Oxygen supply of skeletal muscle in experimental endotoxic shock. Adv Exp Med Biol 169:467–476
36. Astiz M, Rackow EC, Weil MH, Schumer W (1988) Early impairment of oxidative metabolism and energy production in severe sepsis. Circ Shock 26:311–320
37. Guttierrez G, Lund N, Palizas F, et al (1991) Rabbit skeletal muscle PO_2 during hypodynamic sepsis. Chest 99:224–229
38. Rosser DM, Stidwell RP, Jacobson D, Singer M (1996) Cardiorespiratory and tissue oxygen dose response to rat endotoxemia. Am J Physiol 271:H891–H895
39. Vallet B, Lund N, Curtis SE, Kelly D, Cain SM (1994) Gut and muscle tissue PO_2 in endotoxemic dogs during shock and resuscitation. J Appl Physiol 76:793–800
40. Fleckenstein W, Schaffer JA, Heinrich R (1990) Tissue oxygen pressure and transcutaneous oxygen pressure. In: Clinical oxygen pressure measurement II. Blackwell, Berlin, pp 265–278
41. Reinhart K, Bloos F, Konig F, Hannemann L, Kuss B (1990) Oxygen transport related variables and muscle tissue oxygenation in critically ill patients with and without sepsis. Adv Exp Med Biol 277:861–864
42. Kersting T, Reinhart K, Fleckenstein W, Dennhardt R (1985) The effect of dopamine on muscle pO_2 in healthy volunteers and intensive care patients. Eur J Anaesthesiol 2:143–153
43. Lund N, de Asla RJ, Guccione AL, Papadakos PJ (1991) Effects of dopamine and dobutamine on skeletal muscle oxygenation in normoxemic rats. Circ Shock 33:164–170
44. Naumann CP, Ruetsch YA, Fleckenstein W, Fennema M, Erdmann W, Zach GA (1992) pO_2-profiles in human muscle tissue as indicator of therapeutical effect in septic shock patients. Adv Exp Med Biol 317:869–877
45. Boekstegers P, Weidenhofer S, Kapsner T, Werdan K (1994) Skeletal muscle partial pressure of oxygen in patients with sepsis. Crit Care Med 22:640–650
46. Boekstegers P, Weidenhofer S, Pilz G, Werdan K (1991) Peripheral oxygen availability within skeletal muscle in sepsis and septic shock: comparison to limited infection and cardiogenic shock. Infection 19:317–323

Oxygen Electrodes, Optode Microsensing, Near-Infrared Spectroscopy, Spectrophotometry ...

M. Siegemund, M. van Iterson, and C. Ince

Introduction

The introduction of regional measurement techniques has highlighted the inadequacy of classic intensive care monitoring techniques, which assess global hemodynamic and oxygen (O_2) related parameters, to reflect the adequacy of oxygenation of the tissues. Cardiac output (CO), mixed venous O_2 saturation (SvO_2) and derived variables only detect the presence of regional dysoxia if the compromised vascular bed is large enough to influence one of these global measurements. The fact that in septic conditions, despite apparent sufficient oxygen delivery (DO_2) signs of hypoxia and/or metabolic dysfunction persist has focused attention on the processes of underlying microcirculatory oxygenation. Whether tissue distress in states of shock is caused by decreases in intracellular concentration of O_2, leading to a decline in aerobically produced adenosine triphosphate (ATP) or disturbances in cellular metabolic pathways is a source of much debate [1].

Global and regional neuronal and humoral factors, as well as intrinsic metabolic and vascular control systems play a central role in ensuring adequate delivery of oxygenated blood to the tissues [2, 3]. During shock and hypoxemia, where O_2 availability becomes restricted, the tissues will consume as much O_2 as available. In this context, it is useful to specify the term hypoxia as dysoxia; the condition in which the amount of O_2 delivered is insufficient to sustain mitochondrial respiration [4]. In contrast to hemorrhagic shock, where restoration of O_2 transport capacity and global hemodynamics would be the goal of therapy, the correction or supramaximal increase of global variables of DO_2 and O_2 uptake (VO_2) have been shown to be inadequate in the treatment of sepsis [5] and evidence of regional tissue dysoxia remains manifest. Lack of knowledge about basic mechanisms controlling O_2 transport and utilization in the microcirculation, as well as the inadequacy of clinical techniques for assessment of the adequacy of tissue oxygenation, are reasons for the uncertainty about the therapy for different kinds of shock.

In this review we will discuss the clinical and experimental techniques available for the measurement of tissue oxygenation and tissue bioenergetics and their suitability for identifying organs and regions at risk for ischemia and dysoxia as well as their potential impact on therapeutic strategies.

Parameters of Oxygen Transport to Tissue

The measurement of lactate is widely used to assess the prognosis or the response to a specific therapy of critically ill patients [6, 7]. Beside global (shock) or regional (small bowel infarction) causes of anaerobic lactate production, nonhypoxic causes of increased lactate production also can exist. This increase can be caused by, for example, decreased lactate clearance, accelerated aerobic glycolysis (sympathomimetic drugs) or a dysfunction of the enzyme pyruvate-dehydrogenase [8]. Lactate production independent of tissue hypoxia may decrease the prognostic value of the lactate measurement [9]. Intact metabolic abilities of the liver make a significant increase in lactate unlikely, so that individual organ failure may be undetected. For this reason lactic acidosis is a relatively late phenomenon in the course of multiple organ failure in intensive care, occurring when general circulatory failure impairs the function of the liver [10].

SvO_2 can be measured with intermittent blood gas analyses from a pulmonary artery catheter (PAC) or by continuous measurement with a fiberoptic PAC. The SvO_2 is a CO dependent average of the venous effluents from all perfused vascular beds. Therefore, it allows no statement on the adequacy of DO_2 to individual vascular beds and tissues. Vascular beds with a high flow and a low extraction (such as kidney and gut) have greater impact on the SvO_2 than organs perfused with a smaller portion of the CO and high O_2 extraction (such as the heart). Because SvO_2 saturation values are on the steep part of the O_2 dissociation curve the correspondent O_2 partial pressures (PO_2) change on a relatively small scale, and are considerably influenced by pH and temperature. Unfortunately, a critical value of SvO_2 that defines an inadequate regional DO_2 is difficult to determine. Too many factors influence the value of the SvO_2, so that it is of limited value for the assessment of the adequacy of tissue oxygenation [10]. Even the SvO_2 of special organ beds is of little value, because no threshold values have been defined for an adequate oxygenation of tissues with different metabolic activities under certain pathologic conditions. Moreover, in sepsis microcirculatory shunting can cause high levels of SvO_2 to persist, while regional tissue dysoxia can be present (unpublished observations).

Since global measurements of oxygenation and hemodynamics fail to give information on the severity of critical illness and the adequacy of therapeutic interventions, the introduction of local measurements, such as intestinal tonometry, have highlighted the importance of the processes underlying regional tissue oxygenation. The introduction of this new diagnostic technique urges further investigation into the value of critical PO_2 values of the different organ beds, in order to specify the threshold of inadequate tissue oxygenation, e.g., tissue dysoxia. Indeed questions such as "when is tissue PO_2 too low" and "which conditions predestine a low tissue PO_2 to reversible or irreversible tissue damage", remain largely unanswered.

Ideal tissue oximetry methods should provide accurate and reproducible real-time information about DO_2 and VO_2 in specific tissues. In addition oxygenation measurements should be able to discriminate between the arterial and venous microcirculatory and tissue compartment and discern dysoxic, close to normoxic, areas. Furthermore there is the issue of which region to measure because heterogeneity of DO_2 and VO_2 exists at the organ level as well as between organs which worsens during states of shock and sepsis. This implies that the measurement should be made in an organ which is most sensitive to the condition of critical illness, because the heterogeneity in microvascular flow and oxygenation, as well as the different metabolic needs of tissues, make a common critical PO_2 unlikely [10]. For clinical application such an oximeter should ideally be safe, non-invasive and easy to apply.

At the moment, various direct and indirect methods are available, all of which however do not meet the requirements stated above. Direct measurements, such as O_2 electrodes, spectrophotometric techniques and phosphorescence/fluorescence quenching methods serve to measure PO_2 at local or regional levels. The latter ones, however, are only available for research in animals. Indirect methods such as near-infrared (NIR)-spectrophotometry, tonometry and NADH-fluorescence, measure products released during tissue dysoxia in the respiratory chain and in blood.

Oxygen Electrodes

O_2 electrodes can be inserted into tissues or placed on the surface of tissues and organs to measure tissue (micro-) circulatory oxygenation and are based on the Clark electrode [11]. These types of electrodes consist of a noble metal (e.g., silver, gold, and platinum) which reduces O_2 due to a negative polarizing voltage. The current that is generated between the reference electrode (anode) and the measuring electrode (cathode) is proportional to the number of O_2 molecules being reduced on the cathode. In the Clark electrode, both anode and cathode are placed behind an O_2 permeable and electrically insulating membrane. Transport of O_2 occurs due to diffusion from the surrounding tissue with a high O_2 pressure, to the area with an O_2 pressure near zero behind the membrane of the electrode. To obtain reliable measurements, the O_2 consumption of the electrode should be small compared to the local O_2 flux within the tissue [12], otherwise the electrodes have the potential to alter their own environment. The sensitivity of the electrode is determined by the diffusion constant of the electrode, while the surface of the electrode defines the amount of O_2 which combines with hydrogen and generates the current which can be calculated into the PO_2 values after calibration of the current at known O_2 concentrations. This type of electrode has been miniaturized to fit within the tip of a micropipette [13] and has been used to measure the microvascular PO_2 in muscle [14–16]. Microelectrodes however, only measure PO_2 at specific points within a tissue, thereby preventing the evaluation of PO_2 over a wider area. A major limitation of O_2 electrodes is their very limited penetration depth (± 15 µm) [17, 18]. This makes them very sensitive to mechanical movements. A further limitation of O_2 electrodes is, without meaning to sound paradoxical, their sensitivity to O_2. This means that any vessel carrying high PO_2 blood in the neighborhood of the electrode will cause a high value to be read, whereas the surrounding tissue may be hypoxic. Another common limitation of many Clark-type O_2 electrode applications is their disturbed performance in the presence of substances such as halogenated anesthetic gases and nitrous oxide, which may have some influence in clinical and laboratory applications where anesthetic vapors are used [19, 20].

To measure the PO_2 distribution inside the tissue, the tip of the electrode must be inserted into the tissue and thereby will inevitably cause some distortion or disruption of the tissue into which it is inserted. The mechanical forces produced by tip and shaft of the electrode may thus cause structural changes, which may change the local PO_2 [12, 21]. Lubbers and co-workers [22] used a nanostepper, which punctures the tissue by stepwise insertion and withdrawal of the electrode, while the speed of insertion, and the direction as well as the length of the steps is adjustable. With this setup they were able to show the expected heterogeneity and distribution of quantitatively measured PO_2.

Another approach to overcome the local disturbances from tissue reactions is the measurement of correct local PO_2 values before the development of tissue damage. The tissue is punctured very quickly with an O_2 electrode including a gold cathode mounted in an injection canula with a very small outer diameter. The response time of the electrode lies under 500 ms. The needle probe is moved through the tissue with steps consisting of a forward and a backward step. The backward step should revive the tissue from the previous compression caused by the forward motion of the needle. If the desired number of PO_2 recordings has been registered, the probe pulls back completely and the histogram of the PO_2 is calculated [12, 23].

The O_2 electrode can also be applied on the surface of the tissue to avoid tissue damage, which is inflicted by insertion. Further development of the Clark electrode has been the application of "multiwire electrodes". The Mehrdraht Dortmund Oberflächen tissue O_2 electrode is an array of eight individual polarographic electrodes and a silver reference electrode encased in glass and covered with a cellophane and a Teflon membrane, both 12 µm thick, which ensure uniform electrode pressure. The eight measuring points each register PO_2 from non overlapping half-spherical volumes with a radius of approximately 20 µm. The current from these eight electrodes can be read separately. This results in a distribution of O_2 readings over the measured surface with a penetration depth of about ± 15 µm. This method has been applied to measure the O_2 distribution in muscle and intestine in animal studies [24–27]. It is important to note that this distribution is a combination of the spatial distribution under the electrode and the temporal distribution during the measurement [27]. The tissue PO_2 measured under non-pathologic conditions showed a histogram with a normal distribution, which represents the microcirculatory heterogeneity. The values high above the median most likely represent arteriolar or peri-arteriolar PO_2. High pressure applied by the electrode to the tissue may disturb the microcirculatory flow and lead to irregular histograms and low PO_2 readings. Furthermore some types of membrane-covered electrodes used for surface measurements may be sensitive to hydrostatic pressure fluctuation if the membrane is distensible or not tightly applied to the measuring surface.

Tonometry

The introduction of gastric tonometry for measurement of intraluminal carbon dioxide (CO_2) generated by dysoxic intestinal tissue cells can be regarded as a major step forward in monitoring the regional tissue oxygenation in states of shock. Gastric tonometry relies on the principle that CO_2 diffuses freely across tissue and cell membranes. Measurement of luminal PCO_2 by tonometry therefore allows estimation of gut mucosal PCO_2. The classic tonometric technique described by Fiddian-Green [28] for luminal measurement of PCO_2 uses a nasogastric tube with a saline-filled silicon balloon. Measurement of arterial bicarbonate (HCO_3^-) and use of the Henderson-Hasselbalch equation allows, under certain assumptions, the calculation of gut intramucosal pH (pHi). After 30 to 60 minutes of equilibration, the PCO_2 of the intraluminal fluid and the saline are nearly the same. After a measurement time of 30 minutes the equilibration is only 77% complete, so that the PCO_2 values need to be multiplied by 1.24 to compensate for this effect [25]. Conventional blood gas analysis is used to determine the CO_2 content of the saline. A correction factor for incomplete equilibration of the PCO_2 must, therefore be used.

The assumption that the arterial HCO_3^- is in equilibrium with the gut mucosal bicarbonate may not always be correct. Decreased gastric mucosal blood flow in states of shock or therapeutically administered sodium bicarbonate may lead to a significant difference between gastric tissue HCO_3^- and the systemic HCO_3^- and would therefore overestimate the gastric pH_i [29]. The gastric intramucosal PCO_2 (PCO_2i) is a more accurate sign of tissue dysoxia, because it is not directly changed by remote acid-base disturbances. However, the PCO_2i is influenced directly by the systemic arterial PCO_2, which is of obvious importance in critically ill patients where pathologic changes in systemic arterial PCO_2 have direct impact on the gastric PCO_2. Therefore, the gastric-arterial PCO_2 gap has been propagated as a more accurate measurement, because it corrects for systemic abnormalities in CO_2 balance [30].

Whether decreasing intestinal pH_i reflects metabolic acidosis or simply reduced CO_2 off-load by a decrease in splanchnic blood flow, was evaluated by Schlichtig and Bowles [29]. Their study in healthy dogs suggests that the gastric-arterial PCO_2 gap increases from 4–6 mm Hg under normal conditions to 25–35 mm Hg during stagnant gastric blood flow, and that levels above this indicate anaerobic generation of CO_2.

To improve the limitations of classic intestinal tonometry, some new techniques have been developed and introduced in clinical and laboratory practice. Measures of gastric pHi, obtained by sampling gastric juice directly, have been shown by Mohsenifar et al. [31] to be predictive of weaning success in 29 ventilated patients. They found that patients who were not prepared for weaning had substantially reduced gastric intramucosal pHi values. The fact that the patients who were successfully weaned had normal pHi measurements showed that indirect monitoring of the gastric microcirculation may indicate secret cardiovascular insufficiency and an inappropriate phase of weaning from mechanical ventilation.

Three new methods have been introduced for real-time measurement of intestinal PCO_2, by tonometry. Knichwitz and colleagues [32] used a fiberoptic PCO_2 sensor (Paratrend 7, Biomedical Sensors, Highwycombe, UK) originally developed for intravascular blood gas measurements. The fiberoptic PCO_2 sensor in the ileum can precisely and reliably determine intestinal PCO_2, and can quickly and continuously measure changes of the intramucosal PCO_2 during changes in the ventilation pattern of the experimental animals. This catheter also consists of another optical fiber to measure pH and a Clark electrode for PO_2 measurement, which may be of value for additional information.

Another possibility to use the intestinal PCO_2 as an indicator of intestinal microcirculatory perfusion, is the connection of the tonometric catheter to a conventional capnometer (Tonocap, Tonometric Division, Instrumentarium, Helsinki, Finland) [33, 34]. The gas in the tonometric balloon also equilibrates with the PCO_2 in the intestinal mucosa, and in samples of this gas the PCO_2 can be evaluated. Response times to an induced insult are faster than conventional tonometry. After measurement, the air is redirected in the balloon for continuous and automated on-line assessment. The bias, precision and reproducibility of air tonometry *in vitro* are consistent with a clinical reliable device [33]. In a study in mechanically ventilated, septic patients the accuracy of this method was close to that of conventional saline tonometry and the values measured with a cycle time of 10 minutes showed a short response time and correlate very well with conventional tonometry [35].

Tang and coworkers [36] were able to show a prominent increase in gastric intramural PCO_2 during hemorrhagic and anaphylactic shock with miniaturized ion-selective field-effect transistor sensors. By measuring the gastric pH with a miniature glass electrode directly applied to the mucosa, they could show that the calculated intestinal pH, which is based on the assumption that HCO_3^- concentration in the stomach wall and arterial blood are the same, was not fully sustained.

On principle, the same tonometric methods used to determine tissue PCO_2 levels could also be used to measure average tissue PO_2 levels in human patients. A saline perfused dialysis tube may be inserted in tissues to equilibrate with the tissue gases for a period of several hours [37]. The samples produced are analyzed in conventional blood gas machines. For this method, measuring a mean microcirculatory PO_2, as well as for conventional tonometry, the time resolution is a major drawback.

Until now the measurement of intestinal PCO_2 and the derived calculation of pHi is the only regional measurement of microvascular perfusion and oxygenation that is used in clinical practice with therapeutic benefit. This may be an indication that the gut is indeed a suitable and sensitive organ for measurement of microvascular oxygenation during critical illness.

Optode Microsensing

To provide continuous monitoring of oxygenation, ventilatory parameters and acid-base status, intravascular catheters for the measurement of PO_2, PCO_2 and pH on-line have been developed. Their usefulness as reliable alternatives to conventional *in vitro* arterial blood gas analysis in cases of critical blood gas and/or acid-base balance has been shown in patients during long-term application [38]. Optodes quantify analyte concentration by photochemical reactions creating changes in optical properties of indicator substances [39]. The photochemical dyes re-emit light of an altered spectrum after a short flash of an excitation light by emitting a photon during relaxation of electrons to their ground-state position. This lower frequency re-emitted light (fluorescence) will be augmented as the concentration of hydrogen or CO_2 increases or is quenched if O_2 absorbs the energy of the excited electron. The emitted light is transmitted through the optical fiber to a microprocessor to quantify the value changes compared to pre-insertion calibration data [40].

These thin catheters may also be introduced into natural or artificial tissue spaces to measure local blood gas values in tissues. As described above, the usefulness of such catheters has been shown in the measurement of intestinal PCO_2 [32] and for the detection of regional ischemia during cerebral bypass surgery by measuring the tissue PO_2 by means of the included Clark electrode [40].

Near-Infrared Spectroscopy

Near-infrared (NIR) spectroscopy is a non-invasive, optical technique based on the relative transparency of intact biologic tissues to near-infrared light where oxygenated and deoxygenated hemoglobin (Hb), as well as the cytochromes of the mitochondrial respiratory chain, show sharp absorption peaks of light with a wavelength between 550 and 650 nm. The absorption at these characteristic wavelengths, at which maximum absorption occurs, decreases when the cytochromes are in an oxidized state. The terminal cytochrome, cytochrome aa3, has different absorption properties than the other cytochromes with an absorption maximum in the near-infrared region between 800 and 900 nm when the cytochrome is in its oxidized state. Cyotochrome aa3 reduces as much as 90% of the O_2 consumed by tissues during oxidative phosphorylation and limited O_2 availability results in an increase in the reduction level of the cytochrome, thus indicating decreased oxidative metabolism. Monitoring of the redox state cytochrome aa3 could therefore be of particular importance for assessment of pathological impairment of O_2 utilization. Interpretation of near-infrared spectra is however complicated by the uncertainty about the precise contribution of the optical properties of Hb and those of cytochrome aa3 to the measured absorption spectra *in vivo*, as well as of scatter of light by the tissue. This problem has been addressed by Wray et al. [41] who were able to separate the infrared spectra for Hb and cytochrome aa3 in studies done in the rat where blood was replaced by fluorocarbons.

A primary advantage of NIR spectroscopy is that measurement of the absorption of light by tissue and blood makes it possible to quantify the concentration of the chromophores by use of the law of Beer-Lambert, which relates the concentration of a solute to the intensity of light transmitted through solution. Such calculations, however, require knowledge of the length of the optical path traversed by photons. This is unknown since the effective optical path length is much larger than the physical dimensions of the specimen due to lightscattering in the tissue. One method to measure the optical path length in tissue involves the use of the strong absorption of light by water at wavelengths above 900 nm. Knowledge of the concentration of water in tissue permits calculation of the effective optical path length for tissue [41, 42]. It has been found that the optical length of the head, for example, is about four times its physical dimensions.

A different approach makes use of picosecond laser pulses of light sent through the tissue to measure the time of flight of photons through a biological medium. Following propagation through the tissue, a camera detects the photons, and the time necessary for penetration of the tissue is related to the traveling distance. The later a photon is detected, the greater the scattering. This time-intensity profile of photon scattering can be used to estimate the absorption and scattering coefficients of the illuminated tissue [43]. Such measurements have greatly enhanced the accuracy of measurement and allow the quantification of chromophores in tissue as units of concentration.

Most clinical experience with NIR-spectroscopy has been in the field of cerebral oxygenation and cerebral hemodynamics of newborns and infants, because the penetration depth necessary for this age group allows measurement with infrared light [43–45]. It has been shown that changes in arterial O_2 saturation (SO_2) due to breathing abnormalities resulted in a significant fall in oxygenated cerebral Hb and that a concomitant bradycardia even further deteriorates the cerebral oxygenation. An increase of the amount of total Hb in the brain after bradycardia seemed to reflect reactive hyperemia [46]. During deep hypothermic circulatory arrest in pediatric cardiac surgery, NIR-spectroscopy has been used as an indicator of changes in brain oxygenation by measuring the cerebrovascular Hb SO_2 [47].

The use of NIR-spectroscopy in adults during coronary artery bypass surgery, as well as in patients with acute brain disease, has indicated conventional jugular bulb O_2 saturation to be a better monitor of cerebral oxygenation than NIR-spectroscopy [48, 49]. Prough [50] states in an editorial comment that the technique must be improved and refined before it can find a place in the monitoring of adult patients. In contrast, Levy and co-workers [51] find that NIR measurements indeed reflect changes in cerebral oxygenation with a specificity of 60% during ventricular fibrillation, as indicated by electroencephalographic (EEG) evidence of cerebral ischemia. In a recent animal study, NIR spectroscopy could be used to assess the Hb oxygenation and cytochrome oxidase redox state in the lung during hypoxia, histotoxic hypoxia (blockade of cyotochromes) and in hemorrhagic shock by insertion of a fiber bundle via a thoracotomy [52].

Reflectance Spectrophotometry

An alternative approach to absorption of light measurements is the recording and analysis of reflected light. Reflectance spectrophotometry measures whole reflectance spectra or spectra of discrete multiple wavelength. The light coming back from the tissue was in contact with all tissue chromophores and thus the reflected spectra contain information about these substances. Analysis of the backscattered spectra allows calculation of microvascular Hb concentration and can provide information concerning local DO_2, VO_2 and flow.

The Erlangen Microlightguide Spectrophotometer (EMPHO) uses highly flexible lightguides to transmit light from a xenon arc lamp to the tissue [53]. Backscattered light is collected by six surrounding optical fibers, and after passage through a rotating interference bandpass filter, is transmitted to a photomultiplier. This instrument enables measurements of light signals originating from small catchment volumes from the surface of intact, moving organs such as the heart and gut, and allows the resolution of spatial heterogeneities [54]. The device is able to measure Hb, HbO_2, and blood volume at the microcirculatory level. The local O_2 content can be calculated from the Hb content and oxygenation derived form the spectra. Thus, the change in local O_2 content can be determined and, thereby, the VO_2 rate can be estimated [54].

Applied during open heart surgery, this technique has shown improved reflection spectra after completed revascularization [54]. The device was also applied to the fetal scalp during delivery [55]. Although the prognostic value of low scalp tissue oxygenation during delivery is not known, it has been shown that, during delivery, critically low HbO_2 values develop, indicating that the local O_2 reserve is almost exhausted. Sato et al. [56] used the EMPHO to measure intestinal Hb saturation by introducing the flexible lightguide through the working channel of a gastroscope, which provides optical control of the adequate measuring position of the probe. This elegant setup indeed allowed them to measure intestinal oxygenation.

NADH-Fluorescence

O_2 is needed by cells to sustain oxidative phosphorylation in the mitochondria for the production of adenosine triphosphate (ATP) which is necessary for cell metabolism. Metabolic substrates, ADP, inorganic phosphate (P_i) and O_2 are all needed to produce ATP. Due to the central role of oxidative phosphorylation in the metabolism of the cell, methods directed at the measurement of tissue dysoxia (the condition when VO_2 exceeds DO_2) should measure intermediates of oxidative phosphorylation in mammalian tissue cells. The mitochondrial energy state can directly reflect the presence of cellular dysoxia and can be measured and visualized *in vivo* by use of the fluorescent properties of endogenous mitochondrial reduced nicotinamide adenine dinucleotide (NADH). NADH offers one of the main sources of energy transfer from the tricarboxylic acid (TCA) cycle to the respiratory chain in the mitochondria [57, 58]. NADH is situated on the high energy site of the respiratory chain, and during tissue dysoxia, it accumulates because less NADH is oxidized to NAD^+. The redox state of mitochondrial $NADH/NAD^+$ therefore reflects the mitochondrial energy state and is thought to play a regulatory role in the synthesis of ATP [59]. Unlike other intermediates of the respiratory chain, NADH has two absorption maxima at the ultraviolet end of the light spectrum, one at 250 and one at 360 nm, while NAD^+ only has an absorption peak at 250 nm and hardly absorbs light at 360 nm. Thus, like cytochrome aa3, the absorption properties of NAD are dependent on its redox state. NADH however differs from the cytochromes in that the absorbency at 360 nm causes fluorescence at 460 nm. Measurement of the blue fluorescence intensity by spectrophotometry of endogenous mitochondrial NADH *in situ* can, thus, be used as a direct measurement of tissue bioenergetics, since the mitochondrial NADH only increases when the O_2 need of tissue cells exceeds that being delivered by the blood in the microcirculation (unpublished observations). The fluorescent intensity can be imaged using photographic or sensitive video techniques and, thus, can be used to study the regional heterogeneity of tissue dysoxia on organ surfaces *in vitro* and *in vivo* [60–62]. Duboc et al. [63] applied a thin optical fiber over a conventional heart catheter on the endomyocardium during cardiac catheterization in man. After injection of contrast medium into a stenotic coronary artery a transient increase in NADH fluorescence has been shown, which can be interpreted as a marker of ischemia. The NADH fluorescence technique has been incorporated in intravital microscopes for microscopic study of the bioenergetics of cells in the microcirculation [64, 65] and in fluorescence microscopic studies of frozen microsections of freeze biopsies from hearts [66]. Two important limitations of the NADH fluorescence technique for the study of tissue metabolism are, that it is not yet possible to quantify the concentration of NADH from the fluorescence signal and the uncertainty about the contribution of cytosolic NADH to the measured fluorescence.

Pd-Porphyrin Phosphorescence

Wilson and Vanderkooi [67, 68] first introduced a phosphorescence technique for the quantitative measurement of O_2 pressures *in vivo* by use of the O_2-dependent quenching of phosphorescence of Pd-porphyrin. The technique is based upon the principle that a Pd-porphyrin molecule, which has been excited by a pulse of light, can either release this absorbed energy as light (phosphorescence) or transfer the absorbed energy to O_2.

When porphyrin is excited to the first singlet state by light, it is possible to transfer the energy internally to the excited triplet state by changing the electron spin to an unpaired direction without emitting a photon. If the porphyrin is in this excited triplet state and both electrons in the same spin direction collide with an O_2 molecule, the O_2 can absorb the energy from the porphyrin. This event results in a relaxation of the porphyrin to the ground state without emission of photons, the so-called phosphorescence. This process is known as quenching of phosphorescence and results in a shortened phosphorescence decay time and intensity which is dependent on the collision frequency between O_2 and porphyrin. This collision frequency is determined by the amount of O_2 and the chance that a single O_2 molecule causes a quenching event. The relation between the decay time and O_2 concentration is given by the Stern-Volmer relation. Calibration constants associated with the Stern-Volmer relation allow O_2 concentrations to be calculated from the measured decay times [69].

Binding of Pd-porphyrin to a large molecule such as albumin can be used to confine the dye mainly to the vascular compartment. In this way, use of Pd-porphyrin quenching measures predominantly the microvascular O_2 concentration [67, 70]. A phosphorimeter measures O_2 dependent phosphorescence decay following excitation by a pulse of light [65]. Attached to a microscope, the phosphorimeter allows the measurement of PO_2 in single blood vessels of organ microcirculation in Pd-porphyrin infused animals [65, 70–72]. This application has been used to assess the microvascular PO_2 (μPO_2) in hamster and mouse skinfold models [71, 73–78], skeletal muscle [70, 72] and the intestine of rats [65]. Use of sensitive video cameras has enabled imaging of the distribution of μPO_2 on organ surfaces. When used together with the NADH-fluorescence technique (see above), information can be obtained on microvascular O_2 availability as well as tissue bioenergetics. When attached to optical fibers, phosphorimeters allow the measurement of a mean microcirculatory PO_2 on organ surfaces, even in moving organs such as the heart, because direct contact of the probe is not necessary. Such measurements incorporate the μPO_2 of plasma in the capillary and venular blood vessels under the optic fiber over an area of approximately 1 cm^2 to a penetration depth of about 0.5 mm [67]. Our working group also implemented this technique on a microscope and can measure intravascular PO_2 in single capillaries of the microcirculation of anesthetized rats and mice. We compared the Pd-phosphorescence method and the microscopic intravascular measurement in first order arterioles and venules and in capillaries of the ileum for the measurement of the PO_2 in the gut microcirculation of rats at three different inspired O_2 fractions (FiO$_2$). It was shown by simultaneous measurements that the fiber optic technique derived partial pressures correlate well with the capillary and venular PO_2 measured microscopically (unpublished data).

Recently we have developed a multi-fiber phosphorimeter for the simultaneous measurement of μPO_2 in various organs in large animal models of shock and sepsis. Furthermore, a preparation protocol, which makes the Stern-Volmer calibration constants insensitive to pH have also been developed [69]. Fiber phosphorimeters allow measurement of μPO_2 in areas not easily accessible to microscopes and in clinically more relevant animal models. In addition, the pH independence of the decay time is favorable, especially in the microcirculation where changes in the pH are likely to occur and are difficult to measure under pathologic conditions.

In preliminary studies using the multifiber phosphorimeter we have examined the relation between epicardial μPO_2 and the, metabolically less active, gut. Initial results reveal that simultaneously measured epicardial heart μPO_2 is higher than that of other organs and that inotropic stimulation, which causes increased CO and coronary flow, as well as a slight increase of O_2 extraction in the myocardium,

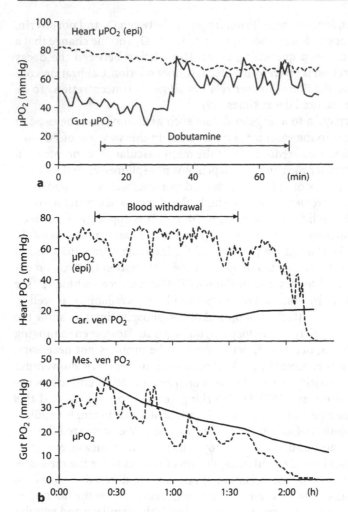

Fig. 1. Comparison between microvascular PO$_2$ (μPO$_2$) of the epimyocardium (epi) and the gut using a multi-fiber phosphorimeter. LAD and mesenteric flow were measured continuously. Cardiac (car) and mesenteric (mes) venous PO$_2$ (ven PO$_2$) were measured by intermittent samples. (a) Inotropic stimulation by dobutamine (stepwise increment of 2 μg/kg/min; cardiac output increased 55%; LAD flow increased 120%) caused a rise in gut μPO$_2$ but had little effect on epicardial heart μPO$_2$. (b) In hemorrhagic shock the gut μPO$_2$ decreased continuously, while the epicardial μPO$_2$ was well preserved. In severe unresuscitated hemorrhagic shock the epicardial μPO$_2$ fell below cardiac venous PO$_2$ indicating functional shunting of epicardial microvascular PO$_2$

had little effect on the epicardial microvascular oxygenation but did cause a large rise in gut μPO$_2$ (Fig. 1a). During hemorrhagic shock, epicardial heart μPO$_2$ was preserved much longer than gut μPO$_2$ and only after a substantial lapse of time without adequate resuscitation did the epicardial μPO$_2$ start to fall while venous PO$_2$ remained unchanged. Shock in advanced stages finally caused epicardial heart μPO$_2$ to fall below venous PO$_2$ values (Fig. 1b). This latter observation demonstrated the presence of functional shunting of the heart microcirculation during severe hypoxemia. These pilot experiments show that epicardial μPO_2 is remarkably well preserved during hemorrhage, and that the gut is an early target organ of shock, possibly the so called "canary of the body" [79]. The data further stress the importance of techniques to measure and compare the microvascular oxygenation at multiple sites.

Reflectance Videophotometry

The microcirculation can be considered to be the most important physiological compartment to monitor the determinants of tissue oxygenation, due to its central role in the etiology of sepsis and shock leading to multiple organ failure. Till now it has only been possible to visualize the microcirculation by use of intravital microscopes in experimental animals in suitable organ beds such as the cremaster muscle or a skinfold model. In man it has only been possible to visualize the microcirculation of the nail bed. A newly developed optical device using reflectance videophotometry (CYTOSCAN™, Cytometrics, Inc., Philadelphia, Pa.) allows on-line microscopic visualization of the microcirculation by use of an image guide and can be applied in humans.

The CYTOSCAN™ instrument is designed for placement on the oral sublingual epithelium or other feasible areas of the body for observation of the microcirculatory system. The instrument consists of a small probe with a halogen light source at a wavelength of 550 nm. Placed over the tip of the probe is a stainless steel cap with a lens mounted in the center. Around the outside of the stainless steel cap is a disposable plastic tube to protect the entire tip. The light is projected through a beam splitter into a series of lenses. The visible light penetrates into the tissue and is reflected back through a unique optical system (patent pending) and is captured by a video camera. Because parts of the incident light are absorbed by Hb, the red blood cells can be seen as dark gray structures on a brighter background on a high-resolution video monitor. With this method, the structure and dimension of vessels are visualized indirectly by their cellular content without a direct image of the vessel walls. In capillaries single erythrocytes and their formation to the so-called "rouleaux" can be observed.

Recently we used this technique to observe the gut microcirculation in pigs during hemorrhagic shock and ischemia reperfusion in a model of aortic cross clamping. During hemorrhage we could observe a decline in the number of perfused vessels together with a decrease of the erythrocyte velocity. After 45 minutes of thoracic aortic cross clamping reperfusion of the ischemic gut showed plugged vessels next to supranormaly perfused ones (Fig. 2). Such clotted vessels may be in part responsible for the so called "no reflow phenomenon" and be expected to contribute to the shunting of the microcirculation. It is expected that this new technique will provide insights into the human microcirculation under conditions of compromised tissue oxygenation and in special diseases affecting the microcirculation.

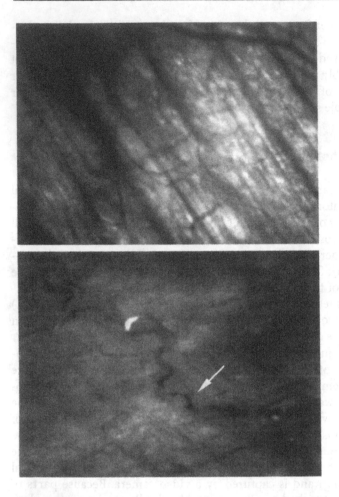

Fig. 2. Reperfusion of the microcirculation on the serosal side of the gut after 45 minutes of thoracic aortic cross clamping. Normal baseline image at the tap. The lower panel shows an image shortly after unclamping the aorta with a reduced number of perfused capillaries and a plugged vessel with clotted non-moving erythrocytes (*arrow*)

Conclusion

The future development of an ideal technique of tissue O_2 measurement should be directed towards an on-line, reliable measurement of tissue oxygenation at the capillary level along with an easy bedside approach for the measurement of a pathologically relevant compartment whose treatment will have a beneficial impact on the course of critical illness. Until such a technique is available, the methods described above, with all their uncertainties and disadvantages must be used to provide further insight into the pathophysiology of O_2 transport to tissue during shock and sepsis. Each single method should be evaluated in terms of which part of the microcirculation is mainly represented and whether each method, indeed reflects signs of tissue dysoxia and oxygen heterogeneity.

In the future, newly developed therapies for the treatment of the different shock states or sepsis should be validated with existing methods, which focus on microcirculatory oxygenation and perfusion. Therefore, the organ beds that show early disturbances of microvascular oxygenation in the distinct disease states should be determined. This information will allow the efficacy of therapies to reduce the heterogeneity of microcirculatory perfusion and dysoxia to be evaluated.

Recently our group has evaluated the application of diaspirin cross-linked Hb (DCLHb) during resuscitation from hemorrhagic shock in anesthetized pigs [80]. Measurement of the gut microvascular oxygen pressure by Pd-porphyrin phosphorescence shows that small volume resuscitation with DCLHb in pigs results in a more sustained improvement of microvascular PO_2, as compared to conventional resuscitation with large volumes of colloid and crystalloid solutions. In contrast to the conventionally resuscitated animals, the DCLHb group shows no significant increase in cardiac output. Figure 3 shows the typical behavior of the μPO_2 during hemorrhage and the subsequent resuscitation with DCLHb. These measurements illustrate the importance of developing such optical techniques for clinical use and can be expected to make an important impact in optimizing treatment strategies for the critically ill patient. The introduction of new vasoactive or vasodilating therapies in septic shock will need to be evaluated in a similar manner, to show the impact of the new approach on the microcirculation.

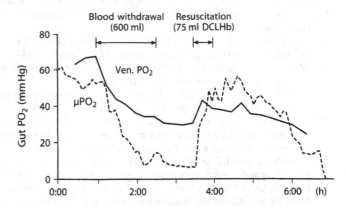

Fig. 3. Hemorrhagic shock and resuscitation with diaspirin cross-linked hemoglobin (DCLHb) in a mechanically ventilated pig. Initially the gut microvascular PO_2 (μPO_2) measured with Pd-porphyrin phosphorescence is similar to the mesenteric venous PO_2 (ven PO_2). During shock, μPO_2 becomes lower than the venous PO_2 creating a characteristic PO_2 gap. The infusion of a 75 ml bolus of DCLHb is already sufficient to restore the μPO_2 of the gut while the mesenteric venous PO_2 only marginally increased

References

1. Gutierrez G (1991) Cellular energy metabolism during hypoxia. Crit Care Med 19:619–626
2. Johnson PC (1986) Autoregulation of blood flow. Circ Res 59:483–495
3. Johnson BA, Weil MH (1991) Redefining ischemia due to circulatory failure as dual defects of oxygen deficits and or carbon dioxide excesses. Crit Care Med 19:1432–1438
4. Robin ED (1980) Of men and mitochondria: coping with hypoxic dysoxia. Am Rev Resp Dis 122:517–531
5. Gattinoni L, Brazzi L, Pelosi P, et al (1995) A trial of goal-oriented hemodynamic therapy in critically ill patients. N Engl J Med 333:1025–1032
6. Bakker J, Gris P, Coffernils M, Kahn RJ, Vincent JL (1996) Serial blood lactate levels can predict the development of multiple organ failure following septic shock. Am J Surg 171:221–226
7. Bakker J, Coffernils M, Leon M, Gris P, Vincent JL (1991) Blood lactate levels are superior to oxygen-derived variables in predicting outcome in human septic shock. Chest 99:956–962
8. Hotchkiss RS, Karl IE (1992) Reevaluation of the role of cellular hypoxia and bioenergetic failure in sepsis. JAMA 267:1503–1510
9. Vincent J-L (1996) End-points of resuscitation: arterial blood pressure, oxygen delivery, blood lactate, or ...? Intensive Care Med 22:3–5
10. Dantzker DR (1993) Adequacy of tissue oxygenation. Crit Care Med 21:S40–S43
11. Clark LC (1956) Monitor and control of blood and tissue oxygen tension. Trans Am Soc Artif Intern Org 2:41–46
12. Lubbers DW (1996) Oxygen electrodes and optodes and their application in vivo. Adv Exp Med Biol 388:13–34
13. Silver IA (1967) Polarography and its biological applications. Phys Med Biol 12:285–299
14. Stein JC, Ellis CG, Ellsworth ML (1993) Relationship between capillary and systemic venous PO_2 during nonhypoxic and hypoxic ventilation. Am J Physiol 265:H537–H542
15. Dulling BR, Berne RM (1970) Longitudinal gradients in periarteriolar oxygen tension: a possible mechanism for the participation of oxygen in local regulation of blood flow. Circ Res 27:669–678
16. Boekstegers P, Weidenhofer S, Kapsner T, Werdan K (1994) Skeletal muscle partial pressure of oxygen in patients with sepsis. Crit Care Med 22:640–650
17. Gutierrez G, Lund N, Acero AL, Marini C (1989) Relationship of venous PO_2 to muscle PO_2 during hypoxemia. Am J Physiol 67:1093–1099
18. Hasibeder W, Germann R, Wolf HJ, et al (1996) Effects of short-term endotoxemia and dopamine on mucosal oxygenation in porcine jejunum. Am J Physiol 270:G667–G675
19. Bates ML, Feingold A, Gold MI (1975) The effects of anesthetics on an in-vivo oxygen electrode. Am J Clin Pathol 64:448–451
20. Tremper KK, Barker SJ, Blatt DH, Wender RH (1986) Effects of anesthetic agents on the drift of a transcutaneous oxygen tension sensor. J Clin Monit 2:234–236
21. Wagner K, Bossen W, Schramm U (1992) Tissue alterations by the penetration of a PO_2 sensing needle probe. Adv Exp Med Biol 317:639–644
22. Lubbers DW, Baumgartl H, Zimelka W (1994) Heterogeneity and stability of local PO_2 distribution within the brain tissue. Adv Exp Med Biol 345:567–574
23. Fleckenstein W, Weiss CH (1984) A comparison of PO_2-histograms from rabbit hindlimb muscles obtained by simultaneous measurements with hypodermic needle electrodes and with surface electrodes. Adv Exp Med Biol 169:447–453
24. Hasjackl M, Luz G, Sparr H, et al (1997) The effects of progressive anemia on jejunal mucosal and serosal tissue oxygenation in pigs. Anesth Analg 84:538–544
25. Fink MP, Cohn SM, Lee PC, et al (1989) Effect of lipopolysacharide on intestinal intramucosal hydrogen ion concentration in pigs: evidence of gut ischemia in a normodynamic model of septic shock. Crit Care Med 17:641–646
26. Vallet B, Lund N, Curtis SE, Kelly D, Cain SM (1994) Gut and muscle tissue PO_2 in endotoxemic dogs during shock and resuscitation. J Appl Physiol 76:793–800
27. van der Meer JT, Wang H, Fink MP (1995) Endotoxemia causes ileal mucosal acidosis in the absence of mucosal hypoxia in a normodynamic porcine model of septic shock. Crit Care Med 23:1217–1226

28. Fiddian-Green RG, Baker S (1987) Predictive value of the stomach wall pH for complications after cardiac operations. Comparison with other monitoring. Crit Care Med 15:153–156

29. Schlichtig R, Bowles SA (1994) Distinguishing between aerobic and anaerobic appearance of dissolved CO_2 in intestine during low flow. J Appl Physiol 76:2443–2451

30. Russel JA (1997) Gastric tonometry: does it work? Intensive Care Med 23:3–6

31. Mohsenifar Z, Hay A, Hay J, Lewis MI, Koerner SK (1993) Gastric intramural pH as a predictor of success of failure in weaning patients from mechanical ventilation. Ann Intern Med 119:794–798

32. Knichwitz G, Roetker J, Bruessel T, Kuhmann M, Mertes N, Moellhoff T (1996) A new method for continuos intramucosal PCO_2 measurement in the gastrointestinal tract. Anesth Analg 83:6–11

33. Kolkman JJ, Zwaarekant LJ, Boshuizen K, Groeneveld AB, Meuwissen SG (1997) In vitro evaluation of intragastric PCO_2 measurement by air tonometry. J Clin Monit 13:115–119

34. Guzman J, Kruse JA (1997) Continuous assessment of gastric intramucosal PCO_2 and pH in hemorrhagic shock using capnometric recirculating gas tonometry. Crit Care Med 25:533–537

35. Heinonen PO, Jousela IT, Blomqvist KA, Olkkola KT, Takkunen OS (1997) Validation of air tonometric measurement of gastric regional concentrations of CO_2 in critically ill septic patients. Intensive Care Med 23:524–529

36. Tang W, Weil MH, Sun S, Noc M, Gazmuri RJ, Bisera J (1994) Gastric intramural PCO_2 as monitor of perfusion failure during hemorrhagic and anaphylactic shock. J Appl Physiol 76:572–577

37. Gys T, van Esbroek G, Hubens A (1991) Assessment of the perfusion in peripheral tissue beds by subcutaneous oximetry and gastric intramucosal pH-metry in elective colorectal surgery. Intensive Care Med 17:78–82

38. Pappert D, Rossaint R, Lewandowski K, Kuhlen R, Gerlach H, Falke KJ (1995) Preliminary evaluation of a new continuous intra-arterial blood gas monitoring device. Acta Anaesthesiol Scand 39:67–70

39. Shapiro BA (1995) Intra-arterial and extra-arterial pH, PCO_2, and PO_2 monitors. Acta Anaesthesiol Scand 39:69–74

40. Hoffman WE, Charbel FT, Abood C, Ausman JL (1997) Regional ischemia during cerebral bypass surgery. Surg Neurol 47:455–459

41. Wray S, Cope M, Delpy DT, Wyatt JS, Reynolds EOR (1988) Characterization of the near infrared absorption spectra of cytochrome aa3 and hemoglobin for non-invasive monitoring of cerebral oxygenation. Biochem Biophys Acta 933:184–192

42. Cope M, Delpy DT, Wray S, Wyatt JS, Reynolds EOR (1988) A CCD spetrophotometer to quantitate the concentration of chromophores in living tissue utilising the absorption peak at 975 nm. Adv Exp Med Biol 248:33–40

43. Rolfe P (1995) Experience with invasive and non-invasive sensors for anaesthesia. Acta Anesthesiol Scand 39:S61–S68

44. Wyatt JS, Cope M, Delpy DT, Wray S, Reynolds EOR (1986) Quantification of cerebral oxygenation and haemodynamics in sick newborn infants by near infrared spectrophotometry. Lancet 8:1063–1066

45. Ince C, Bruining HA (1991) Optical spectroscopy for measurement of tissue hypoxia. In: Vincent J-L (ed) Update in intensive care and emergency medicine. Springer Verlag, Berlin, pp 161–171

46. Wickramasinghe YABD, Livera LN, Spencer SA, Rolfe P, Thorniley M (1992) Plethysmographic validation of near infrared spectroscopic monitoring of cerebral blood volume. Arch Dis Child 67:407–411

47. Kurth CD, Steven JM, Nicolson SC (1995) Cerebral oxygenation during pediatric cardiac surgery using deep hypothermic circulatory arrest. Anesthesiology 82:74–82

48. Tateishi A (1995) Qualitative comparison of carbon dioxide-induced change in near-infrared spectroscopy versus jugular venous oxygen saturation in adults with acute brain disease. Crit Care Med 23:1734–1738

49. Sapire KJ, Gopinath SP, Farhat G, et al (1997) Cerebral oxygenation during warming after cardiopulmonary bypass. Crit Care Med 25:1655–1662

50. Prough DS (1995) Cerebral near-infrared spectroscopy: ready for prime time? Crit Care Med 23:1624–1626
51. Levy WJ, Levin S, Chance B (1995) Near-infrared measurement of cerebral oxygenation. Anesthesiology 83:738–746
52. Noriyuki T, Ohdan H, Yoshioka S, Miyata Y, Asahara T, Dohi K (1997) Near-infrared spectroscopic method of assessing the tissue oxygenation state of living lung. Am J Respir Crit Care Med 156:1656–1661
53. Frank KH, Kessler M, Appelbaum K, Duemmler W (1989) The Erlangen micro-lightguide spectrophotometer EMPHO 1. Phys Med Biol 34:1883–1900
54. Frank K, Kessler M, Appelbaum K, Zuendorf J, H-P A, Siebenhaar G (1990) In situ monitoring of organs. In: Vincent J-L (ed) Update in intensive care and emergency medicine. Springer Verlag, Berlin, pp 145–159
55. Hoper J, Kessler M, Frank K, et al (1991) Monitoring of intracapillary HbO$_2$ in foetal scalp during delivery. In: Erdmann W, et al (eds) Oxygen Transport to tissue XIV. Plenum Press, New York, pp 485–489
56. Sato N, Kamada T, Shichiri M, Kawanao S, Abe H, Hagihara B (1989) Measurement of hemoperfusion and oxygen sufficiency in humans. Gastroenterology 76:814–819
57. Chance B (1976) Pyridine nucleotide as an indicator of the oxygen requirements for energy-linked functions of mitochondria. Circ Res 38:31–38
58. Ashruf JF, Coremans JM, Bruining HA, Ince C (1995) Increase of cardiac work is associated with decrease of mitochondrial NADH. Am J Physiol 269:H856–H862
59. Balaban RS (1990) Regulation of oxidative phosphorylation in the mammalian cell. Am J Physiol 258:C377–C389
60. Coremans JMMC, Ince C, Bruining HA, Puppels G (1997) (Semi-)quantitative analysis of NADH fluorescence images in blood-perfused heart. Biophys J 72:1849–1860
61. Ince C, Ashruf JF, Avontuur JA, Wieringa PA, Spaan JA, Bruining HA (1993) Heterogeneity of the hypoxic state in rat heart is determined at capillary level. Am J Physiol 264:H294-301
62. Avontuur JA, Bruining HA, Ince C (1995) Inhibition of nitric oxide synthesis causes myocardial ischemia in endotoxemic rats. Circ Res 76:418–425
63. Duboc D, Toussaint M, Donsez D, et al (1986) Detection of regional myocardial ischaemia by NADH laser fluorimetry during human left heart catheterisation. Lancet 2:522
64. Toth A, Pal M (1996) Are there oxygen-deficient regions in resting skeletal muscle? Am J Physiol 270:H1933–H1939
65. Sinaasappel M, van Iterson M, Ince C (1996) In vivo application of Pd-porphine for measurement of oxygen concentration in the gut. In: Kohen E, Hirschberg JG (eds) Analytical use of fluorescent probes in oncology. Plenum Press, New York, pp 91–96
66. Vetterlein F, Prange M, Lubrich D, Pedina J, Neckel M, Schmidt G (1995) Capillary perfusion pattern and microvascular geometry in heterogeneous hypoxic areas of hypoperfused rat myocardium. Am J Physiol 268:H183–H194
67. Wilson DF, Pastuszko A, DiGiacomo JE, Pawlowski M, Schneiderman R, Delivoria-Papadopoulos M (1991) Effect of hyperventilation on oxygenation of the brain cortex of newborn piglets. J Appl Physiol 70:2691–2696
68. Vanderkooi JM, Maniara G, Green TJ, Wilson DF (1987) An optical method for measurement of dioxygen concentration based upon quenching of phosphorescence. J Biol Chem 262:5476–5482
69. Sinaasappel M, Ince C (1996) Calibration of Pd-porphyrin phosphorescence for oxygen concentration measurements in vivo. J Appl Physiol 81:2297–2303
70. Shonat RD, Johnson PC (1997) Oxygen tension gradients and heterogeneity in venous microcirculation: a phosphorescence quenching study. Am J Physiol 272:H2233–H2240
71. Kerger H, Saltzman DJ, Menger MD, Messmer K, Intaglietta M (1996) Systemic and subcutaneous microvascular PO$_2$ dissociation during 4-h hemorrhagic shock in conscious hamsters. Am J Physiol 270:H827–H836
72. Zheng L, Golub AS, Pittman RN (1996) Determination of PO$_2$ and its heterogeneity in single capillaries. Am J Physiol 271:H365–H372
73. Torres Filho IP, Kerger H, Intaglietta M (1996) PO$_2$ measurements in arteriolar networks. Microvasc Res 51:202–212

74. Torres Filho IP, Intaglietta M (1993) Microvessel PO_2 measurements by phosphorescence decay method. Am J Physiol 265:H1434–H1438
75. Intaglietta M, Johnson PC, Winslow RM (1996) Microvascular and tissue oxygen distribution. Cardiovasc Res 32:632–643
76. Kerger H, Torres Filho IP, Rivas M, Winslow RM, Intaglietta M (1995) Systemic and subcutaneous microvascular oxygen tension in conscious Syrian golden hamsters. Am J Physiol 268: H802–H810
77. Kerger H, Tsai AG, Saltzman DJ, Winslow RM, Intaglietta M (1997) Fluid resuscitation with O_2 vs. non-O_2 carriers after 2 h of hemorrhagic shock in conscious hamsters. Am J Physiol 272:H525–H537
78. Kerger H, Saltzman DJ, Gonzales A, et al (1997) Microvascular oxygen delivery and interstitial oxygenation during sodium pentobarbital anesthesia. Anesthesiology 86:372–386
79. Dantzker DR (1993) The gastrointestinal tract: the canary of the body? JAMA 270: 1247–1248
80. van Iterson M, Sinaasappel M, Hansen HR, et al (1997) Microvascular gut oxygenation measured by Pd-porphyrin phosphorescence during severe hemorrhagic shock and resuscitation with DCLHb in pigs. J Crit Care 1:S131 (Abst)

Blood and Blood Substitutes as Oxygen Carriers

The Optimal and Critical Hemoglobin in Health and Acute Illness

D. R. Spahn

Introduction

The optimal hemoglobin (Hb) may be regarded as the Hb concentration at which a specific organ functions at peak performance. The optimal Hb concentration is sought to achieve near maximum organ function while avoiding untoward side effects of too low or too high Hb concentrations. Alternatively, the optimal Hb may also be regarded as the Hb concentration at which in terms of organ function the best ratio of benefit to risk of too low and too high Hb concentrations is achieved.

The optimal Hb, therefore, is different in trained athletes for whom maximum oxygen consumption (VO_2) and maximum muscle strength is crucial, in ordinary people who wish to accomplish their daily activity without rapid fatigue, dyspnea or other debilitating side effects of anemia, and in patients suffering from an acute illness, in particular when undergoing a surgical procedure for whom it is important that minimal allogeneic blood transfusions are given due to associated side effects. In surgical patients the optimal Hb may furthermore vary at different periods of their illness, i.e., intraoperatively versus postoperatively and during rehabilitation. The aim of this article is to outline some current knowledge regarding the optimal Hb in these different conditions admitting that this overview cannot be comprehensive nor include all possible situations.

Optimal Hemoglobin for Maximum Oxygen Consumption and Exercise Capacity

There are several reports documenting a significant correlation between increasing Hb concentration and an improvement in maximum VO_2 and exercise capacity [1–8]. A true optimal Hb, however, is difficult to define in athletes since information is largely lacking about the Hb concentration above which maximum VO_2 and exercise capacity would decrease again. In animal experiments, however, it has been demonstrated that rainbow trout reach a peak in maximum VO_2 at a hematocrit (Hct) of approximately 42% and maximum VO_2 decreased with further increases in Hct up to 55% [1]. Interestingly, the optimal Hct for maximum VO_2 was considerably higher than the physiologic normal Hct range in rainbow trout of 23–33%.

Treatment of chronic anemia in humans has beneficial effects not only on maximum VO_2 and maximum exercise capacity, but a striking improvement in overall quality of life has also been noted in several studies, as recently reviewed by Levin [4]. Gradual correction of renal anemia with recombinant human erythropoietin therapy progressively increased maximum VO_2 and exercise capacity [2–7]. Interestingly, the increase in maximum VO_2 is relatively less than the increase in Hb concentration due to recombinant human erythropoietin therapy in most studies. This may be due to a reduced leg blood flow after correction of anemia [7] and reversal of the anemia related compensatory increase in cardiac output (CO) [5]. In patients with anemia and coronary artery disease, partial correction of anemia (increase of Hb from 7.9 ± 0.7 to 10.4 ± 1.1 g/dL) not only increased exercise capacity but also reduced exercise-induced ST segment depression [2]. This beneficial effect on myocardial O_2 balance might not be entirely limited to the increased arterial O_2 content (CaO_2) with higher Hb levels, but might also, in part, be related to the fact that the heart rate at maximum exercise level decreases with increasing Hb levels [5]. Defining optimal Hb levels is again difficult since partial correction of rather severe anemia (Hb of 5–7 g/dL) to Hb levels of approximately 10–11 g/dL is accompanied by a progressive increase in maximum VO_2, maximum exercise capacity and general quality of life. A more complete correction of anemia therefore might be associated with an even greater improvement in maximum VO_2 and maximum exercise capacity. Nevertheless it appears that for daily activity and submaximal exercise, a Hb of at least 10 g/dL is beneficial. This, however, does not exclude the possibility that higher Hb levels could enhance exercise capacity even more.

Optimal Hemoglobin for Surgical Patients

In surgical patients, the focus is not maximum VO_2 or maximum exercise capacity, but, rather, the goal of perioperative management is to avoid allogeneic blood transfusions due to associated side effects [9, 10]. Minimizing allogeneic blood transfusions is not only important to decrease the transmission of blood born pathogens such as human imunodeficiency virus (HIV), hepatitis B and C viruses, cytomegalovirus and potentially even prion diseases [11]. Minimizing allogeneic blood transfusions also minimizes the immunosuppression of the recipient of an allogeneic blood transfusion [12], associated with a 3–10 fold increase in postoperative infections [13–16], prolonged hospitalization [17] and increased costs [18, 19]. Furthermore, minimizing allogeneic blood transfusions also decreases the chance of an AB0 incompatible blood transfusion, and last but not least, an increasing number of well-informed patients wish not to receive allogeneic blood transfusions. For the perioperative period defining minimal Hb levels, thus, may be more clinically relevant than defining optimal Hb levels.

Also, conceptually defining the optimal Hb level in the perioperative period is difficult. The optimal Hb level might be defined as the Hb level at which the organism or a specific organ performs optimally. The problem with such a definition is that it is very difficult to define optimal performance of an organism or a specific organ. In the absence of signs of regional ischemia, overall VO_2 could be a parameter to assess such an optimization. Since, however, VO_2 has been shown to be relatively stable over a wide range of Hb levels in surgical patients [9, 20–32], VO_2 would appear not to be well-suited parameter for assessing the optimal Hb level.

The critical Hb level can be defined more easily as the Hb level below which oxygen delivery (DO_2) to the entire organism, a specific organ or a specific part thereof, becomes insufficient, resulting in global or regional ischemia. For perioperative surgical patients defining the critical Hb level thus may be more realistic and clinically more relevant considering the serious side effects of allogeneic blood transfusions.

Despite a relatively clear definition of a critical Hb, it is relatively difficult to define the critical Hb in any given surgical patient, in particular, since the critical Hb appears to be an individual value [33]. Nevertheless it is possible to summarize the knowledge concerning critical Hb levels for patients of specific age groups, for patients with specific pre-existing disease, for different organs and for different perioperative periods, i.e., the intraoperative versus the postoperative period. In the entire discussion of critical Hb levels, normovolemia is always assumed even when not specifically mentioned. Maintaining normovolemia is of paramount significance when low Hb values are tolerated [9, 34]; actually maintaining normovolemia is more important the lower the Hb level.

Critical Hemoglobin in Children

There are two studies investigating tolerance to extreme hemodilution in children [35, 36]. Haberkern et al. [35] hemodiluted children of age 3 to 20 years preoperatively and re-transfused only at a Hct of 12–14%. Despite this rather marked degree of hemodilution, no lactic acidosis developed in the perioperative period. Fontana et al. [36] also performed preoperative hemodilution. Subsequent surgical blood loss was replaced with asanguinous colloid as long as mean arterial pressure (MAP) was greater than 60 mmHg, cardiac index (CI) was higher than $2.2 \, L \cdot min^{-1} \cdot m^{-2}$, mixed venous Hb O_2 saturation (SvO_2) was above 60%.

The autologous blood was re-transfused when one of the parameters was lower than the above transfusion triggers, or when the operation was finished. Only one transfusion was triggered by a SvO_2 below 60%. All other autologous transfusions were administered at the end of the operation. The lowest Hb reached in this group of pediatric surgical patients ranged from 2.1–4.5 g/dL with a mean of 3.0 ± 0.8 g/dL. The children compensated the extreme decrease in arterial O_2 carrying capacity due to such extremely low Hb values completely by increases in CI and O_2 extraction [36]. Again, no lactic acidosis developed at the nadir Hb value experienced by each individual pediatric patient [36]. The critical Hb value in anesthetized children thus appears to be in the range of 3–4 g/dL.

Adults, in general, also tolerate quite extreme degrees of acute hemodilution remarkably well. Weiskopf et al. [37] recently demonstrated that acute isovolemic hemodilution from a Hb of 13.1 ± 0.2 g/dL to 5.0 ± 0.1 g/dL was well tolerated and fully compensated by awake adult surgical patients and volunteers of 19 to 69 years of age. The observed compensatory mechanisms were increases in CO and O_2 extraction resulting in maintained VO_2 and lack of lactic acidosis at a Hb level of 5.0 ± 01 g/dL.

Critical Hemoglobin in the Elderly

The hemodilution tolerance of elderly patients is controversial. Some studies report an increase in CO in elderly patients [9, 21] during hemodilution, while others do not [9, 38]. In a recent study [21], we found that elderly patients, age 66 to 88 years, fully compensate the decrease in arterial O_2 carrying capacity due to low Hb levels by increases in CI and O_2 extraction. Myocardial ischemia was not observed at maximum hemodilution with a mean Hb of 8.8 ± 0.3 g/dL [21]. Furthermore, age (range: 38–81 years) was found not to influence the individual compensatory increase in CI and O_2 extraction in response to progressive hemodilution from 12.6 ± 0.2 to 9.9 ± 0.2 g/dL in patients with severe coronary artery disease prior to coronary artery bypass graft (CABG) surgery [20]. However, Viele and Weiskopf, [39] found that in Jehovah's Witnesses, mortality was increased in patients with a nadir Hb of less than 5 g/dL, in particular in patients older than 50 years. In contrast, even a temporary Hb of 1.1 g/dL was survived by a 58 year old patient suffering from massive blood loss in tumor surgery [34]. The critical Hb level in elderly patients, thus, is difficult to define but in general appears to be below 9 g/dL provided normovolemia is well maintained. This conclusion is confirmed by a recent study by Carson et al. [40]. These authors found in 8787 consecutive hip fracture patients aged 60 years and older (mean of 80 ± 9 years) that 30 day and 90 day mortality were similar in transfused and non-transfused patients after adjusting for trigger Hb level, cardiovascular disease and other risk factors for death, and concluded that blood transfusion at a Hb level of 8.0 g/dL and higher does not affect mortality in the aged surgical population [40]. In fact 30 day mortality was lower in non-transfused patients in the trigger Hb range of 8–10 g/dL in which 2474 (56%) of 4452 patients received a blood transfusion. This report again highlights the remarkable hemodilution tolerance of aged surgical patients and a certain ineffectiveness of allogeneic blood transfusions as suggested by Fitzgerald et al. [41] based on studies in DO_2 dependent rats.

Critical Hemoglobin in Patients with Coronary Artery Disease

The critical Hct is higher in the presence of coronary artery disease. In dogs with a single 90–95% experimental coronary artery stenosis, regional myocardial systolic and diastolic dysfunction were only found at a Hb of 6 g/dL [42]. In turn, hemodilution to a Hb of 7.5 g/dL was tolerated without alterations in regional myocardial function in the myocardial territory supplied by the stenosed coronary artery [42]. In dogs with experimental single vessel coronary artery disease, the critical Hb, thus, appears to be 6–7 g/dL. In dogs with two proximal 90–95% coronary artery stenoses (left anterior descending and circumflex coronary arteries), a critical Hb of approximately 9 g/dL was observed [43]. The lowest tolerable Hct thus appears to be critically influenced by the severity of coronary artery disease [9, 43]. The remarkable tolerance of low Hct values in subjects with coronary artery disease is based, in part, on an increase of transtenotic coronary flow during hemodilution [42, 43].

Finally, relatively low Hb levels (9.9 ± 0.2 g/dL) are also well tolerated by patients with severe coronary artery disease prior to CABG surgery [20]. Even patients with severe left main coronary artery stenosis (75 ± 9%) tolerated hemodilution to a Hb value of approximately 11 g/dL without electrocardiograph (EKG) signs of myocardial ischemia, arrhythmias or hemodynamic instabilities [44]. Although the exact level is unknown at the present time, the critical Hb is below 10 g/dL even in patients with coronary artery disease. An important finding in this regard is the fact that should hemodilution-induced myocardial dysfunction occur, minimal blood transfusion will alleviate dysfunction promptly [34, 42]

Critical Hemoglobin in Patients with Compromised Cardiac Contractility

The influence of pre-existing contractile dysfunction on hemodilution tolerance and critical Hb is incompletely understood at the present time. Estafanous at al. [45] found that rats with severe disopyramide-induced myocardial depression responded with a blunted increase in CI to hemodilution as compared with control animals. Hemodilution was performed to a Hct of approximately 23%. Rats with mild disopyramide-induced myocardial depression, however, responded to hemodilution similarly to control animals. Kobayashi et al. [46] described hemodilution tolerance in rats with large (healed) myocardial infarctions. The increase in CI was similar in animals with myocardial infarctions as in control animals during moderate hemodilution to a Hct of 30%. During advanced hemodilution (Hct of 20%), animals with previous myocardial infarction exhibited a smaller increase in CI when compared with control animals. It thus appears that both the degree of myocardial dysfunction and the achieved Hct, influence the compensatory mechanisms during hemodilution and thus the critical Hct. Interestingly, left ventricular ejection fraction (range: 26–83%) was found not to influence the individual compensatory increase in CI and O_2 extraction in response to progressive hemodilution from 12.6 ± 0.2 to 9.9 ± 0.2 g/dL in patients with severe coronary artery disease prior to CABG surgery [20]. Also, patients with severe mitral regurgitation and a left ventricular ejection fraction of 61 ± 3% increased their CI and O_2 extraction in response to acute normovolemic hemodilution from 13.0 ± 0.4 g/dL to 10.3 ± 0.4 g/dL prior to mitral valve replacement or reconstruction surgery [47]. Interestingly, patients with sinus rhythm and patients with atrial fibrillation increased CI and O_2 extraction similarly during hemodilution [47]. With the potential exception of extremely compromised cardiac contractility, cardiac contractility appears to only moderately influence hemodilution tolerance and critical Hb may be less than 10 g/dL.

Critical Hemoglobin for the Brain

Even extreme hemodilution from a Hct of $42 \pm 3\%$ to Hct of 6–11% was well tolerated by normal cats [48]. During extreme hemodilution the calculated DO_2 to the brain was maintained and no suppression of spontaneous cortical electrocorticogram evoked primary cortical potentials were observed, and high energy phosphate concentrations were maintained. However, elderly patients as well as patients scheduled for cardiac and vascular surgery often have generalized arteriosclerosis and thus may also have carotid artery stenoses. As in coronary artery disease, the concern is that DO_2 to the brain is compromised with low Hct values in patients with carotid artery stenosis. The only relevant study in this field was performed in dogs [49]. Kee and Wood [49] produced a progressive carotid artery stenosis, first at the native Hct of $40 \pm 1\%$, and again after isovolemic hemodilution to a Hct of $32 \pm 0\%$. Hemodilution increased (transtenotic) blood flow at all degrees of carotid artery stenoses, the increase was even exaggerated at the most severe carotid artery stenoses (90% and 95%). The increase in blood flow fully compensated the decrease in arterial O_2 content during hemodilution resulting in a maintained (transstenotic) O_2 delivery. Should these findings be extrapolated to the clinical situation, the critical Hb in patients with carotid artery stenoses may be below 10 g/dL. This is in keeping with studies documenting a beneficial effect of therapeutic hemodilution to a Hct of 30–35% in terms of long term outcome in patients suffering from acute ischemic stroke [50–52]. Furthermore, should hemodilution-induced neurologic dysfunction occur, minimal blood transfusion is expected to alleviate neurologic dysfunction promptly [53].

Critical Hemoglobin for the Liver and Splanchnic Organs

Nöldge at al. [54] studied hemodilution tolerance of the liver and the small intestine in pigs during progressive hemodilution from a Hct of $30 \pm 1\%$ to a Hct of $14 \pm 1\%$. They found similar compensatory mechanisms in these splanchnic organs as are generally observed in the entire organism, namely an increase in organ blood flow and an increase in O_2 extraction [54], resulting in a maintained VO_2 at low Hct levels. Additionally, surface O_2 tension (PO_2) was measured. In both organs, a normal PO_2 histogram, characterized by the lack of PO_2 readings in the very low range was observed at a Hct of $30 \pm 1\%$ and $20 \pm 1\%$. In contrast, a widening of the PO_2 distribution, including low surface PO_2 values was measured at a Hct of $14 \pm 1\%$. The authors [54] concluded that the critical Hct for liver and small intestine in the pig was close to a value of $14 \pm 0\%$. Extrapolation of these data to humans is fraught with difficulties, in particular due to the difference in native Hct values in pigs of approximately 30%, versus humans with native Hct of approximately 40%. Even hypothesizing that a 50% decrease in Hb could be critical for the liver and splanchnic organs may be problematic, considering the many patients intraoperatively hemodiluted below a Hb of 6–7 g/dL who very rarely if ever exhibit signs of compromised DO_2 to these organs. This is exemplified by a recent case report [34] of a 58 year old patient who was inadvertently hemodiluted to a nadir Hb of 1.1 g/dL due to massive blood loss in tumor surgery, and did not show any elevation of liver enzymes or any gastrointestinal dysfunction. The critical Hb for the liver and the splanchnic organs thus remains to be determined in humans.

Optimal Hemoglobin: Intraoperative versus Postoperative Period

Intraoperatively, low Hb values are remarkably well tolerated by a variety of high risk patients (see above). This might not necessarily be the case in the postoperative period. Nelson et al. [55] reported an increased incidence of cardiac complications such as myocardial infarction, unstable angina and cardiac deaths in patients following peripheral vascular surgical procedures with a Hct below 28% as compared with a group of patients with a Hct value higher than 28% [55]. Intuitively, this appears reasonable considering the lower VO_2, the better arterial saturation and the better control of heart rate and blood pressure during anesthesia. However, there were also several important differences between the groups. The patients retrospectively assigned to the anemic group (Hct less than 28%) with more cardiac complications postoperatively tended to be older (74 ± 10 vs. 64 ± 9 years), have longer operations (420 ± 116 vs. 314 ± 92 in) and had more ischemic events in the preoperative Holler EKG monitoring (39 vs. 7%). Besides having a lower Hct the first morning after the operation, these patients thus had other important risk factors for an adverse cardiac outcome. Nevertheless, it is conceivable that the critical Hct level might be higher postoperatively than intraoperatively due to a higher VO_2 and a less stringent postoperative heart rate and blood pressure control. Prospective studies are needed to specifically investigate this important issue.

Optimal Hemoglobin in Intensive Care Medicine

In intensive care medicine an optimal Hb level might be defined in three ways. First, by an improved outcome at a higher Hb level as compared with a lower Hb level; second, by correction of a (lactic) acidosis by an increase in the Hb concentration; and third, by an increase in VO_2 with elevation of the Hb level.

There are several studies investigating the effect of blood transfusions on DO_2 and VO_2 in a variety of patient groups treated in an intensive care unit (ICU) (Table 1). DO_2 consistently increased with elevated Hb concentrations. VO_2, however, increased only in subsets of 4 of 14 studies (32 of 205 patients). In all other studies, VO_2 did not increase due to blood transfusion (Table 1). The Hb concentration prior to transfusion (range 8.1–11.0 g/dL), the age of patients, presence or absence of an elevated lactate concentration prior to a transfusion, or nature of the underlying critical illness does not allow us to predict in which situation a blood transfusion is more likely to increase VO_2. Particularly puzzling is the predictive value of the lactate concentration prior to a blood transfusion. In one study [22], septic patients with elevated lactate levels increased their VO_2 due to a

Table 1. Effect of blood transfusions on oxygen delivery and oxygen consumption

Author	Year	N	Hbb [%]	Hba [%]	ΔDO_2 [%]	ΔVO_2 [%]	Lactate	Diagnosis
Shah et al. [23]	1982	8	9.2±0.3	10.1±0.3	∅	∅	normal	Trauma
Gilbert et al. [22]	1986	7	9.4±1.5	11.4±2.4	+34	∅	normal	Sepsis
		10	8.1±2.0	11.2±1.2	+33	+17	elevated	Sepsis
Kahn et al. [24]	1986	15	10.9±0.8	12.5±0.8	+ 6	∅	nr	Resp. failure
Conrad et al. [25]	1990	19	8.3±0.3	10.7±0.3	+29	∅	elevated	Sepsis
Dietrich et al. [26]	1990	19	8.4±0.3	10.7±0.3	+29	∅	nr	Sepsis
		14	8.3±0.3	10.5±0.3	+28	∅	nr	Cardiac shock
Lucking et al. [60]	1990	7	9.3±1.4	12.4±0.7	+30	+40	nr	Ped. sepsis
Mink et al. [27]	1990	8	10.2±0.8	13.2±1.4	+37	∅	nr	Ped. sepsis
Ronco et al. [61]	1990	5	10.9±1.2	13.0±1.3	+22	+11	nr	Resp. failure
Ronco et al. [28]	1991	17	11.0±1.2	13.1±0.9	+20	∅	normal	Resp. failure
Steffes et al. [29]	1991	10	9.3±1.2	10.5±1.1	+21	+22	normal	Sepsis
		17	9.3±1.1	10.8±1.5	+18	∅	elevated	Sepsis
Seear et al. [30]	1993	8	8.4±1.4	9.9±1.7	+28	∅	normal	Ped. card. surg.
Lorente et al. [31]	1993	16	9.6±0.3	11.6±0.3	+21	∅	nr	Sepsis
Gramm et al. [32]	1996	19	8.4±0.2	10.1±0.2	∅	∅	normal	Sepsis

N = number of patients studied; Hbb = Hb before blood transfusion; Hba = Hb hemoglobin after blood transfusion; ΔDO_2 = difference in oxygen delivery due to a blood transfusion; ΔVO_2 = difference in oxygen consumption due to a blood transfusion; ∅ = no significant change; nr = not reported; Resp. failure = respiratory failure; Ped. = pediatric; card. surg. = cardiac surgery.

blood transfusion, but not septic patients with a normal pre-transfusion lactate level. In contrast, in another study [29] only septic patients with a normal lactate level increased VO_2 due to a blood transfusion, and not patients with an elevated lactate level beforethe blood transfusion. In yet other studies [25, 26], the pre-transfusion lactate level did not discriminate between patients with and without an increase in VO_2 due to a blood transfusion. The pre-transfusion lactate level thus cannot consistently predict the response of VO_2 due to a blood transfusion.

The relative lack of effect of blood transfusion on VO_2 may be explained by the fact that VO_2 in most of these patients was probably not DO_2 dependent prior to the transfusions. The extra DO_2 capacity offered by the supplemental Hb therefore did not (retrospectively) unmask a compromised VO_2 due to low DO_2. Therefore, VO_2 did not increase after the blood transfusion. A second explanation may be that the blood transfused was stored several weeks before transfusion and therefore had only a limited capacity to improve VO_2. Indeed, Fitzgerald et al. [41] recently demonstrated that only fresh blood (stored 3 days) but not blood stored for 28 days was able to restore VO_2 in a rat model of compromised VO_2 due to low DO_2.

A potential effect of the Hb level on long term mortality has been investigated in several recent studies [57–59]. In a prospective randomized study the impact of a relatively low Hb target range of 7–9 g/dL with a transfusion trigger of <7.5

g/dL and a relatively high Hb target range of 10–12 g/dL with a transfusion trigger of < 10.5 g/dL were compared [57]. The two treatment groups were identical on admission to the ICU and had identical outcomes as assessed by the incidence of organ failures and 30 and 120 day mortality. Accordingly, the authors [57] concluded "… a more restrictive approach to the transfusion of red blood cells may be safe in critically ill patients". Indeed, it appears fair to conclude that in a range of 8–11 g/dL, the Hb concentration does not affect outcome to a clinically relevant degree.

Besides this prospective randomized study, there is a descriptive study [58] asking the question. "Does transfusion practice affect mortality in critically ill patients?" A total of 4470 surgical and trauma patients were included in a very complex data analysis. In this analysis, patients were categorized according to admission acute physiology and chronic health evaluation (APACHE) score (≤ 20 vs. > 20), pre-transfusion Hb (< 9.5 g/dL vs. 9.5–12.5 g/dL), and presence or absence of coexisting cardiovascular disease. Any of the following was considered as coexisting cardiovascular disease: Presence of coronary artery disease, history of myocardial infarction, congestive heart failure, cardiogenic shock, rhythm disturbance, cardiac arrest, or postoperative after a cardiovascular procedure. Analyzing all patients, the authors [58] found that patients who died in the ICU were transfused red cells more frequently than survivors (43% vs. 28%). However, there was one single subgroup of 202 patients (4.5% of 4470 patients) with an APACHE score > 20, a pre-transfusion Hb < 9.5 g/dL and a coexisting cardiovascular disease, in whom mortality was different with respect to the number of packed red cells transfused: No transfusion was associated with a mortality of 55%, 1–3 units with a mortality of 35%, 4–6 units with a mortality of 32% and more than 6 units with a mortality of 60%. However, in a far greater group of 970 patients with an APACHE score < 20 and a pre-transfusion Hb < 9.5 g/dL mortality increased monotonically with increasing numbers of units of packed red cells transfused from 14% in non-transfused patients to 27% in patients transfused with more than 6 units irrespective of the presence of a coexisting cardiac disease. Nevertheless, the overall conclusion was: "… anemia increases the risk of death in critically ill patients with cardiac disease" [58]. Interestingly, it was the same group of authors that came to the opposite conclusion in their prospective randomized trial [57].

Another retrospective cohort study assessed outcome in adult patients refusing blood transfusions for religious reasons [59]. The authors found that first, patients with an initial Hb > 12 g/dL had a lower mortality than patients with an admission Hb of < 6 g/dL; second, patients with a major blood loss had a higher mortality than patients with a minor blood loss; and third, the presence of a coexisting cardiovascular disease generally compromises outcome. This study cannot (although it will) be interpreted to indicate that low Hb levels are generally associated with a higher perioperative mortality; the only conclusion from this study is that the combination of low preoperative Hb, high surgical blood loss and refusal of blood transfusion may be dangerous to your health. Interestingly, the same first author later found in 8787 consecutive hip fracture patients with a mean age of 80 ± 9 years, that 30 day and 90 day mortality were similar in transfused and non-transfused patients after adjusting for trigger Hb level, cardiovascular disease and other risk factors for death and concluded that blood transfusion at a Hb level of 8.0 g/dL and higher does not affect mortality in the aged surgical population [40]. In fact 30 day mortality was lower in non-transfused patients in the trigger Hb range of 8–10 g/dL in which 2474 (56%) of 4452 patients received a blood transfusion [40].

Based on this information, it is very difficult to determine an optimal or critical Hb for critically ill patients. In most patients, the critical Hb level appears to be below 8–9 g/dL.

Conclusion

Partially correcting severe anemia to a Hb level of approximately 10 g/dL is beneficial to improve submaximal exercise capacity, symptoms of coronary artery disease and to alleviate debilitating symptoms of severe anemia and thus to improve quality of life. Supranormal Hb levels enable higher maximum VO_2 and improved exercise capacity in athletes. In surgical patients, definition of optimal Hb levels is extremely difficult. Due to the considerable side effects of allogeneic blood transfusions, definition of critical Hb levels appears more clinically relevant. When normovolemia is well maintained, the critical Hb for elderly patients is less than 9 g/dL and for patients with coronary artery disease or compromised cardiac contractility the critical Hb is less than 10 g/dL. Postoperatively, the critical Hb is higher than intraoperatively. For most critically ill patients the critical Hb may be less than 8–9 g/dL. The critical Hb remains an individual value and no generally applicable number can be provided.

References

1. Gallaugher P, Thorarensen H, Farrell AP (1995) Hematocrit in oxygen transport and swimming in rainbow trout (Oncorhynchus mykiss). Respir Physiol 102:279–292
2. Hase H, Imamura Y, Nakamura R, Inishi Y, Machii K, Yamaguchi T (1993) Effects of rHuEPO therapy on exercise capacity in hemodialysis patients with coronary artery disease. Jpn Circ J 57:131–137
3. Robertson HT, Haley NR, Guthrie M, Cardenas D, Eschbach JW, Adamson JW (1990) Recombinant erythropoietin improves exercise capacity in anemic hemodialysis patients. Am J Kidney Dis 15:325–332
4. Levin NW (1992) Quality of life and hematocrit level. Am J Kidney Dis 20 (Suppl 1):16–20
5. Metra M, Cannella G, La Canna G, et al (1991) Improvement in exercise capacity after correction of anemia in patients with end-stage renal failure. Am J Cardiol 68:1060–1066
6. Lundin AP, Akerman MJ, Chesler RM, et al (1991) Exercise in hemodialysis patients after treatment with recombinant human erythropoietin. Nephron 58:315–319
7. Marrades RM, Roca J, Campistol JM, et al (1996) Effects of erythropoietin on muscle oxygen transport during exercise in patients with chronic renal failure. J Clin Invest 97:2092–2100
8. Suzuki M, Tsutsui M, Yokoyama A, Hirasawa Y (1995) Normalization of hematocrit with recombinant human erythropoietin in chronic hemodialysis patients does not fully improve their exercise tolerance abilities. Artif Organs 19:1258–1261

9. Spahn DR, Leone BJ, Reves JG, Pasch T (1994) Cardiovascular and coronary physiology of acute isovolemic hemodilution: a review of nonoxygen-carrying and oxygen-carrying solutions. Anesth Analg 78:1000–1021
10. Walker RH (1987) Special report: transfusion risks. Am J Clin Path 88:374–378
11. Morris K (1997) WHO reconsiders risks from Creutzfeldt-Jakob disease. Lancet 349:1001
12. Landers DF, Hill GE, Wong KC, Fox IJ (1996) Blood transfusion-induced immunomodulation. Anesth Analg 82:187–204
13. Jensen LS, Andersen AJ, Christiansen PM, et al (1992) Postoperative infection and natural killer cell function following blood transfusion in patients undergoing elective colorectal surgery. Br J Surg 79:513–516
14. Jensen LS, Kissmeyer Nielsen P, Wolff B, Qvist N (1996) Randomised comparison of leucocyte-depleted versus buffy-coat-poor blood transfusion and complications after colorectal surgery. Lancet 348:841–845
15. Jensen LS, Hokland M, Nielsen HJ (1996) A randomized controlled study of the effect of bedside leucocyte depletion on the immunosuppressive effect of whole blood transfusion in patients undergoing elective colorectal surgery. Br J Surg 83:973–977
16. Heiss MM, Mempel W, Jauch KW, et al (1993) Beneficial effect of autologous blood transfusion on infectious complications after colorectal cancer surgery. Lancet 342:1328–1333
17. Murphy P, Heal JM, Blumberg N (1991) Infection or suspected infection after hip replacement surgery with autologous or homologous blood transfusions. Transfusion 31:212–217
18. Healy JC, Frankforter SA, Graves BK, Reddy RL, Beck JR (1994) Preoperative autologous blood donation in total-hip arthroplasty. A cost-effectiveness analysis. Arch Pathol Lab Med 118:465–470
19. Jensen LS, Grunnet N, Hanberg Sorensen F, Jorgensen J (1995) Cost-effectiveness of blood transfusion and white cell reduction in elective colorectal surgery. Transfusion 35:719–722
20. Spahn DR, Schmid ER, Seifert B, Pasch T (1996) Hemodilution tolerance in patients with coronary artery disease who are receiving chronic beta adrenergic blocker therapy. Anesth Analg 82:687–694
21. Spahn DR, Zollinger A, Schlumpf RB, et al (1996) Hemodilution tolerance in elderly patients without known cardiac disease. Anesth Analg 82:681–686
22. Gilbert EM, Haupt MT, Mandanas RY, Huaringa AJ, Carlson RW (1986) The effect of fluid loading, blood transfusion, and catecholamine infusion on oxygen delivery and consumption in patients with sepsis. Am Rev Respir Dis 134:873–878
23. Shah DM, Gottlieb ME, Rahm RL, et al (1982) Failure of red blood cell transfusion to increase oxygen transport or mixed venous PO_2 in injured patients. J Trauma 22:741–746
24. Kahn RC, Zaroulis C, Goetz W, Howland WS (1986) Hemodynamic oxygen transport and 2,3-diphosphoglycerate changes after transfusion of patients in acute respiratory failure. Intensive Care Med 12:22–25
25. Conrad SA, Dietrich KA, Hebert CA, Romero MD (1990) Effect of red cell transfusion on oxygen consumption following fluid resuscitation in septic shock. Circ Shock 31:419–429
26. Dietrich KA, Conrad SA, Hebert CA, Levy GL, Romero MD (1990) Cardiovascular and metabolic response to red blood cell transfusion in critically ill volume-resuscitated nonsurgical patients. Crit Care Med 18:940–944
27. Mink RB, Pollack MM (1990) Effect of blood transfusion on oxygen consumption in pediatric septic shock. Crit Care Med 18:1087–1091
28. Ronco JJ, Phang PT, Walley KR, Wiggs B, Fenwick JC, Russell JA (1991) Oxygen consumption is independent of changes in oxygen delivery in severe adult respiratory distress syndrome. Am Rev Respir Dis 143:1267–1273
29. Steffes CP, Bender JS, Levison MA (1991) Blood transfusion and oxygen consumption in surgical sepsis. Crit Care Med 19:512–517
30. Seear M, Wensley D, MacNab A (1993) Oxygen consumption-oxygen delivery relationship in children. J Pediatr 123:208–214
31. Lorente JA, Landin L, De-Pablo R, Renes E, Rodriguez-Diaz R, Liste D (1993) Effects of blood transfusion on oxygen transport variables in severe sepsis. Crit Care Med 21:1312–1318
32. Gramm J, Smith S, Gamelli RL, Dries DJ (1996) Effect of transfusion on oxygen transport in critically ill patients. Shock 5:190–193

33. Leone BJ, Spahn DR (1992) Anemia, hemodilution, and oxygen delivery. Anesth Analg 75: 651–653
34. Zollinger A, Hager P, Singer T, Friedl HP, Pasch T, Spahn DR (1997) Extreme hemodilution due to massive blood loss in tumor surgery. Anesthesiology 87: 985–987
35. Haberkern M, Dangel P (1991) Normovolaemic haemodilution and intraoperative autotransfusion in children: experience with 30 cases of spinal fusion. Eur J Pediatr Surg 1: 30–35
36. Fontana JL, Welborn L, Mongan PD, Sturm P, Martin G, Bunger R (1995) Oxygen consumption and cardiovascular function in children during profound intraoperative normovolemic hemodilution. Anesth Analg 80: 219–225
37. Weiskopf RB, Viele MK, Feiner J, et al (1998) Human cardiovascular and metabolic response to acute, severe isovolemic anemia. JAMA 279: 217–221
38. Rosberg B, Wulff K (1981) Hemodynamics following normovolemic hemodilution in elderly patients. Acta Anaesthesiol Scand 25: 402–406
39. Viele MK, Weiskopf RB (19943 What can we learn about the need for transfusion from patients who refuse blood? The experience with Jehovah's Witnesses. Transfusion 34: 396–401
40. Carson JL, Duff A, Berlin JA, et al (1998) Perioperative blood transfusion and postoperative mortality. JAMA 279: 199–205
41. Fitzgerald RD, Martin CM, Dietz GE, Doig GS, Potter RF, Sibbald WJ (1997) Transfusing red blood cells stored in citrate phosphate dextrose adenine-1 for 28 days fails to improve tissue oxygenation in rats. Crit Care Med 25: 726–732
42. Spahn DR, Smith RL, Veronee CD, et al (1993) Acute isovolemic hemodilution and blood transfusion: Effects on regional function and metabolism in myocardium with compromised coronary blood flow. J Thorac Cardiovasc Surg 105: 694–704
43. Spahn DR, Smith LR, Schell RM, Hoffman RD, Gillespie R, Leone BJ (1994) Importance of severity of coronary artery disease for the tolerance to normovolemic hemodilution. Comparison of single-vessel versus multivessel stenoses in a canine model. J Thorac Cardiovasc Surg 108: 231–239
44. Herregods L, Moerman A, Foubert L, et al (1997) Limited intentional normovolemic hemodilution: ST segment changes and use of homologous blood products in patients with left main coronary artery stenosis. J Cardiothorac Vasc Anesth 11: 18–23
45. Estafanous FG, Smith CE, Selim WM, Tarazi RC (1990) Cardiovascular effects of acute normovolemic hemodilution in rats with disopyramide-induced myocardial depression. Basic Res Cardiol 85: 227–236
46. Kobayashi H, Smith CE, Fouad-Tarazi FM, Wicker P, Estafanous GF (1989) Circulatory effects of acute normovolaemic haemodilution in rats with healed myocardial infarction. Cardiovasc Res 23: 842–851
47. Spahn DR, Seifert B, Pasch T, Schmid ER (1998) Haemodilution tolerance in patients with mitral valve regurgitation. Anaesthesia 53: 20–24
48. Bauer R, Iijima T, Hossmann KA (1996) Influence of severe hemodilution on brain function and brain oxidative metabolism in the cat. Intensive Care Med 22: 47–51
49. Kee DB, Wood JH (1991) Experimental isovolemic haemodilution-induced augmentation of carotid blood flow and oxygen transport through graded carotid stenoses. Neurol Res 13: 205–208
50. The Hemodilution in Stroke Study Group (1989) Hypervolemic hemodilution treatment of acute stroke. Results of a randomized multicenter trial using pentastarch. Stroke 20: 317–323
51. Koller M, Haenny P, Hess K, Weniger D, Zangger P (1990) Adjusted hypervolemic hemodilution in acute ischemic stroke. Stroke 21: 1429–1434
52. Strand T (1992) Evaluation of long-term outcome and safety after hemodilution therapy in acute ischemic stroke. Stroke 23: 657–662
53. Shahar A, Sadeh M (1991) Severe anemia associated with transient neurological deficits. Stroke 22: 1201–1202
54. Nöldge GF, Priebe HJ, Bohle W, Buttler KJ, Geiger K (1991) Effects of acute normovolemic hemodilution on splanchnic oxygenation and on hepatic histology and metabolism in anesthetized pigs. Anesthesiology 74: 908–918

55. Nelson AH, Fleisher LA, Rosenbaum SH (1993) Relationship between postoperative anemia and cardiac morbidity in high-risk vascular patients in the intensive care unit. Crit Care Med 21:860–866
56. Marik PE, Sibbald WJ (1993) Effect of stored-blood transfusion on oxygen delivery in patients with sepsis. JAMA 269:3024–3029
57. Hebert PC, Wells G, Marshall J, et al (1995) Transfusion requirements in critical care. A pilot study. Canadian Critical Care Trials Group. JAMA 273:1439–1444
58. Hebert PC, Wells G, Tweeddale M, et al (1997) Does transfusion practice affect mortality in critically ill patients? Transfusion Requirements in Critical Care (TRICC) Investigators and the Canadian Critical Care Trials Group. Am J Respir Crit Care Med 155:1618–1623
59. Carson JL, Duff A, Poses RM, et al (1996) Effect of anaemia and cardiovascular disease on surgical mortality and morbidity. Lancet 348:1055–1060
60. Lucking SE, Williams TM, Chaten FC, Metz RI, Mickell JJ (1990) Dependence of oxygen consumption on oxygen delivery in children with hyperdynamic septic shock and low oxygen extraction. Crit Care Med 18:1316–1319
61. Ronco JJ, Montaner JS, Fenwick JC, Ruedy J, Russell JA (1990) Pathologic dependence of oxygen consumption on oxygen delivery in acute respiratory failure secondary to AIDS-related Pneumocystis carinii pneumonia. Chest 98:1463–1466

Hemoglobin-Based Artificial Oxygen Carriers (HBOC): Classification and Historical Overview

G. Kemming, O. Habler, and K. Messmer

Introduction

Oxygen (O_2) is essential for mammalian life. While single cell organisms receive O_2 by diffusion from the surrounding aqueous milieu, evolutionary higher species had to develop systems that transport O_2 from the site of uptake towards the tissues, where it is consumed. Species beyond a critical body mass transport O_2 in a closed circulatory system by means of a polydisperse multifunctional fluid: blood. Having passed the alveolocapillary membrane, O_2 is carried in blood in two forms: the larger part chemically "bound" to hemoglobin (Hb) by van der Vaal's interactions within red blood cells (RBCs), and a minor art physically dissolved in plasma. While the sum of O_2 in these two transport states defines the total O_2 content of blood, the total amount of O_2 delivered to the tissues within a defined period of time (DO_2) is determined by the product of cardiac output (CO) and arterial O_2 content (CaO_2). In the case of anemia, a reduction in CaO_2 can be temporarily compensated by two mechanisms: a rise in CO, providing constant DO_2 over a large hematocrit (Hct) range, and a rise in O_2 extraction by the tissues, when in fact DO_2 is reduced (Hct $< 20\%$). When these physiological compensatory mechanisms become exhausted, DO_2 cannot meet the actual O_2 demand of the tissues (critical oxygen content), hence the only remedy will be the augmentation of CaO_2 by hyperoxic ventilation, transfusion of RBCs, or administration of an artificial O_2 carrier.

Transfusion of human homologous blood in this situation involves certain risks, most of them being adverse to the patient (e.g., transfusion-associated infection, incompatibility due to clerical error, immunosuppression) [1]. Transfusion of homologous packed RBCs is hampered by several logistic issues, e.g., supply and storage [2], and, most importantly, prehospital stabilization of patients experiencing massive hemorrhage has to be achieved without having red cells available for transfusion. For these reasons a safe and effective artificial O_2 carrier is desirable in order to reduce transfusion-associated risks and to guarantee unlimited supply for improvement of trauma care. The desire for such a safe and effective substitute for blood dates back at least to the 17th century [3].

Artificial O₂ Carriers

According to the two modes of O_2 transport, either chemical binding to Hb or physical dissolution in plasma, O_2 content may be increased by artificial O_2 carriers. Two types of artificial O_2 carriers were developed: perfluorocarbon-based artificial O_2 carriers transporting O_2 in a physically dissolved form like plasma, and Hb-based compounds transporting O_2 bound cooperatively by van der Vaal's interactions. Figure 1 depicts the characteristic interrelationship between O_2 partial pressure (PO_2) and percentage O_2 saturation of Hb as well as the interrelationship between PO_2 and CaO_2 for Hb-based artificial O_2 carriers (HBOC) in comparison to human whole blood and plasma.

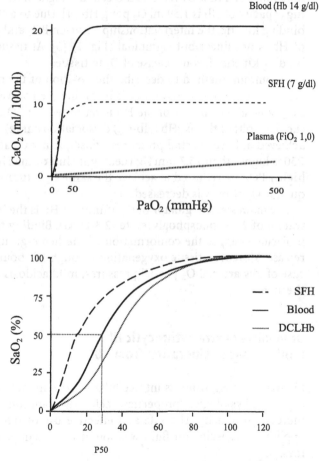

Fig. 1. Oxygen dissociation curves for stroma-free hemoglobin (SFH), native human blood and diaspirin cross-linked hemoglobin (DCLHb). The corresponding oxygen partial pressures at half-maximum oxygen saturation of hemoglobin (p50) are 12–14 mm Hg, 27 mm Hg, and 29–35 mm Hg, respectively for the named hemoglobins

Intraerythrocytic Hb: Physiological Properties

Adult human Hb (HbA) consists of four protein chains, one α- and one β-chain forming a tightly bound dimer, two $\alpha\beta$-dimers form the more loosely bound $\alpha_2\beta_2$-tetramer. Each tetramer carries one heme-group (protoporphyrin including Fe^{2+}). Depending on the absence or presence of reversibly bound O_2, two quarternary structures are possible, each corresponding either to the fully deoxygenated (T, tense) or to the fully oxygenated (R, relaxed) state. These two conformations provide different affinities for O_2, and as O_2 molecules are sequentially bound, the O_2 affinity of Hb increases with the transition from deoxy to oxystate. This change in affinity is called cooperativity and enhances the O_2 uptake of Hb within the lungs and O_2 offloading to tissues. One mol of Hb is able to bind a maximum of 4 mol O_2 With its molecular weight of 64458.8 Dalton, the O_2 binding capacity of Hb is 1.39 ml O_2 per g Hb [4]. Due to a characteristic four step O_2 binding kinetic, the interrelationship between PO_2 and percentage O_2 saturation of Hb is not linear but sigmoidal (Fig. 1) [5]. At tissue PO_2 (~ 40 mm Hg), O_2 binding kinetics favour release of O_2 to tissue.

A common method to describe the position of the oxyHb equilibrium curve along the physiologic PO_2 range is by giving the P50-value. P50 is defined as the PO_2 value at which 50% of the Hb is saturated with O_2. If the P50 is diminished (i.e., left shift of the oxyHb (Hb-O_2) dissociation curve), the same O_2 saturation is achieved at lower partial pressures, consequently O_2 affinity is increased. If the P50 is higher than 26.7 mm Hg (i.e., right shift of the Hb-O_2 dissociation curve), higher PO_2 are required to achieve the same O_2 saturation at a given PO_2, consequently O_2 affinity is decreased.

The main steric regulator of O_2 affinity of Hb is the intraerythrocytic concentration of 2,3-diphosphoglycerate (2,3-DPG). Binding to the β-chains of the Hb molecule changes the conformation of the heme-group, thereby facilitating O_2 release. Moreover, tissue oxygenation through Hb-bound O_2 is enhanced in the case of low arterial O_2 partial pressures, mild acidosis (Bohr effect) and hyperthermia.

Unmodified Extra-rythrocytic Hb: Implications of Liberation from RBCs

Liberation of Hb from its intracellular environment leads to subsequent changes in its physiological properties, including compromised O_2 transport and an increase in toxicity. The safe and effective use of free Hb as an intravenously applicable resuscitation fluid was found to be hampered by the following factors:

1) Free intravascular Hb is bound to haptoglobin and phagocytosed with a half-life of 10 to 30 minutes by cells of the reticuloendothelial system (RES). When the haptoglobin binding capacity is saturated, about half the free Hb still circulating is excreted by the kidneys [6].

2) When Hb is isolated from RBCs, the tetramer of two α- and two β-chains spontaneously dissociates into αβ-dimers or α- and β- monomers [7], thereby reducing the molecular weight from approximately 64 kD to 32 kD or 16 kD. The molecular weight of dimers and monomers is below kidney threshold, therefore they are rapidly excreted in the urine [6, 8].

3) Due to the Hb-tetramer dissociation outside the RBCs, the number of molecules contributing to plasmatic osmotic pressure rises. Infusion of free Hb solutions at concentrations higher than 7 g/dl [9] would, therefore, lead to osmotic overload.

4) Outside the RBC, the O_2 binding cooperativity of Hb is reduced due to the lack of 2,3 DPG. The O_2 dissociation curve is shifted to the left [10] and the high O_2 affinity of unmodified Hb prevents adequate release of O_2 to the tissues.

5) Free Hb is cytotoxic. Mechanisms include complement activation [11], free O_2 radical generation and a rise of catalytically active iron concentration [12]. Precipitating Hb dimers [8, 13] and red cell stroma debris [11] in the ascending part of the loop of Henle contribute to renal failure following intravenous administration of free Hb.

6) Free Hb increases mean arterial pressure (MAP) [14]. Together with a lack of increase in CO on infusion of free Hb this is indicative for vasoconstriction [15–18]. Possible underlying mechanisms for this phenomenon are: scavenging of nitric oxide (NO) by free Hb [19]; increased release of endothelin or upregulation of endothelin-receptors; sensibilization of adreno-receptors; and direct vasoconstrictive properties of Hb [20].

History of Hb-Based O_2 Carriers

Hb was first isolated by crystallization in 1862 by Felix Hoppe-Seyler [21]. Naunyn [22] conducted the first experiments with Hb products, setting the stage for subsequent animal research work. Von Starck [23] in 1898 followed by Sellards and Minot [24] in 1916 were the first to give intravenous injections of RBC lysates to human volunteers.

It was Amberson et al. in 1934 [25, 26], who systematically described the biologic activity of unmodified Hb as an artificial O_2 carrier in an experimental setup. In a unique experiment he demonstrated the efficacy of stroma free Hb as a blood substitute to allow complete exchange transfusions in cats [25]. His Hb solution consisted of lysed RBCs. The cats survived total exsanguination for a short period of time without overt organ dysfunction: The potential of Hb-solutions as a blood substitute was proved. In the following years Amberson's group employed Hb-lysates in patients for the treatment of different forms of anemia [14]. In an impressive case report, Amberson et al. [14] described the outcome of a young woman suffering from major post partum bleeding. After exhaustion of all compatible homologous blood, life threatening anemia was treated with intravenous infusion of an unmodified Hb-solution. The infusion of 300 ml of free Hb (infusion rate 30 ml/min) instantaneously reversed shock and awakened the previously somnolent cyanotic, hypotensive patient. Infusion of free Hb was repeated to a total amount of 2 300 ml (i.e., 250 g Hb). All aforementioned side-effects of free Hb were noticed in this patient (i.e., vasoconstriction, short duration of action, renal toxicity). At the time of infusion a severe pyrogenic reaction was observed; the patient died a few days later in uremia.

During the following decades, intensive research work was initiated with the aim of reducing the obvious adverse effects of free Hb. These efforts resulted in numerous modifications of the Hb molecule and in the development of a variety of different products. Rabiner and coworkers [11] proved in 1967 that contamination of Hb solutions with red cell stroma debris was responsible for many of the side effects encountered after intravenous administration. Stepwise purification of Hb lysates through hemolysis, dialysis, cation exchange filtration and/or crystallization led to highly purified Hb preparations [27], so-called stroma-free Hb (SFH) [28]. Renal toxicity and complement activation seemed to be lesser problems.

SFH is usually prepared by lysis of RBCs and washing with pyrogen free water. A series of filtration steps permits complete elimination of the RBC membrane residuals (stroma) from the Hb solution. This is followed by heat treatment and viral inactivation. The properties of this unmodified, tetrameric or stripped Hb solution are summarized in Table 1.

In comparison to previous compounds, SFH presented the following advantages: The absence of antigen-carrying RBC-membrane allows for SFH infusion without previous crossmatching; extensive heat treatment excludes the risk of infection; oncotic activity of the solution results in good properties as a volume replacement fluid; the Hb contained in the preparation provides sufficient O_2 transport characteristics even when breathing room air.

The most important disadvantages of SFH solutions, however, were still present:
1) high O_2 affinity due to leftward-shift of O_2 dissociation curve for the lack of 2,3-DPG (see P50, Table 1),
2) short intravascular half-life [29],
3) low Hb-concentration [17] and
4) renal toxicity [30].

Table 1. Properties and parameters of stroma-free Hb (SFH) and human whole blood. (From [28] with permission)

Properties	SFH	Whole blood
Hb concentration (g/dl)	6–8	12–14
O_2 -carrying capacity (vol%)	8–11	16–19
Binding coefficient (ml O_2/g Hb)	1.30	1.30
P50 (mm Hg) (PCO$_2$ 40 mm Hg, pH 7,40)	12–14	26–28
MetHb (%)	< 2	< 1
Colloid osmotic pressure (mm Hg)	18–25	18–25
Osmolarity (mOsm)	290–310	290–310

Despite these limitations SFH showed efficacy as a blood substitute in different animal models [15].

The specifications and adverse effects of SFH discussed indicate, that in order to provide a safe and effective HBOC, the following requirements have to be met:

1) further purification of the SFH solution,
2) reduction of O_2 affinity,
3) stabilization of Hb-molecule, thereby prolonging intravascular half-life, reducing renal toxicity and, allowing preparation of higher concentrated solutions,
4) finding of sources for Hb supply, other than human RBC,
5) control of Hb-induced vasoconstriction.

Classification of (SFH)-Hb-Modifications

Research work addressing these topics resulted in distinct modifications of SFH. The problem of O_2 affinity of the tetramer was tackled by modifying the 2,3-DPG binding site. The majority of modification strategies tried to increase the stability of SFH by chemically cross-linking the Hb-tetramer inter- or intramolecularly. Polymerization of Hb-tetramers and conjugation to large molecules as well as encapsulation of the Hb-molecule in order to mimic RBC properties were further strategies. The results were: stabilized tetrameric molecules, polymerized SFH, conjugated SFH and encapsulated SFH [31]. Examples of the different modifications are listed in Table 2.

Benesch and Benesch [32] studied in detail the impact of 2,3-DPG on O_2 affinity, finally showing, that 2,3-DPG's specific binding site on the Hb molecule can be occupied by various ligands including pyridoxal-5-phosphate (PLP). This structural modification resulted in a reduction of the high O_2 affinity of SFH in the absence of 2,3-DPG [32]. Since the N-terminal valine is blocked by PLP, CO_2 transport of SFH-PLP is limited [33]. The first *in vivo* experiments with SFH-PLP were carried out by Jesch et al. [29,34] and Messmer et al. [35,36]. Pyridoxalation of the 2,3-DPG binding site lowers the O_2 affinity but neither prevents dissociation of the tetramer nor prolongs plasma half-life. Therefore, further modifications were necessary.

Crosslinking of two Hb subunits, as shown by Bunn et al. in 1969 [6–8], leads to prolonged half-life by prolonged persistence of the tetrameric structure outside the red cell membrane. Single stabilized tetramers are obtained by modification with agents that form site-specific covalent links between αβ-dimers. These agents stabilize the tetramer preventing its spontaneous dissociation and reduce the O_2 affinity of the molecule. DBBF (bis 3,5-dibromosalicylfumarate) crosslinks between α99–α99 amino acid residues, resulting in a P50 of 28 mm Hg [33] and a plasma half-life of about 3 hours (Table 2) [37]. NFPLP (nor-2-formylpyridoxal 5'-phosphate) crosslinks between β1–β82 amino acid residues. DBBF as well as NFPLP reduce O_2 affinity and stabilize the tetramer [38, 39]. When crosslinking with DBBF is carried out on oxygenated Hb, the bond is established between β-

Table 2. Classifcation of SFH-modifcations. (Modified from [31] with permission)

Product	Chemical agent	Class	Location of linkages
Intramolecular	bis (3,5) dibromosalicylfumarate	DBBF $\alpha\alpha$-Hb	Lys G6(99)α_1 – Lys G6(99)α_2
Crosslinked Hb	bis (3,5) dibromosalicylfumarate	DBBF $\beta\beta$-Hb	Lys E6(82)β_1 – Lys E6(82)β_2
Tetramers	nor-2-formylpyridoxal 5′-phosphate	NFPLP $\beta\beta$-Hb	Val NA1(1)β_1 – Lys EF6(82)β_2
Genetically Crosslinked Hb	Glycine; 2 α-chains contiguous with each other	rHb 1.1	α_1 – α_2 N-terminus – C-terminus
Polymerized	Glycoaldehyde	Poly-SFH	Intra-/extratetramerically
Hb-tetramers	Glutaraldehyde o-Raffinose		
Externally	Polyethyleneglycol	Hb-conjugate	intra/extratetramerically
Conjugated	Dextran		
Hb tetramers	Polyoxyethylene		
Liposome	Polyoxyethylene-2 cethylether	non-phospholipid	none
Encapsulated	Cholesterol	LEH (BRIJ)	
Hb-tetramers	Distearoyl phosphatidycholine	Phospholipid	
(LEH)	Monosialoganglioside Cholesterol Vitamin E	LEH	

lysin residues. This crosslinking-product has a much higher O_2 affinity than that of deoxygenated Hb. Crosslinking of lysin 82 of the β-chain with DBBF does not interfere with CO_2 transport.

Genetically engineered crosslinking of the molecule is the most advanced technique for creating stable Hb-tetramers. Functional human Hb expressed from recombinant human DNA could be produced in bacteria (*Escherichia coli* [40]), yeast (saccharomyces cerevisiae [41]) and plants (tobacco [42]). In the *E. coli* approach the introduction of a new crosslink was successful. During this process two α chain genes are introduced into the *E. coli* genome such that when they are transcribed, a single gene product results in which one α chain is contiguous with the other. The resulting molecule is a di-α-peptide, fused N-terminus to C-terminus over glycine. The molecular weight is 64 kD, and the molecule does not dissociate into dimers [31].

Polymerization of free Hb molecules is another approach to reduce osmotic activity and increase intravascular half-life. Such preparations contain oligomers of crosslinked Hb or polymers of Hb chains [43–46]. Polymerization of Hb creates both intra- and intermolecular multiple crosslinks, yielding heterogeneous, polymeric Hb derivates with varying molecular weights up to 512 kD. As ligands glutaraldehyde [45] and glycoaldehyde [47] have been used without, however, achieving a lowered O_2 affinity of the polymerized Hb. This requires an additional modification by pyridoxalation (PLP) [48] or NFPLP as described above [38]. Another crosslinker, open-ring-raffinose, polymerizes Hb while reducing O_2 affinity of the molecule [49]. A major concern about polymerization, is the fact that it lowers P50 and cooperativity of the molecule. Furthermore, these solutions are unstable under storage conditions reflected by an increasing concentration of metHb [33, 50].

In conjugated Hbs, modifying molecules are bound on the surface of the Hb tetramer [51] in the absence of specific binding sites. Macromolecules to produce SFH-conjugates include albumin, dextran [52], polyvinylpyrrolidone [53], polyoxyethylene or polyethylene glycol [54]. All these substances have very high molecular weights and are easy to obtain. Conjugation of the tetramer is another strategy to avoid glomerular filtration and prolong the intravascular half-life of SFH. Additionally the hydration shell around the Hb-tetramer is increased, restricting the reaction of the molecule with other substances in the cell-free environment. Reaction with these macromolecules stabilizes the Hb tetramer, but an additional step, for example, modification with PLP or inositol hexaphosphate is required to lower O_2 affinity. The mentioned polymers are not easily excreted and polyvinylpyrrolidone is not used clinically anymore for safety reasons after episodes of renal insufficiency occurred [33].

Encapsulation of Hb (SFH)

Encapsulation of Hb in order to mimic an intraerythrocytic environment was a first attempt to reduce osmotic activity and to enhance intravascular half-life, as shown by Chang in 1957 using liposomes for encapsulation of Hb (unpublished observations). This approach is challenging, because Hb must be encapsulated in a high concentration (normal intraerythrocytic Hb concentration, Hb_c: 32 g/dl), and the "artificial RBCs" have to be sterile and endotoxin-free. Apart from merely adding Hb to the liposomes, Hb-modifications or other substances, e.g., steric regulators like 2,3-DPG, can be co-encapsulated [55], which allows modulation of O_2 affinity. Co-encapsulation of enzymes (methemoglobin reductase [56], superoxide dismutase, catalase[57]) may reduce metHb formation and probably lipid peroxidation.

Liposome encapsulated SFH (LEH) [58] presents several advantages as compared to SFH and SFH compounds. First, the artificial membrane protects the Hb molecule from oxidative agents outside the artificial cell. Second, the membrane protects the vascular endothelium from Hb-associated toxicity, which results from heme loss, generation of free O_2 radicals and scavenging of endothelial NO. Moreover, encapsulation significantly increases the intravascular persistence of the Hb-tetramer, polymer or conjugate. Furthermore, encapsulation reduces the osmotic activity of the Hb-molecule, allowing higher Hb concentrations and thereby higher O_2 carrying capacity. Lastly encapsulated Hb can be freeze-dried for storage. The main disadvantage is the complicated and costly production process, hampering large-scale production of encapsulated Hb. Materials to imitate the bilayer-membrane of a RBC include phospholipid and non phospholipid components (Table 2). Most liposomes which have been used for encapsulation of Hb were based on double chain phospholipids and sterols (Table 2). The presence of cholesterol is considered essential since it reduces the tendency of particles to fuse, either to each other or to natural membranes, and increases the elasticity of the vesicles.

The choice of the specific phospholipid to be used in the artificial membrane will determine critical properties such as surface charge, stability of the liposome and RES activation [31]. Disadvantages of phospholipid LEH include [37]: LEH clearance by RES uptake leading to activation of the RES and cytokine release; LEH-accumulation within liver and spleen; and a transient blockade of the RES after single high-dose administration of LEH. Another drawback of LEH is the complicated and expensive production process. Presently no LEH-product is under clinical investigation in humans.

Some of the problems associated with the encapsulation of Hb into phospholipid liposomes could be avoided by encapsulation into lipid solutions of polyoxyethylene-2-cetyl ether and cholesterol (2/3 to 1/3 vol. ratio). The properties of the resulting particles are similar to the abovementioned, but development is still in its infancy. Non-phospholipid liposomes could offer a promising alternative to the phospholipid approach for large-scale production of an O_2 carrier because of their much lower production costs [31].

The most recent artificial RBCs are Hb nanocapsules. They are formed by supersonic activation of Hb molecules. During the activation, superoxide cross-links are created. The resulting O_2 carrier has adequate O_2 affinity, sufficient O_2 carrying capacity, is stable at $4\,°C$ over 6 months storage. While it has promising properties, there is little known at this time, as no experimental or clinical investigations have been conducted.

Sources for SFH

The production of large amounts of artificial O_2 carriers based on human Hb might be a problem [33] due to limited availibility of outdated human blood. Alternatives might be
1) bovine Hb,
2) human Hb expressed from recombinant DNA in microorganisms or plants,
3) human Hb derived from large transgenic mammalians,
4) hemoglobin from non-vertebrates.

Several solutions currently under investigation are based on bovine Hb as an O_2 carrier [43, 51, 59]. Bovine Hb presents several advantages over human Hb. Apart from its nearly unlimited availibility, modulation of O_2 affinity is not dependent on 2,3-DPG as a steric regulator [60], but on chloride ions [61], which are present in adequate concentration (90–100 mmol/l) in human blood. The chloride concentration in human blood results in a physiological P50 of about 28–33 mm Hg.

Additionally, a stronger Bohr effect in bovine Hb augments DO_2 to tissues with low pH [2]. Thus, the modification of bovine Hb has just to prevent dissociation of the molecule. Although bovine- Hb based products have been shown to be effective in different experimental [43] and clinical protocols, the positive features of this compound are outweighed by one major concern: the use of bovine Hb as artificial O_2 carrier is overshadowed by the potential transmission of bovine spongiform encephalitis (BSE) [62]. As long as knowledge about interspecies transmission of diseases is inadequate, caution is advised. However, in contrast to conventional human blood products, both human and bovine Hb-based artificial O_2 carriers can be rigorously sterilized, which should minimize the potential risk of infection.

Genetically engineered Hb expressed from recombinant human DNA might be another possible source for HbOCs. Human Hb has been expressed in bacteria (*Escherichia coli* [40]), yeast (saccharomyces cerevisiae [41]) and plants (tobacco [42]) as mentioned previously. Furthermore transgenic mice and swine were created that produce 80% of their Hb from incorporated human DNA [63–65]. Moreover, with genetic engineering techniques, new functional and physical properties can be introduced into the molecule. As described above the introduction of a glycine link between two α-chains expressed on modified *E. coli* DNA creates a stable tetramer not dissociating into dimers. Moreover, this rHb1.1 compound contains a naturally occuring β-globin mutation, Hb Presbyterian, which reduces the O_2 affinity to a P50-value of 32 mm Hg.

A most remarkable gentically enigneered Hb molecule is "Hb-Scuba" containing information from crocodile DNA. In crocodiles, O_2 affinity is regulated by bicarbonate ions instead of 2,3-DPG. The accumulation of bicarbonate ions as a metabolic end product reduces O_2 affinity and increases the fraction of O_2 offloaded to tissues. This effect allows crocodiles to stay under water for a long time without breathing. The gene-locus containing this information could be located

Table 3. Plasma half-life and P50 of human erythrocytes stroma-free hemoglobin (SFH) and different modifications of SFH. (Modified from [17] and [33] with permission)

Product	Plasma half-life	P50 (37°C) [mm Hg]
Erythrocytes	120 days	26,5
Erythrocytes without 2,3-DPG	–	12
Stroma-free Hb	60'	12–14
Hb-pyridoxal 5'-phosphate (SFH-PLP)	60'	18–20
Lys α$_1$- α$_2$ crosslinked Hb	180'	28
Poly-Hb	10–30 h	12–14
Poly-Hb -pyridoxal 5'-phosphate (SFH-PLP)	10–30 h	18–20
Dextran-Hb-conjugate	20–60 h	24–26
Liposome encapsulated Hb	10–40 h	26
Hb, bovine	60–100'	26
Poly-Hb, bovine	Hours	50–60 (22 at 15°C)

and integrated into human recombinant DNA. Hb Scuba's properties do not differ from those of native crocodile Hb [66]. Genetic engineering of the Hb-molecule can be expected to be one of the most important research areas in the field of HBOCs. At present, limitations of genetically engineered Hb encompass purification needs and considerable costs, that to date do not allow production of required quantities. The involvement of transgenic animals with sufficiently high body mass and blood volume might enable the provision of the required large quantities of Hb. A first step is the production of human Hb in transgenic swine [65, 67].

Another possible Hb-source for HBOCs might be the natural high molecular weight dodecameric Hb produced by *Lumbricus terrestris*, the common earthworm (LtHb). LtHb is the earthworm's extracellular circulating Hb (MW ~4·10³ kD). At neutral pH-values LtHb exhibits oxygen affinity and cooperativity similar to that of human Hb. In an experimental setup, LtHb induced no apparent physical or behavioural changes after partial exchange transfusions in mice and rats [68]. However, whether LtHb might become a cost effective source for large-scale production of HBOC remains questionable.

As a result of intense research most of the major inconveniences of Hb liberated from the RBC environment, e.g., the short plasma half-life, high O_2 affinity and osmotic activity as well as adverse effects of SFH solutions, can be reduced or overcome by different combinations of the modified Hb preparations that have been developed. Plasma half-life and P50-value of modified SFH-preparations are listed in Table 3.

After purification of RBC-lysates and development of stroma-free Hb-solutions a variety of structural modifications has been introduced to the Hb molecule. Some have been combined to improve the properties of HBOCs in order to make them suitable for intravenous application in humans. The O_2 carrying solutions presently under clinical investigation are listed in Table 4.

Table 4. Currently available Hb modifications. (From [2] with permission)

Product	Source	Trademark	Manufacturer
Polyoxyethylene glycol conjugated Hb	human	none	Apex Bioscience Inc.USA
Diaspirin cross-linked Hb	human	HemAssist™	Baxter Healthcare Corp. USA
Glutaraldehyde polymerized Hb	bovine	Hemopure™	Biopure Corporation USA
Polyoxyethyleneglycol conjugated Hb	bovine	none	Enzon Corp. USA
O-raffinose cross-linked and polymerized Hb	human	Hemolink™	Hemosol Inc. Canada
Pyridoxalated and glutaraldehyde polymerized Hb	human	Polyheme™	Northfield Laboratories Inc. USA
Recombinant human Hb	*E. coli*	Optro™	Baxter Healthcare Corp. Somatogen Inc. USA

Combination of HBOC with other Fluids

Combinations of different compounds were created with two aims: to reduce unwanted side effects with unchanged efficacy, and to increase the efficacy of a compound.

In a recent study, de Figueiredo and coworkers [69] investigated the combination of hypertonic acetate and $\alpha\alpha$-crosslinked human hemoglobin (HAHb). Hypertonic acetate, a small volume resuscitation fluid with vasodilator properties was shown to restore CO and global VO_2 promptly when infused in animals undergoing arterial hemorrhage to a MAP of 40 mm Hg [70]. Combination of hypertonic acetate with the vasoconstrictive HBOC compound should be effective in resuscitation from hemorrhagic shock without overshooting vasoconstriction. Six hemorrhaged pigs were resuscitated with HAHb (4 ml/kg BW), presenting a modest increase in CO and mixed venous oxygen saturation (SvO_2) following therapy. However, pulmonary hypertension previously observed with infusion of HBOC [18], was still markedly increased with administration of HAHb. Two animals experienced episodes of severe hypotension and a fall in CO accompanied by pulmonary hypertension. Although the combination of both compounds produced a more pronounced increase in CO than $\alpha\alpha$-crosslinked Hb alone, the concept failed to succeed due to unpredictable side effects of the combination.

Rabinovici and coworkers [71] studied the effects of small volume resuscitation with hypertonic saline 7,5% (HTS) in combination with LEH in a model of lethal hemorrhagic shock. After removal of 70% of blood volume, Sprage-Dawley rats (n = 10/group) were resuscitated with either HTS (5 ml/kg), LEH (5 ml/kg), HTS/LEH (5 ml/kg), Ringer's Lactate (3:1 blood loss) or solely breathing 100% oxygen without fluid resuscitation. Treatment with LEH/HTS reversed hypotension, tissue hypoxia and base excess and markedly improved 24 h survival. No other therapy investigated by the authors ameliorated the shock state or increased survival. The dispersion of LEH in HTS lead to an increase of methemoglobin concentration (by 7%) and to reversible *in vitro* liposome aggregation. Dilution of HTS to lower sodium concentrations reversed liposome aggregation. Rabinovici's study showed that the combination LEH/HTS allows efficient resuscitation from severe hemorrhagic shock. LEH/HTS may be superior to either single component. Yet, prior to the administration of such combinations in humans, stable ready-for-use solutions with defined specifications must be developed and extensively tested.

The history and classification of HBOCs shows that different types of compounds might qualify for blood replacement in acute major hemorrhage or perioperative anemia. The combination of HBOC with other compounds in order to improve efficacy or reduce side effects appears possible. However, clinical trials with HBOCs were prematurely terminated, when side effects, consisting of renal failure despite adequate hydration and elevation of pancreatic enzyme activity, emerged after application of Hb solutions [72]. NO-scavenging is still an unsolved problem and control of vasoconstriction remains questionable.

Conclusion

Integration of Hb compounds into the therapeutic regimen of hemorrhagic shock is premature, for both questionable efficacy and for safety reasons. Whether any of these compounds will be beneficial for patients presenting with acute normovolemic or hypovolemic anemia will have to be elucidated in clinical outcome studies. Of critical importance will finally be the risk and cost issues of Hb compounds as compared to human RBC-concentrates.

References

1. Habler OP, Messmer K (1997) Avoidance of allogeneic transfusion in surgery. Anaesthetist 46:915–926
2. Waschke KF, Quintel M, Kerger H, Lenz C (1997) Oxygen-carrying blood substitutes. Infusionsther Transfusionsmed 24:114–120
3. Winslow RM (1995) Blood substitutes: A moving target. Nature Med 1:1212–1215
4. Braunitzer G (1963) Molekulare Struktur der Hämoglobine. Nova Acta Acad Caesar Leop Carol 26:471
5. Nunn JF (1993) Oxygen. In: Nunn JF (ed) Nunn's applied respiratory physiology. Butterworth-Heinemann Ltd, Oxford, pp 247–305
6. Bunn HF, Jandl JH (1969) The renal handling of hemoglobin. II. Catabolism. J Exp Med 129:925–934
7. Bunn HF (1969) Subunit dissociation of certain abnormal human hemoglobins. J Clin Invest 48:126–138
8. Bunn HF, Esham WT, Bull RW (1969) The renal handling of hemoglobin. I. Glomerular filtration. J Exp Med 129:909–923
9. Moss GS, Gould SA, Seghal HL, Seghal LR (1984) Hemoglobin solution – from tetramer to polymer. Surgery 95:249–255
10. DeVenuto F, Friedman HI, Neville JR, Peck CC (1979) Appraisal of hemoglobin solution as a blood substitute. Surg Gynecol Obstet 149:417–436
11. Rabiner SF, Helbert JR, Lopas H, Friedman LH (1967) Evaluation of a stroma-free hemoglobin for use as a plasma expander. J Exp Med 126:1127–1142
12. Biro GP, Ou C, Ryan-MacFarlane C, Anderson PJ (1995) Oxyradical generation after resuscitation of hemorrhagic shock with blood or stroma-free hemoglobin solution. Biomater Artif Cells Immobil Biotechnol 23:631–645
13. Baker SB de C, Dawles RLF (1964) Experimental hemoglobinuric nephrosis. J Pathol 87:49–56
14. Amberson W, Jennings JJ, Rhode M (1949) Clinical experience with hemoglobin-saline solutions. J Appl Physiol 1:469–489
15. Moss GS, De Woskin R, Rosen AL (1976) Transport of oxygen and carbon dioxide by hemoglobin-saline solution in the red-cell free primate. Surg Gynecol Obstet 142:357–362
16. Hauser CJ, Kaufmann C, Frantz R, Shippy C, Schwartz S, Shoemaker WC (1982) Use of crystalline hemoglobin as replacement of red blood cell mass. Arch Surgery 117:782–786
17. Keipert PE (1992) Properties of chemically cross-linked hemoglobin solutions designed as temporary oxygen carriers. In: Erdmann W, Bruley DF (eds) Oxygen transport to tissue (XIV). Plenum Press, New York, pp 453–464
18. Hess JR, Macdonald VW, Brinkley WW (1993) Systemic and pulmonary hypertension after resuscitation with cell-free hemoglobin. J Appl Physiol 74:1769–1778
19. Schultz SC, Grady B, Cole F, Hamilton I, Burhop K, Malcolm DS (1993) A role for endothelin and NO in the pressor response to cross-linked hemoglobin. J Lab Clin Med 122:301–308
20. Macdonald RL, Weir BKA (1991) A review of hemoglobin and the pathogenesis of cerebral vasospasm. Stroke 22:971–982

21. Hoppe-Seyler F (1862) Über das Verhalten des Blutfarbstoffes im Spektrum des Sonnenlichtes. Arch Pathol Anat Physiol 23:446–452
22. Naunyn B (1873) Untersuchungen über Blutgerinnung im lebenden Thiere und ihre Folgen. Arch Exp Pathol Pharmacol 1:1–17
23. von Starck G (1898) Über Hämoglobin Injektionen. Münch Med Wochenschr 14:69–113
24. Sellards AW, Minot, GR (1916) Injection of hemoglobin in man and its relation to blood destruction, with especial reference to the anemias. J Med Res 34:469–494
25. Amberson WR, Flexner J, Steggerda FR, Mulder AG, Tendler MJ, Pankrata P, Laug EP (1934) On the use of Ringer-Locke solutions containing hemoglobin as a substitute for normal blood in mammals. J Cell Comp Physiol 5:359–382
26. Mulder AG (1934) Oxygen consumption with hemoglobin-Ringer. J Cell Comp Physiol 5:383–397
27. Moss GS, De Woskin R, Cochin A (1973) Stroma-free hemoglobin. I. Preparation and observation of in vitro changes in coagulation. Surgery 74:198–203
28. Gould SA, Moss GS (1996) Clinical development of human polymerized hemoglobin as a blood substitute. World J Surg 20:1200–1207
29. Jesch F, Endrich B, Messmer K (1976) Oxygen transport and hemodynamics of stroma-free hemoglobin solutions. Adv Exp Med Biol 75:105–112
30. Savitzky JP, Doczi J, Black J, Arnold JD (1978) A clinical safety trial of stroma-free hemoglobin. Clin Pharmacol Ther 23:73–80
31. Winslow RM (1996) Blood substitute oxygen carriers designed for clinical applications. In: Winslow RM, Vandegriff KD, Intaglietta M (eds) Blood substitutes: new challenges. Birkhäuser, Basel, Boston, pp 60–73
32. Benesch R, Benesch RE (1967) Effects of organic phosphates from human erythrocytes on the allosteric properties of haemoglobin. Biochem Biophys Res Commun 26:162–167
33. Förster H (1997) Künstlicher Blutersatz. Chirurg 65:1085–1094
34. Jesch F, Hobbhahn J, Endrich B, Peters W, Messmer K (1976) Improved in vivo oxygen delivery from stroma-free hemoglobin by pyridoxilation. Pflügers Arch Physiol 362: R16 (Abst)
35. Messmer K, Jesch F, Endrich B, Peters W (1976) Oxygen supply by stroma free hemoglobin (SFH). Fed Proc 35:526 (Abst)
36. Messmer K, Jesch F, Endrich B, Hobbhahn J, Peters W, Schoenberg M (1979) Tissue PO$_2$ during reanimation with hemoglobin solutions. Eur Surg Res 11:161–171
37. Rabinovici R, Rudolph RS, Ligler FS (1990) Liposome encapsulated hemoglobin: An oxygen carrying fluid. Circ Shock 32:1–17
38. Benesch R, Benesch RE (1981) Preparation and properties of hemoglobin modified with derivates of pyridoxal. Method Enzymol 76:147–159
39. Snyder SR, Welty EV, Walder RY (1987) HbXL99a: A hemoglobin derivate that is crosslinked between the alpha-subunits is useful as a blood substitute. Proc Natl Acad Sci 84:7280–7284
40. Hoffman SJ, Looker DL, Roehrich JM, et al (1990) Expression of fully functional tetrameric human hemoglobin in Escherichia coli. Proc Natl Acad Sci 87:8521–8525
41. Wagenbach M, O'Rourke K, Vitez L, et al (1991) Synthesis of wild type and mutant human hemoglobins in Saccharomyces cerevisiae. Biotechnology 9:57–61
42. Dieryck W, Pagnier J, Poyart C (1997) Human hemoglobin from transgenic tobacco. Nature 386:29–30
43. Vlahakes GJ, Lee R, Jacobs EE Jr (1990) Hemodynamic effects and oxygen transport properties of a new blood substitute in a model of massive blood replacement. J Thorac Cardiovasc Surg 100:379–388
44. Sehgal LR, Rosen AL, Gould SA (1983) Preparation and in vitro characteristics of polymerized pyridoxylated hemoglobin. Transfusion 23:158–162
45. Sehgal LR, Gould SA, Rosen AL (1984) Polymerized pyridoxylated hemoglobin: A red cell substitute with normal oxygen capacity. Surgery 95:433–438
46. Sehgal LR, Sehgal HL, Rosen AL (1988) Characteristics of polymerized pyridoxylated hemoglobin. Biomater Artif Cells Artif Org 16:173–183
47. MacDonald SL, Pepper DS (1994) Hemoglobin polymerization. Methods Enzymol 231: 287–308

48. Bakker JC, Berbers GAM, Bleeker WK (1992) Preparation and characterization of cross-linked and polymerized hemoglobin solutions. Biomater Artif Cells Immobil Biotechnol 20:511–524
49. Hsia JC (1991) O-Raffinose polymerized hemoglobin as a red blood cell substitute. Biomater Artif Cells Immobil Biotechnol 19:402
50. Lenz G, Bissinger U (1994) Modifizierte Hämoglobinlösungen als künstliche Sauerstoffträger. Infusionsther Transfusionsmed 21:63–67
51. Nho K, Glower D, Bredehoeft S, Shankar H, Shorr R, Abuchowski A (1992) PGE-bovine hemoglobin: safety in a canine dehydrated hypovolemic-hemorrhagic shock model. Biomater Artif Cells Immobil Biotech 20:511–524
52. Tam SC, Blumenstein J, Wong JT (1976) Soluble dextran-hemoglobin complex as a potential blood substitute. Proc Natl Acad Sci 73:2128–2132
53. Schmidt K (1979) Polyvinylpyrrolidon-gebundenes Hämoglobin als ein Sauerstoff übertragender Blutersatzstoff. Klin Wochenschr 57:1169–1175
54. Yabuki A, Yamaji K, Ohki H, Iwashita Y (1990) Characterization of a pyridoxilated hemoglobin-polyoxyethylene conjugate as a physiologic oxygen carrier. Transfusion 30:516–520
55. Waschke KF (1995) Modified hemoglobins as oxygen carrying blood substitutes. Anaesthetist 44:1–12
56. Ogata Y, Goto H, Kimura T, Fukui H (1997) Development of neo red cells (NRC) with the enzymatic reduction system of methemoglobin. Artif Cells Blood Substit Immobil Biotechnol 25:417–427
57. Chang TMS (1997) Recent and future developments in modified hemoglobin and microencapsulated hemoglobin as red blood cell substitutes. Artif Cells Blood Substit Immobil Biotechnol 25:1–24
58. Djordjevich L, Ivankovich AD (1988) Progress in development of synthetic erythrocytes made by encapsulation of hemoglobin. Adv Exp Med Biol 238:161–170
59. Feola M, Gonzalez H, Canizaro PC (1983) Development of a bovine stroma-free hemoglobin as a blood substitute. Surg Gynecol Obstet 157:399–408
60. Bunn HF (1971) Differences in the interaction of 2,3-diphosphoglycerate with certain mammalian hemoglobins. Science 172:1049–1050
61. Fronticelli C, Bucci E, Orth C (1984) Solvent regulation of oxygen affinity in hemoglobin. J Biol Chem 259:10841–10844
62. Dormont D (1996) Transmission of spongiform encephalopathy agents or prions. Med Maladies Infect 26:455–464
63. Greaves DR, Fraser P, Vidal MA, Ropers D, Luzzato L, Gosveld F (1990) A transgenic mouse model of sickle cell disorder. Nature 343:183–185
64. Ryan TM, Townes TM, Reilly MP, Asateera T, Palmiter RD, Brinster RL, Behringer RR (1990) Human sickle cell hemoglobin in transgenic mice. Science 247:566–568
65. Logan JS, Martin MJ (1994) Transgenic swine as a recombinant production system for human hemoglobin. Methods Enzymol 231:435–445
66. Komiyama NH, Miyazaki G, Tame J, Nagai K (1995) Transplanting a unique allosteric effect from crocodile into human hemoglobin. Nature 373:244–246
67. O'Donnell JK, Martin MJ, Logan JS, Kumar R (1993) Production of human hemoglobin in transgenic swine; an approach to a blood substitute. Cancer Detect Prevent 17:307–312
68. Hirsch RE, Jelicks LA, Wittenberg BA, Dhananjaya KK, Shear HL, Harrington JP (1997) A first evaluation of the natural high molecular weight polymeric lumbricus terrestris hemoglobin as an oxygen carrier. Artif Cells Blood Substit Immobil Biotechnol 25:429–444
69. De Figueiredo LF, Elgjo GI, Mathru M, Rocha e Silva M, Kramer GC (1997) Hypertonic acetate-αα hemoglobin for small volume resuscitation of hemorrhagic shock. Artif Cells Blood Substit Immobil Biotechnol 25:61–73
70. Nguyen TT, Zwischenberger JP, Watson WC, et al (1995) Hypertonic acetate dextran achieves high-flow low-pressure resuscitation of hemorrhagic shock. J Trauma 38:602–608
71. Rabinovici R, Rudolph AS, Vernick J, Feuerstein C (1993) A new salutary resuscitative fluid: liposome encapsulated hemoglobin/hypertonic saline solution. J Trauma 35:121–126
72. Fox JL (1994) Assessing blood substitutes. Biotechnology 12:231–232

Hemoglobin Solutions: Effects on Tissue Oxygenation

O. Habler and K. Messmer

Introduction

Artificial oxygen (O_2) carriers are intended to increase the reduced O_2 carrying capacity of blood in severe anemia. Preconditions essential to meet this demand are rapid and maximal O_2 uptake by the artificial O_2 carrier during passage through the pulmonary capillary bed, the ability to reach the area of O_2 demand, i.e., the microcirculatory system within different organs, and the easy delivery of transported O_2 to tissues following the O_2 partial pressure (PO_2) gradient between blood and tissues. The compound of choice needs also to be non-antigenic, non-infectious and void of organ toxicity or pharmacodynamic effects which could *per se* limit its potential use.

It is not surprising that it was isolated, purified (stroma free) hemoglobin (Hb) as the 'natural' O_2 carrier, which was first tested for efficacious tissue oxygenation in experimental and clinical investigations [1]. In an early case-report [1], dating from 1949, the american physiologist William Amberson described the effects observed after infusion of a self-made human Hb solution in a young, obstetric patient. After exhaustion of all available homologous blood, this patient who suffered from uncontrolled hemorrhage after incomplete delivery, received a total of 2 300 ml of the solution, containing ~ 250 gram of purified human Hb. Despite extreme anemia, reflected by hematocrit (Hct) values between 5.5 and 7% over a period of 30 hours, the patient remained conscious, spontaneously breathing and hemodynamically stable, indicating that the O_2 demand of vital tissues, e.g., myocardium and brain, must have been met. Amberson concluded from his observations that "this patient lived because of the Hb dissolved in plasma, which supplemented the oxygen capacity of the intracorpuscular hemoglobin". Amberson's solution was immature in terms of purification and chemical stability and the young woman died on the 9th day after the first infusion, from uremia due to renal insufficiency.

Since these early observations, serious efforts have been made by researchers and pharmaceutical companies to develop safe and effective Hb preparations suitable for intravenous infusion in anemic patients in whom blood transfusion is impossible because of medical or logistic problems. Briefly, some of the main disadvantages of first generation Hb based oxygen carriers (HBOC), i.e., low Hb concentration, high O_2 affinity of free Hb, rapid dissociation of the Hb tetramer into dimers and monomers, renal toxicity and vasoconstriction, have been overcome by chemical modification of the native Hb molecule. Second generation HBOCs are free of red blood cell membrane fragments, which formerly caused renal insufficiency and coagulopathy. Intramolecular cross-linking of Hb α-subunits (reduction of spontaneous dissociation), polymerization of single Hb molecules or conjugation to macromolecules (reduction of glomerular membrane passage) have led to prolonged intravascular half-life of free Hb, reduction of renal toxicity and attenuation of the vasoactive properties of stroma free Hb. Furthermore stabilization of the molecule allows for administration of more concentrated solutions without the risk of osmotic overload of the organism.

In this chapter we discuss the main results of experimental studies investigating the effects of Hb solutions on tissue oxygenation. We focus on recent publications and those compounds currently under clinical investigation.

HBOCs in Hemorrhagic Shock

The cornerstones of hemorrhagic shock management are control of bleeding and rapid normalization of intravascular volume to restore tissue perfusion and adequate O_2 delivery (DO_2).

HBOCs seem to be appropriate resuscitation fluids in the case of hemorrhagic shock for the following reasons:
1) HBOCs can be provided as iso- or hyperoncotic solutions and hence may act as true O_2 carrying plasma expanders;
2) beside the volume expanding effect, vasoconstrictor properties of free Hb might contribute to hemodynamic stabilization during fluid resuscitation, provided however, that local DO_2 is not curtailed due to vasoconstriction and blood flow redistribution within the microcirculation.

Tissue oxygenation during shock treatment with HBOCs has been monitored directly by use of O_2 sensitive electrodes or fluorescence-quenching optodes, and indirectly by monitoring of parameters like O_2 consumption (VO_2), mixed venous O_2 saturation (SvO_2), arterial base deficit and plasma lactate concentration.

The HBOCs most extensively investigated in this respect are:
1) diaspirin-crosslinked hemoglobin – DCLHb, a 10% solution of human αα-crosslinked Hb (Hemassist™, Baxter, Round Lake, Ill, USA)
2) glutaraldehyde-polymerized bovine hemoglobin - PBH (Hemopure™, Biopure Corp, Boston, Mass, USA)
3) o-raffinose crosslinked and polymerized human hemoglobin (Polyheme™, Northfield Lab, USA).

Comparison of HBOCs with control solutions void of O_2 carrying capacity, yielded controversial results (Table 1). Powell et al. [18] measured subcutaneous O_2 tension (PO_2) by use of a fluorescence-quenching optode in thiopental-anesthetized rats submitted to a hemorrhage of 30% of estimated blood volume.

Table 1. Hemoglobin based oxygen carriers

Author	Species	Hemor-rhage (% of EBV)	HBOC	Parameters investigated	Comparison to control solution[a]
Powell et al. [18]	Rat	~30	10% DCLHb	Subcutaneous PO$_2$, central venous SO$_2$	No differences
Frankel et al. [8]	Rat	~32	10% DCLHb	Gut mucosal PO$_2$ (pmO$_2$), base excess (BE), small intestinal histology	No differerences in pmO$_2$ and BE, normal gut histology only in DCLHb animals
Bosman et al. [2]	Dog	~38	11% polymerized bovine Hb	DO$_2$, VO$_2$ (calculated), mixed venous SO$_2$ (SvO$_2$), O$_2$ extraction	No differences
DeAngeles et al. [5]	Sheep	~43–58	10% DCLHb	VO$_2$ (measured!), BE, lactate	Faster BE restoration in DCLHb group, otherwise no differences
Schultz et al. [19]	Rat	~50	7% DCLHb	BE, central venous SO$_2$	Superiority of DCLHb
Nolte et al. [16]	Hamster	~50	10% DCLHb	Skeletal muscle PO$_2$	Superiority of DCLHb
Sprung et al. [24]	Dog	~63	4% and 8% pyridoxilated human Hb	BE, VO$_2$ (calculated), lactate	Restoration to baseline levels; but no real control solution
Chang et al. [3]	Rat	~67	o-raffinose polymerized human Hb	Long term survival (14 days)	Superiority of PolyHb

[a] Only resuscitation fluids without oxygen carrying capacity were considered "control" solutions

Within an observation period of 120 min, monitoring of subcutaneous PO$_2$ revealed no statistically significant differences between 10% DCLHb (1:1 exchange of shed blood), albumin oncotically matched to DCLHb (1:1 exchange of shed blood), whole blood (1:1 exchange of shed blood) and Ringer's lactate (3:1 exchange of shed blood) (Fig. 1a). Additionally, no differences were found concerning central venous oxygen saturation (Fig. 1b).

The parameters subcutaneous PO$_2$ and central venous desaturation reflect both tissue perfusion and oxygenation. The absence of a significant difference between DCLHb and albumin seems due to the inadequacy of the model and less to an insufficient O$_2$ carrying capacity of DCLHb. As the authors [18] state in their discussion, base deficit did not change significantly in response to hemorrhage, thus indicating that shock was not severe enough to allow demonstration of the superiority of any O$_2$ carrying solution over conventional colloids.

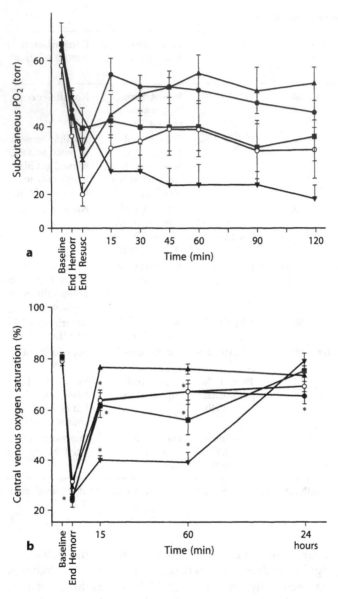

Fig. 1. Subcutaneous PO_2 (fluorescence quenching optode) (Fig. 1a) and central venous O_2 saturation (Fig. 1b) at baseline, in shock and after infusion of different resuscitation fluids in rats ●: 10% DCLHb; ○: albumin; ■: Ringer's lactate; ▲: blood; ▼: no resuscitation. *: $p<0.05$ compared with treatment group baseline. (Modified from [18] with permission)

The study of Frankel et al. [8] faced the same problem: although a ~ 32% hemorrhage in pentobarbital/ketamin anesthetized rats led to a significant increase in base deficit, both 10% DCLHb and albumin restored base excess and gut mucosal PO_2 (fluorescence-quenching optode) without differences between groups (Fig. 2).

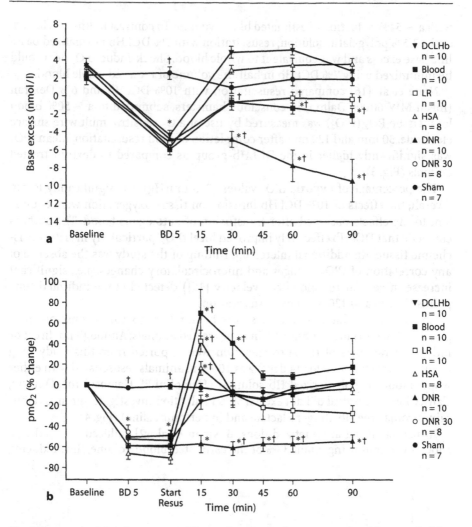

Fig. 2. Base excess (a) and gut mucosal O₂ tension (PmO₂, fluorescence quenching optode, **b**) at baseline, shock and 15–90 min after infusion of different resuscitation fluids. LR: Ringer's lactate, HSA: human albumin, DNR: no resuscitation. *: p < 0.01 significant change from baseline; †: p < 0.01 significant change from DCLHb. (Modified from [8] with permission)

Nevertheless, small bowel histology revealed that DCLHb treated animals presented significantly less damage than animals of all other groups. Thus, despite the absence of differences between groups in ability to restore base excess and PO₂, the authors [8] conclude that DCLHb was superior in preserving reperfusion injuries after hemorrhage-induced ischemia.

The findings reported by Powell et al. [18] and Frankel et al. [8] indicated the need of a more severe shock model in order to confirm a potential superiority of HBOCs as compared to non-HBOCs. Consequently, Schultz et al. [19] bled conscious rats until a target base deficit of 13 ± 1 mmol/l was reached, coinciding with a ~ 54% reduction of estimated blood volume. In contrast to Ringer's lactate and a 3.5% polygelatin solution, resuscitation with 7% DCLHb normalized baseline base excess and was equivalent to whole blood. Shock-induced O_2 debt could be minimized using 7% DCLHb in half the volume of required whole blood.

Nolte et al. [16] compared resuscitation with 10% DCLHb and 6% Dextran (mean MW 60000 Dalton) in conscious hamsters, submitted to a ~ 50% blood loss. Tissue PO_2 (tPO_2) was measured by use of a O_2 sensitive multiwire surface electrode. 30 min and 120 min after completion of fluid resuscitation, mean tPO_2 was significantly higher in the DCLHb-group as compared to dextran treated animals (Fig. 3).

The percentage of hypoxic tPO_2 values (0–5 mm Hg) was significantly lower. Overall, the effects of 10% DCLHb infusion on tissue oxygenation were equivalent to the effects observed after transfusion of autologous blood. The authors conclude that DCLHb effectively improved local tPO_2, particularly in critically ischemic tissue. An additional interesting finding of the study was the absence of any correlation of tPO_2 changes and microcirculatory changes (i.e., significant increase in venular red blood cell velocity [15]) detected at the indicated time points (i.e., 30 and 120 min post resuscitation).

Chang et al. [3] induced a more severe hemorrhage (67%) in conscious rats, giving 100% mortality within 30 min in untreated animals. Although no direct or indirect parameters of tissue oxygenation were reported from this study, long term survival (followed for 14 days) was 100% in animals resuscitated with either whole blood or polymerized Hb solution (Hemolink™, Hemosol Inc, Ontario, Can), whereas survival did not exceed 50% in all other investigated groups (albumin, stroma-free Hb, Ringer's lactate and hypertonic saline) (Fig. 4).

In pentobarbital anesthetized dogs, Bosman et al. [2] induced hemorrhagic shock by withdrawing about 38% of the estimated blood volume, thus reducing

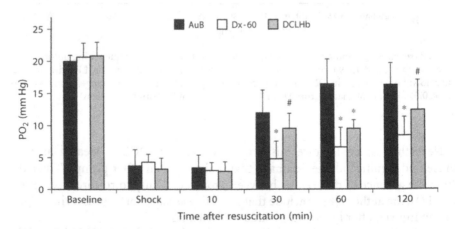

Fig. 3. Mean local tissue PO_2 response (O_2 sensitive electrode) in striated skin muscle before (baseline), during and after severe hemorrhagic shock in conscious hamsters followed by resuscitation with autologous blood (Aub), dextran 60 (Dx-60) and 10% DCLHb. *: $p < 0.05$ versus AuB; #: $p < 0.05$ versus Dx-60. (Modified from [16] with permission)

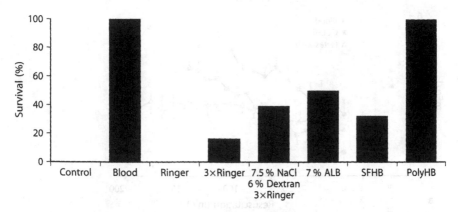

Fig. 4. Effects of one single replacement transfusion on long term survival (followed for 14 days) in a lethal hemorrhagic rat model. (From [3] with permission)

mean arterial pressure (MAP) to 40 mm Hg. After 30 min of shock, animals were resuscitated with an amount equal to the shed blood volume of either isooncotic 6% hydroxyethylstarch (HES) or an isooncotic 11% solution based on polymerized, bovine Hb (PBH, B. Braun Melsungen AG, Melsungen, FRG). Concerning parameters of tissue oxygenation, i.e., DO_2, VO_2, SvO_2 and O_2 extraction, no statistically significant differences were found between groups. While resuscitation with 6% HES led to dilutional anemia (Hb 7.6 g/dl) with compensatory increases in heart rate and cardiac output (CO), resuscitation with 11% PBH increased total Hb concentration to 11.6 g/dl without compensatory hemodynamic changes. The use of hyperbaric oxygenation [6] or infusion of high-viscous dextran [9] respectively, indicates that it is more likely the dilutional decrease in blood viscosity than the decreased arterial oxygen content which causes the increase in CO during normovolemic hemodilution. It can be assumed that whole blood viscosity after administration of 6% HES and 11% PBH is similar; it must have been the increase of arterial oxygen content which made compensatory increases in heart rate and CO unnecessary. This theory is supported by our own findings [10] in a canine hemodilution model where a large content of physically dissolved O_2 achieved via hyperoxic ventilation partially neutralized the hemodynamic compensation initiated by extreme hemodilution (Hct 21%).

Bosman et al. [2] calculated VO_2 as the product of arterio-venous O_2 content difference and CO, accepting the methodologic problem that Hb solutions are potentially able to blunt CO increases by their vasoconstrictor property. Calculated VO_2 might therefore lag behind an already ongoing increase of real O_2 uptake by tissues. In contrast, De Angeles et al. [5] measured VO_2 by analysis of expired spirometric gas in a hemorrhagic shock model in conscious sheep (43–58% blood loss, target base deficit -5 to -10 mmol/l), resuscitated by either 10% DCLHb or 6% HES. These authors [5] found that CO was not significantly different between both groups, despite dilutional anemia (Hct $\sim$ 12%) in the HES treated animals. Although baseline VO_2 was significantly higher in the DCLHb treated group as compared to control (6% HES), an increase of VO_2 was not noted dur-

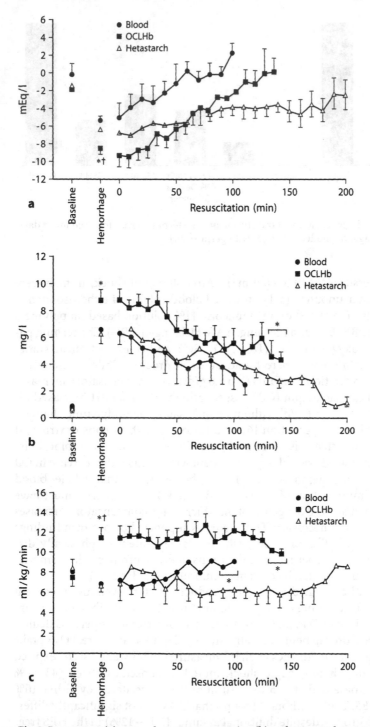

Fig. 5. Base excess (**a**), serum lactate concentration (**b**) and measured oxygen consumption (**c**) at baseline shock and after resuscitation with blood, DCLHb and hydroxyethylstarch (HES) in conscious sheep. †: $p < 0.05$ significantly different from autologous blood; *: $p < 0.05$ significantly different from HES. (Modified from [5] with permission)

ing infusion of the 10% DCLHb solution (Fig. 5c). Base deficit however had been restored with both resuscitation fluids (Fig. 5a). The only difference between groups, was the significantly faster restoration of base deficit using DCLHb and might be explained by the low pH of the HES solution itself. The reduction of shock induced lactacidosis was equivalent in both groups (Fig. 5b). In conclusion, obvious advantages of DCLHb over HES were not encountered in this severe shock model.

HBOCs in Hemodilution

Any fluid resuscitation from hypovolemic shock finally results in dilution of the remaining whole blood. In contrast, during acute normovolemic hemodilution (ANH), blood is withdrawn from the body and simultaneously replaced by an isooncotic colloid (1:1 exchange ration) or isotonic crystalloid solution (1:3 exchange ratio). When normovolemia is strictly preserved, ANH may be extended to very low Hct levels ($\sim 9\%$) in healthy subjects without the risk of tissue hypoxia [7]. With further dilutional reduction of Hct, the compensatory mechanisms providing adequate O_2 support to tissues, i.e., increase of CO and O_2 extraction, become exhausted, and finally VO_2 decreases. The Hct level below which VO_2 becomes DO_2-dependent is defined as the 'critical' Hct and varies between 6.5% [11] and 13% [4], depending on species, anesthesia, inspired oxygen fraction (FiO_2) and core body temperature. Preoperative ANH has been proved effective in reducing homologous blood transfusion in surgical patients [13, 14, 17], even in the case of advanced age [23] and impaired ventricular function [22]. Since the target Hct of ANH predicts the amount of collectable blood and, as a consequence, the efficacy of ANH, it is evident, that from a theoretical point of view hemodilution with HBOCs might allow for extension of ANH to much lower Hct levels. The pre-condition is, however, once again that Hb solutions effectively contribute to tissue oxygenation under these circumstances (Table 2).

Nolte et al. [16] performed isovolemic hemodilution in conscious hamsters (target Hct 30%) using a 10% DCLHb solution and compared tPO$_2$ (O_2 sensitive multiwire surface electrode) in striated skin muscle to a control group hemodiluted with 6% Dextran. Exchange transfusion with DCLHb resulted in a $\sim 20\%$ reduction of baseline tPO$_2$. This decrease in tpO$_2$ was more pronounced than in the dextran group ($\sim 9\%$ reduction) (Fig. 6).

The authors [16] speculate that both the vasoconstrictor action of DCLHb as well as a specific modulation of vasomotor frequency, resulting in increased hydraulic resistance, could be responsible for this phenomenon. The findings of Nolte et al. [16] are supported by the results of Tsai et al. [27] obtained in a very similar animal model (hamster skinfold preparation). Tissue PO$_2$ was measured with the phosphorescence decay technique based on the O_2-dependent quenching of phosphorescence emitted by albumin-bound metalloporphyrins. Phosphorescence lifetime decreases in proportion to the local PO$_2$. In analogy to Nolte et al. [16], Tsai et al. [27] found that a 70% reduction of Hct by isovolemic exchange of whole blood with either dextran (MW 70 000 Dalton) or 15% DCLHb,

Table 2. Hemoglobin based oxygen carriers as diluents for normovolemic hemodilution

Author	Species	Target hematocrit (%)	HBOCS	Parameters investigated	Comparison to control solution[a]
Nolte et al. [16]	Hamster	30	10% DCLHb	Skeletal muscle PO_2	Inferiority of DCLHb
Tsai et al. [27]	Hamster	70% reduction of baseline Hct	15% $\alpha\alpha$-cross-linked Hb	Skeletal muscle PO_2	No difference
Slanetz et al. [21]	Sheep	5–6	13% polymerized bovine Hb	DO_2, VO_2 (calculated), mortality	Superiority of Hb solution
Sielenkämper et al. [20]	Rat[b]	DO_2 dependency of VO_2 at Hb 3.9 g/dl	10% DCLHb	DO_2, VO_2 (measured!), central venous SO_2 O_2 extraction, lactate	Increase in VO_2 and O_2 extraction, decrease in lactate, but: no real control solution.
Horn et al. [12]	Dog[c]	~25	13% polymerized bovine Hb	DO_2, VO_2 (calculated), O_2 extraction, lactate, skeletal muscle PO_2	Superiority of Hb solution concerning skeletal muscle PO_2
Standl et al. [25]	Dog	~10	13% polymerized bovine Hb	DO_2, VO_2(calculated), O_2 extraction, lactate, skeletal muscle PO_2	Superiority of Hb solution concerning skeletal muscle PO_2
Standl et al. [26]	Dog	2–5	13% polymerized bovine Hb	DO_2, VO_2 (calculated), O_2 extraction, skeletal muscle PO_2	Superiority of Hb solution concerning skeletal muscle PO_2

a Only resuscitation fluids without oxygen carrying capacity were considered "control" solutions

b Before starting the hemodilution protocol, sepsis was induced by cecal ligation and perforation

c Measurements were performed during 95% stenosis of the popliteral artery

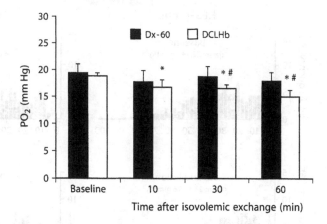

Fig. 6. Mean local tissue PO_2 response (O_2 sensitive electrode) in striated skin muscle before (baseline), and after isovolemic exchange transfusion of either dextran 60 (Dx-60) or DCLHb. *: $p < 0.05$ versus baseline; #: $p < 0.05$ versus Dx-60. (Modified from [16] with permission)

led to a significant decrease of tPO_2 (dextran: 33% decrease of tPO_2; DCLHb: 47% decrease of tPO_2; no statistically significant difference). The following underlying mechanisms of this phenomenon were discussed: lowered blood viscosity after infusion of DCLHb resulting in decreased shear stress at arteriolar vessel walls and consecutive decrease of endogenous vasodilator release (i.e., nitric oxide (NO), prostacyclin); scavenging of NO by free Hb; and autoregulatory mechanisms due to high arteriolar PO_2 levels. Together, these mechanisms are supposed to result in arteriolar vasoconstriction with reduction of functional capillary density and consequently impaired tissue oxygenation.

In contrast to these rather unfavorable results, Slanctz et al. [21] demonstrated in conscious, splenectomized sheep, that an initial ANH to Hct 12–15% using 6% HES as diluent could be extended to Hct 5–6% by further use of a 13% polymerized bovine Hb solution (Biopure Corp, Boston, Mass, USA) without any changes in DO_2 or VO_2. Although comparison to a real control group, i.e., ANH to Hct 5–6% with 6% HES exclusively, is missing in this study, it is undoubted that in conscious animals breathing room air the critical Hct would have been reached at such low levels.

Sielenkämper et al. [20] hemodiluted conscious septic rats with plasma until critical DO_2 was reached. VO_2 was measured by gas analysis of the in- and outflow of an airtight box. During a subsequent exchange transfusion with 10% DCLHb, VO_2 was completely restored, although no simultaneous increase in DO_2 could be registered. This, at first view controversial finding, was discussed as due to a redistribution of macro- and microcirculatory blood flow away from not fully supply-dependent organ parts towards more supply-dependent areas, and a facilitated O_2 release to the tissues and thus augmented O_2 extraction in DCLHb treated animals.

Beside reduction of Hct towards critical levels, another possible method to create critical DO_2 to tissues is the controlled reduction of organ blood flow by

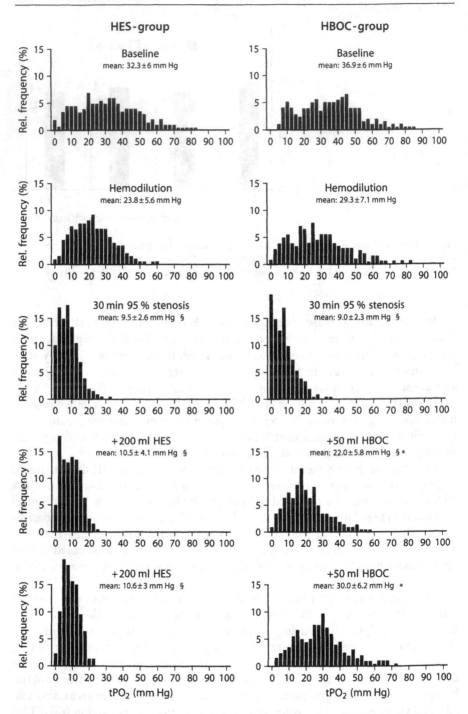

Fig. 7. Pooled histograms of skeletal muscle tissue oxygen tension (tPO$_2$, needle electrode) during isovolemic hemodilution, arterial stenosis and infusion of hydroxyethylstarch (HES) or 13% polymerized bovine hemoglobin (HBOC). *: $p < 0.05$ versus HES; §: $p < 0.05$ versus baseline. (Modified from [12] with permission)

vessel stenosis. After initial hemodilution to Hct 25% using Ringer's lactate, Horn et al. [12] induced a 95% stenosis of the popliteal artery in midazolam/fentanyl anesthetized dogs. This decrease of organ blood flow resulted in a 86% decrease of hind limb VO_2. Subsequent to a top-load infusion of 400 ml 6% HES or 100 ml of a 13% bovine Hb solution (Biopure Corp, Boston, Mass, USA) skeletal muscle tissue oxygenation (gastrocnemius muscle) was measured by use of an O_2 sensitive needle probe. Despite identical popliteal arterial flow, DO_2, VO_2 and serum lactate levels, skeletal muscle tPO_2 was significantly higher in the HBOC group (Fig. 7).

This was explained by facilitated O_2 extraction from HBOCs due to its right-shifted O_2 dissociation curve (P50 34 mm Hg). Similar results are reported by Standl et al. [25], who hemodiluted dogs to Hct 10% using 6% HES and administered subsequently either autologous blood (Hb 9 g/dl) or 13% bovine Hb to increase total Hb concentration by 1, 2 and 3 g/dl. Again, no differences were detected between groups concerning global tissue oxygenation parameters DO_2, VO_2 and serum lactate concentrations. However due to superior O_2 extraction, skeletal muscle tPO_2 (sartorius muscle, polarographic needle probe) was significantly higher in the HBOC group. After the final HBOC infusion, contribution of the bovine Hb to total CaO_2 was 47%.

In an even more extreme protocol, the same group [26] performed ANH to Hct levels as low as 2–5% in fentanyl/midazolam anesthetized dogs using the same 13% bovine Hb solution as diluent. tPO_2 was measured in skeletal muscle (gastrocnemius muscle) by use of a O_2 sensitive needle electrode and compared to a second animal group hemodiluted with 6% HES. While whole body VO_2 surprisingly did not differ between groups, other parameters reflecting tissue oxygenation, e.g., base excess, skeletal muscle VO_2 or tPO_2 were significantly higher in the group hemodiluted with bovine Hb (Fig. 8). The calculated contribution of bovine Hb to total arterial content was 82% at Hct 2%.

Conclusion

Second generation Hb solutions are able to transport and deliver O_2 to the tissues. Proof of their efficacy mainly depends on the suitability of the chosen experimental model. Since Hb solutions may be administered in large doses, and do not require ventilation with high FiO_2, they are useful resuscitation fluids in the emergency treatment of hemorrhagic shock. Although the vasoconstrictive action of free Hb might have pressure stabilizing effects in this context, the influence of this pharmacologic property on microcirculation, tissue perfusion and oxygenation is not yet understood.

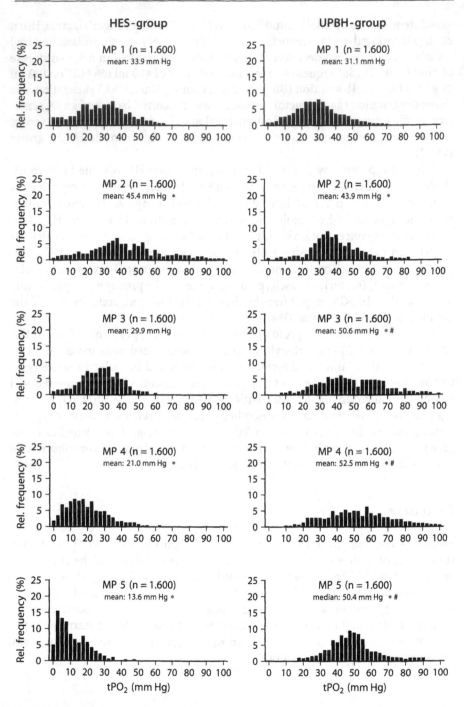

Fig. 8. Pooled histograms of skeletal muscle tissue PO_2 (tPO_2, gastrocnemius muscle) at baseline (MP 1), during initial ANH to Hct 20% (diluent: Ringer's lactate; MP 2), and after blood exchange to Hct 15% (MP 3), 10% (MP 4) and 5% (MP 5, group 1) and 2% (MP 5, group 2) with 6% hydroxyethylstarch (HES) or 13% polymerized bovine hemoglobin (UPBH). *: $p < 0.05$ versus MP 1; #: $p < 0.05$ versus HES. (Modified from [26] with permission)

References

1. Amberson W, Jennings JJ, Rhode M (1949) Clinical experience with hemoglobin-saline solutions. J Appl Physiol 1:469–489
2. Bosman RJ, Minten J, Lu HR, Van Aken H, Flameng W (1992) Free polymerized hemoglobin versus hydroxyethyl starch in resuscitation of hypovolemic dogs. Anesth Analg 75:811–817
3. Chang T, Varma R (1992) Effect of a single replacement of one ringer lactate, hypertonic saline/dextrane, 7 g% albumin, stroma-free hemoglobin, o-raffinose polyhemoglobin or whole blood on the long term survival of unanesthetized rats with lethal hemorrhagic shock after 67% acute blood loss. Biomater Art Cells Immob Biotech 20:503–510
4. Crystal GJ (1988) Coronary hemodynamic response during local hemodilution in canine hearts. Am J Physiol 254:H525–H531
5. DeAngeles DA, Scott AM, McGrath AM, Korent VA, Rodenkirch LA, Conhaim RL, Harms BA (1997) Resuscitation from hemorrhagic shock with diaspirin cross-linked hemoglobin, blood or hetastarch. J Trauma 42:406–412
6. Dedichen H, Race D, Schenk WG (1967) Hemodilution and concomitant hyperbaric oxygenation. J Thorac Cardiovasc Surg 53:341–348
7. Fontana JL, Welborn L, Mongan PD, Sturm P, Martin G, Bünger R (1995) Oxygen consumption and cardiovascular function in children during profound intraoperative normovolemic hemodilution. Anesth Analg 80:219–225
8. Frankel HL, Nguyen HB, Shea-Donohue T, Aiton LA, Ratigan J, Malcolm DS (1996) Diaspirin cross-linked hemoglobin is efficacious in gut resuscitation as measured by a GI tract optode. J Trauma 40:231–241
9. Gelin LE, Bergentz SE, Helander CG (1968) Hemodynamic consequences from increased viscosity of blood. In: Copley AL (ed) Hemorheology. Pergamon Press, Oxford,pp 722–728
10. Habler OP, Kleen MS, Hutter JW, et al (1998) Effects of hyperoxic ventilation on hemodilution induced changes in anesthetized dogs. Transfusion 38:135–144
11. Haisjackl M, Luz G, Sparr H, et al (1997) The effects of progressive anemia on jejunal mucosal and serosal tissue oxygenation in pigs. Anesth Analg 84:538–544
12. Horn E-P, Standl T, Wilhelm S, Jacobs E, Freitag U, Schulte am Esch J (1997) Bovine hemoglobin increases skeletal muscle oxygenation during 95% artificial arterial stenosis. Surgery 121:411–418
13. Kahraman S, Altunkaya H, Celebioglu B, Kanbak M, Pasaglu I, Erdem K (1997) The effect of acute normovolemic hemodilution on homologous blood requirements and total estimated red blood cell volume lost. Acta Anaesthesiol Scand 41:614–617
14. Monk TG, Goodnough LT, Brecher ME, Pulley DD, Colberg JW, Andriole GL, Catalona WJ (1997) Acute normovolemic hemodilution can replace preoperative autologous blood donation as a standard of care for autologous blood procurement in radical prostatectomy. Anesth Analg 85:953–958
15. Nolte D, Botzlar A, Pickelmann S, Bouskela E, Messmer K (1997) Effects of diaspirin-cross-linked hemoglobin (DCLHb) on the microcirculation of striated skin muscle in the hamster: a study of safety and toxicity. J Lab Clin Med 130:314–327
16. Nolte D, Steinhauser P, Berger S, Härtl R, Messmer K (1997) Effects of diaspirin-cross-linked hemoglobin (DCLHb) on local tissue oxygen tension in striated skin muscle: an efficacy study in the hamster. J Lab Clin Med 130:328–338
17. Olsfanger D, Fredman B, Goldstein B, Shapiro A, JedeikinR (1997) Acute normovolemic haemodilution decreases postoperative allogeneic blood transfusion after total knee replacement. Br J Anaesth 79:317–321
18. Powell CC, Schultz SC, Burris DG, Drucker WR, Malcolm DS (1995) Subcutaneous oxygen tension: a useful adjunct in assessment of perfusion status. Crit Care Med 23:867–873
19. Schultz SC, Hamilton IN, Malcolm DS (1993) Use of base deficit to compare resuscitation with lactated ringer"s solution, haemacel, whole blood and diaspirin cross-linked hemoglobin following hemorrhage in rats. J Trauma 35:619–626
20. Sielenkämper AW, Chin-Yee IH, Martin CM, Sibbald WJ (1997) Diaspirin crosslinked hemoglobin improves systemic oxygen uptake in oxygen supply-dependent septic rats. Am J Respir Crit Care Med 156:1066–1072

21. Slanetz PJ, Lee R, Page R, Jacobs EE, LaRaia PJ, Vlahakes GJ (1994) Hemoglobin blood substitutes in extended preoperative autologous blood donation: An experimental study. Surgery 115:246–254
22. Spahn DR, Schmid ER, Seifert B, Pasch T (1996) Hemodilution tolerance in patients with coronary artery disease who are receiving chronic beta-adrenergic blocker therapy. Anesth Analg 82:687–694
23. Spahn DR, Zollinger A, Schlumpf RB, Stöhr S, Seifert B, Schmid ER, Pasch T (1996) Hemodilution tolerance in elderly patients without known cardiac disease. Anesth Analg 82: 681–686
24. Sprung J, Mackenzie CF, Barnas GB, et al (1995) Oxygen transport and cardiovascular effects of resuscitation from severe hemorrhagic shock using hemoglobin solutions. Crit Care Med 23:1540–1553
25. Standl T, Horn P, Wilhelm S, et al (1996) Bovine hemoglobin is more potent than autologous red blood cells in restoring muscular tissue oxygenation after profound isovolemic haemodilution in dogs. Can J Anesth 43:714–723
26. Standl TG, Reeker W, Redmann G, Kochs E, Werner C, Schulte am Esch J (1997) Haemodynamic changes and skeletal muscle oxygen tension during complete blood exchange with ultrapurified polymerized bovine hemoglobin. Intensive Care Med 23:865–872
27. Tsai AG, Kerger H, Intaglietta M (1998) Microcirculation consequences of blood substitution with hemoglobin solutions. In: Rudolph AS, Rabinovici R, Feuerstein GZ (eds) Red blood cell substitutes. Marcell Dekker, New York, pp 69–78

Effect of Diaspirin Crosslinked Hemoglobin on Systemic and Regional Blood Circulation

A. Gulati

Introduction

Blood has several functions which include the transport of oxygen (O_2) and maintenance of tissue oxygenation. Severe loss of blood results in a hypovolemic state and ultimately leads to depletion of O_2 delivering capability [1]. Biologically significant hemorrhage may be defined as a blood loss sufficient to impair O_2 transport [2–4]. The major physiological effects of hemorrhage are anemia and hypovolemia, leading to drastic alterations in blood flow to vital organs [5]. Persistent hypoperfusion of organ systems is responsible for ultimate organ failure even after reperfusion [6]. Hemoglobin (Hb) therapeutics have been proposed as an effective treatment of hemorrhagic shock.

Effective and well tolerated O_2 carrying Hb therapeutics could be life saving for trauma victims and has become a major goal of many research groups within industry, academic centers, and the military. O_2 carrying Hb therapeutics have numerous advantages over conventional blood transfusions. They can be produced in large volumes, stored for prolonged periods (about one year or more), administered rapidly and without need for cross matching, and can withstand effective viral inactivation procedures [7, 8]. Hb therapeutics are a new generation of "O_2 carriers" or "O_2 therapeutics" which in pre-clinical studies exhibit efficacy in the treatment of several disease conditions, such as hypovolemic shock, septic shock, myocardial infarction, stroke, burns, cardiopulmonary bypass, nosocomial infections, and wound healing. A number of Hb therapeutic agents have passed significant phase I safety hurdles and are now in phase II or phase III patient testing.

Diaspirin crosslinked Hb (DCLHb) is a modified Hb solution derived from human erythrocytes. DCLHb is prepared by cross-linking between the α-subunits of Hb, within the Hb tetramer by means of a reaction with the diaspirin compound, bis(3,5-dibromosalicyl) fumarate. DCLHb is purified by heat pasteurization to inactivate any contaminating viruses and precipitate undesirable proteins. DCLHb possesses biochemical stability and exhibits greater intravascular retention than unmodified Hb. It is slowly metabolized to low molecular weight compounds which are eliminated through the urine and feces. DCLHb does not require cross-matching or typing prior to administration, is less viscous than whole blood, and may be better able to carry O_2 through narrowed vessels to ischemic tissues due to the smaller size of the Hb molecule relative to erythrocytes. DCLHb is devoid of white cells and other blood components which are known to contribute to ischemic tissue injury by releasing cytotoxic products. DCLHb does not elicit inflammatory reactions in sheep and monkeys, nor does it interfere with the coagulation cascade, or the reticuloendothelial system (RES).

Cardiovascular Effects of DCLHb

Studies [9, 10] have been conducted in male Sprague-Dawley rats to determine the effect of DCLHb on regional circulation and systemic hemodynamics using a radioactive microsphere technique. Systemic hemodynamics, distribution of cardiac output (CO), regional blood flow and vascular resistance were determined before (baseline) and 15, 30 and 60 min after the administration of 400 mg/kg, iv of DCLHb [9, 10]. Infusion of an equal volume of Ringer's lactate did not produce a significant change in systemic hemodynamics or regional circulation. DCLHb produced an increase in the mean arterial blood pressure (MAP) which lasted for more than 60 min. Heart rate, CO and stroke volume were not significantly affect-

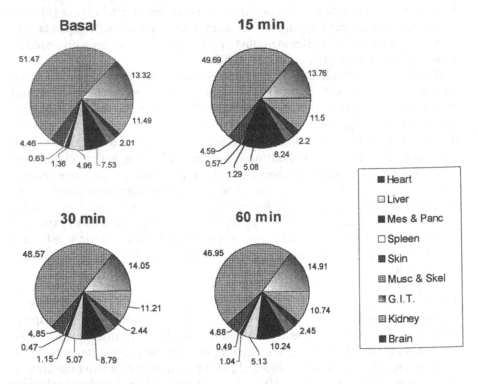

Fig. 1. The percent change in regional blood flow in rats 60 min following administration of DCLHb 10% solution (4 ml/kg, iv). There was a significant increase in blood flow to visceral organs like the heart, brain, GIT and portal system, while a marked decrease in blood flow to the musculoskeletal system was observed with DCLHb in normal rats. (Mes+Pan = Mesentery and pancreas; uns skel = musculoskeletal system)

ed, while total peripheral resistance was increased after the administration of DCLHb. DCLHb produced significant increases in blood flow to the heart, gastrointestinal tract (GIT), portal system and skin. Although the blood flow to the kidney, brain and musculoskeletal system was not significantly affected by DCLHb, there was a marked increase in the vascular resistance in the musculoskeletal system. However, vascular resistance was not altered in the heart, brain, GIT, portal system, kidney or skin. The percentage of CO received by visceral organs such as the heart, GIT and portal system was increased, while a marked decrease in the percentage of CO to the musculoskeletal system was observed with DCLHb. These data suggest that the increase in blood flow to visceral organs is due to a redistribution of the CO. Furthermore, the increase in vascular resistance to the musculoskeletal system appears to be responsible for the redistribution of blood flow away from the musculoskeletal system towards visceral organs. Since about 54% of the CO in the rat goes to the musculoskeletal system, a small decrease in the percentage of CO to the musculoskeletal system can account for a marked increase in the blood flow to other organs receiving a smaller percentage of CO. Results obtained from several studies conducted in our laboratory [9, 10] have been pooled (N = 31) to show the effect of DCLHb (Fig. 1) on regional blood flow in normal rats.

Efficacy of DCLHb in Hemorrhagic Shock

Identification and control of bleeding and restoration of intravascular volume is the mainstay of initial resuscitation therapy in the hemorrhaged patient. In order to prevent tissue damage and multiple organ failure and to improve survival [11, 12], it is necessary to rapidly restore O_2 delivery (DO_2) and tissue perfusion. Initial volume restoration followed by transfusion with allogeneic donor blood is still the conventional treatment for hemorrhagic shock [13]. Unfortunately, there are several limitations to the use of blood, such as the time required for typing and cross-matching, which may be critical, the potential for adverse reactions and immune suppression, transmission of human immunodeficiency virus (HIV) [14] and hepatitis [15], storage and delivery problems and limited supply [13, 16]. Although resuscitation with hypervolemic isotonic crystalloid solutions has been commonly used to treat hemorrhagic shock, there is a resurgence in the evaluation of its usefulness due to the high volumes necessary for resuscitation and poor survival rate [17, 18]. Hypertonic solutions (7–7.5% NaCl) in small volumes, either alone or in combination with hyperoncotic colloids, have been effectively used in animal models of hemorrhage and in clinical trials [19, 20]. Nevertheless, the need still exists for developing low volume resuscitative fluids which would overcome the limitations of allogeneic blood transfusion and in addition, would possess excellent O_2 carrying capacity.

In situations simulating clinical settings, DCLHb administered at 50–100% of shed blood volume, was found to be an effective resuscitative fluid following hemorrhage in rats [21–23]. The efficacy of DCLHb was comparable to that of autologous blood and superior to that of Ringer's lactate. DCLHb maintained cardiac and renal functions after partial or complete exchange transfusions [24] and restored mean arterial pressure (MAP), CO and plasma lactate levels [25, 26] after hemorrhage in swine. In rats trained to complete a water alley maze and subjected to hemorrhagic shock, resuscitation with DCLHb did not result in significant degradation in performance [27]. DCLHb infused at 25% of shed blood volume was found to reduce the base deficit observed following hemorrhage in rats [28].

Studies on the efficacy of DCLHb in hemorrhagic resuscitation have demonstrated improvements in base deficit [26, 29], transcutaneous O_2 tension [21], subcutaneous O_2 tension [23], cardiac and renal functions [24], and CO, stroke volume and plasma lactate levels [26].

The systemic and regional circulatory effects of a 10% w/v solution DCLHb (20%, iv of shed blood volume, SBV) and Ringer's lactate (20% of SBV as control) were studied in hemorrhaged rats using a radioactive microsphere technique [30, 31]. Hemorrhage significantly decreased MAP, CO, and stroke volume, and increased total peripheral resistance. In addition, hemorrhage significantly decreased regional blood flow to all tissues and decreased whole body O_2 consumption (VO_2). Control rats that were administered Ringer's lactate (20% of SBV, iv)

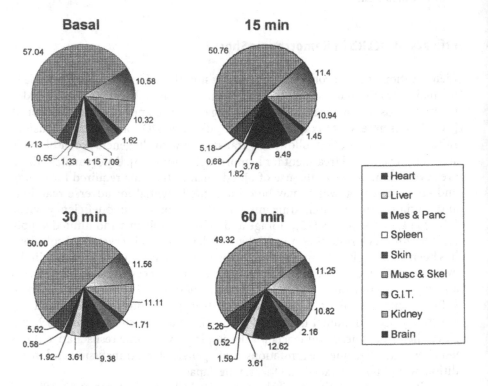

Fig. 2. The effect of DCLHb (400 mg/kg, iv) on the percent change in regional blood flow of severely hemorrhaged rats. Hemorrhage significantly decreased regional blood flow to all tissues. Resuscitation with DCLHb 10% solution (4 ml/kg, iv) produced a significant improvement in regional blood flow

did not show improvements in systemic hemodynamics, regional blood flow or VO_2. However, resuscitation with DCLHb (20% of SBV) produced significant improvements in systemic hemodynamics, regional blood flow and VO_2 (Fig. 2). The mean survival time for Ringer's lactate (20% of SBV, iv) treated hemorrhaged rats was 63 min, while resuscitation with DCLHb significantly increased the survival time (152 min for 20% of SBV) [30, 31].

Further studies [31, 32] were carried out in hemorrhaged rats to determine the efficacy of DCLHb in restoring blood flow to vital organs such as brain and kidney. Blood perfusion of the brain and kidney, concentration of moving red blood cells (CMBC) and red blood cell velocity were determined using laser Doppler flowmetry (Perimed, Model Periflux 4001). Hemorrhage significantly decreased blood pressure ($-53.2 \pm 2.9\%$), arterial blood pH, PCO_2 and total Hb (THb), and increased arterial PO_2. Furthermore, a significant decrease in the brain ($-20.2 \pm 3.27\%$) and renal ($-73.6 \pm 3.39\%$) blood perfusion was observed following hemorrhage. Resuscitation with Ringer's lactate (4 ml/kg, iv) did not produce improvements in blood pressure, arterial blood pH, PO_2, PCO_2, THb or renal perfusion and a further decrease in brain perfusion ($-27.3 \pm 2.6\%$) was observed. In contrast, resuscitation with DCLHb (400 mg/kg, iv) produced significant improvements in blood pressure, arterial blood pH, PO_2, PCO_2, and perfusion to both the brain ($9.0 \pm 0.3\%$) and kidney ($36.5 \pm 10.7\%$) [31, 32], thus suggesting that small volume resuscitation with DCLHb is effective in restoring blood flow to vital organs such as the brain and kidney.

Pharmacological Mechanisms Involved in the Action of DCLHb

Hb solutions have been shown to increase MAP and to cause a redistribution of blood flow. Numerous studies have been performed to determine the mechanism by which Hb therapeutic agents alter cardiovascular function. The involvement of adrenergic receptors [18, 33–35], endothelin (ET) [10, 30, 36, 37], nitric oxide (NO) [30, 37–39] and calcium channels [39] in the cardiovascular responses to DCLHb have been implicated.

Adrenergic Mechanism

In one of the few studies of this type [40] which have been performed to determine the mechanism of action of cell-free Hb solutions, the constrictor responses of hind limb perfusion in rats to angiotensin II and 5-HT after exchange transfusion with pyridoxalated Hb polyoxyethylene conjugate (PHP), were not found to be altered by the presence of the Hb solution. However, the responses to norepinephrine were significantly augmented in PHP transfused rats [40]. Using a rat model, we [33] have found that DCLHb increases the sensitivity of vascular α-adrenoceptors to catecholamines and prazosin, an α-adrenoceptor blocker, has been found to decrease the pressor effect induced by DCLHb [18]. Severe hypotension following hemorrhage is known to decrease the sensitivity of the cardiovascular system to catecholamines [41] and cause an irreversible loss of arteriolar tone [42]. It has been demonstrated that hemorrhagic shock is characterized by a hyporesponsiveness to phenylephrine, an α-adrenergic agonist [43]. Therefore, increasing the sensitivity of vascular α-adrenergic receptors in the presence of DCLHb [33] may be responsible at least in part, for the efficacy of DCLHb as a resuscitation solution. Studies are ongoing to address this possibility.

Nitric Oxide Mechanism

Several studies indicate that the cardiovascular actions of DCLHb are mediated through NO. Besides O_2, NO is also bound by Hb and may be converted to nitrate through interaction with the heme group [44]. Binding of NO by cell-free Hb may be responsible in part, for the pressor effect of these solutions. Severe hemorrhagic hypotension causes hyporeactivity of the cardiovascular system to catecholamines which is mediated by an increase in NO synthase (NOS) activity and release of NO [45]. Endogenous NO mediates most of its actions through cyclic guanosine monophosphate (cGMP) [46] and the hyporeactivity to vasoconstrictors following hemorrhage could be due to an increased production of NO and cGMP as a result of enhanced activity of NOS [45]. Excessive levels of NO and cGMP during severe hemorrhage lead to a loss of vascular tone, hyporeactivity of blood vessels to vasoconstrictors, hypotension, cardiovascular collapse, and ultimately death. In theory, scavenging of excess NO by DCLHb would decrease the concentration of cGMP, thus contributing to restoration of the vascular tone, vascular responsiveness and hemodynamic stability. To test the hypothesis that DCLHb is efficacious in the treatment of hemorrhagic shock because of its NO-scavenging ability, DCLHb was administered in hemorrhaged rats pre-treated with L-NAME [30]. In rats pre-treated with L-NAME, the DCLHb induced an increase in base deficit, and VO_2 was attenuated. Pre-treatment with L-NAME also attenuated the DCLHb induced increase in MAP and improvement in blood flow to the brain, GIT, kidneys, mesentery and pancreas, skin, and musculoskeletal system. If removal of increased NO formed following hemorrhage is responsible for the therapeutic effect of DCLHb, L-NAME should have potentiated the beneficial effects of DCLHb under hemorrhagic conditions. In contrast, L-NAME attenuated the beneficial effects of DCLHb [30]. Many studies [47–49] using L-NAME have also shown that it does not improve systemic hemodynamics of hemorrhaged rats [47], swine [48] or rabbits [49]. The results of our studies [50] also suggest that L-NAME is ineffective in resuscitation of hemorrhaged rats.

Endothelin Mechanism

Elevation of plasma ET-1 concentration has been reported following hemorrhage in rats [51, 52] and dogs [53]. In normal rats, the circulating ET-1 level is low and ET-1 is preferentially released toward the abluminal side of the endothelial cells. Hemorrhage leads to an increase in plasma ET-1 concentration due to an increase in the synthesis or release of ET-1 as a consequence of hemodynamic changes, or as a result of activation of stress hormones or the coagulation cascade. Alternatively, the decrease in blood flow to the kidneys and lungs that occurs during hemorrhage may cause decreased clearance of ET-1. We [30] have found that hemorrhage produces a significant increase in plasma ET-1 levels in rats. DCLHb also significantly increases plasma ET-1 levels, though this increase is significantly less than that seen with hemorrhage [30]. These results are in agreement with another report in which an oxyhemoglobin solution was found to increase ET-1 concentration in cultured bovine pulmonary artery endothelial cells following platelet-mediated stimulation [54]. Studies with ET receptor antagonists suggest that ET is involved in the pressor effects of DCLHb, and may be important in the efficacy of DCLHb as a resuscitative fluid. The DCLHb induced increase in MAP, total peripheral resistance and blood flow to the brain and musculoskeletal system was significantly attenuated by FR139317 (an ETA receptor antagonist). Furthermore, pre-treatment with FR139317 significantly attenuated the beneficial effects of DCLHb during hemorrhage. The DCLHb induced decrease in base deficit, and increase in VO_2 and survival time that were observed in hemorrhaged rats after resuscitation with DCLHb were attenuated by FR139317, suggesting that release of ET-1 may be important in the resuscitative effect of DCLHb. Interestingly, neither L-NAME nor FR139317 altered the DCLHb in-

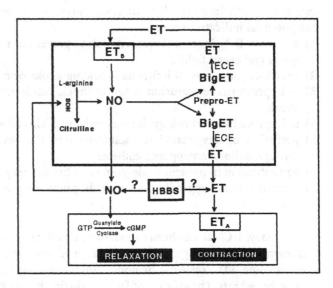

Fig. 3. The role of endothelin (ET) and nitric oxide (NO) in maintaining the homeostatic mechanisms in the wall of blood vessels. ET produces vasoconstriction by inducing smooth muscle contraction due to its action on ET_A-type receptors located on the smooth muscle cells. This is counterbalanced by the action of NO on guanylate cyclase, increasing the production of cGMP, which produces relaxation of the smooth muscles. The production of NO is also regulated by ET acting on ET_B-type receptors located on the luminal side of endothelial cells. It is our hypothesis that both ET and NO contribute to the pathophysiology of hemorrhagic shock. Following severe hemorrhage loss of vascular tone occurs due to an increase in NO and cGMP levels and the body tries to compensate for this by increasing circulating ET levels

duced improvement in blood flow to the heart. It was recently shown that, in normal rats, ET receptors in the heart are different from those found in other vascular beds [55]. It may be possible that under hemorrhagic conditions this distinction is maintained.

DCLHb has been found to both increase ET-1 plasma concentration [10, 36] and to scavenge NO [56]. The restoration of arteriolar tone observed after DCLHb infusion could be a result of both of these effects. However, the results with L-NAME suggest that NO scavenging may not play a significant role in the efficacy of DCLHb, since L-NAME pre-treatment attenuated the beneficial effects of DCLHb in hemorrhaged rats. In contrast, FR139317 (an ET_A receptor antagonist) did attenuate the beneficial effects of DCLHb, suggesting that the increase in plasma ET-1 concentration following hemorrhage and resuscitation is important in restoring hemodynamic stability in hemorrhaged rats (Fig. 3). These results suggest that ET release is important in the beneficial effects of DCLHb in hemorrhaged rats whereas NO scavenging may be less involved.

Conclusion

Hb therapeutics will likely provide O_2 carrying capabilities in the management of critical care patients. A variety of potential applications of DCLHb, a Hb therapeutic currently in phase III testing, are currently under investigation. Some of the potential indications are:
1) to restore DO_2, in trauma resuscitation to prevent or reverse shock and subsequent end organ failure
2) to reduce the degree of ischemia following stroke or myocardial infarction
3) to improve tissue perfusion in septic shock, cardiogenic shock, post-surgical shock
4) to improve blood rheology during crisis in sickle cell anemia
5) perfusion of oxygenated Hb solutions into the occluded coronary artery through balloon angioplasty catheters
6) hemodilution in patients undergoing elective surgery
7) extracorporeal oxygenation as in cardiopulmonary bypass and organ perfusion.

In summary, DCLHb has been shown to be an effective resuscitation solution for treatment of hemorrhagic shock. DCLHb produces significant improvements in survival time, VO_2, systemic hemodynamics, and regional blood circulation in hemorrhaged rats. The efficacy of DCLHb during hemorrhage has been attributed to its ability to transport O_2; however, it has also been demonstrated that the ability of DCLHb to produce significant alterations in hemodynamics also contributes toward its efficacy. The role of NO and ET in hemorrhagic shock has been examined. It was found that following hemorrhage, an increase in NO and ET-1 occurs. The removal of NO by DCLHb assists in decreasing the toxicity due to NO, while an increase in ET-1 following hemorrhage appears to be a compensatory response which is augmented by DCLHb.

References

1. Dracker RA (1995) The development and use of oxygen-carrying blood substitutes. Immunol Invest 24:403–410
2. Shoemaker WC, Montgomery ES, Kaplan E, et al (1973) Physiologic patterns in surviving and non-surviving shock patients. Arch Surg 106:630–636
3. Bassin R, Vladick BC, Kim SI, Shoemaker WC (1971) Comparison of two hemorrhagic shock models with clinical hemorrhage. Surgery 69:722–730
4. Hauser CJ, Shoemaker WC (1982) Hemoglobin solutions in the treatment of hemorrhagic shock. Crit Care Med 10:283–287
5. Prough DS, Whitney JM, Taylor CL, Deal DD, DeWitt DS (1991) Small volume resuscitation from hemorrhagic shock in dogs: effects on systemic hemodynamics and regional blood flow. Crit Care Med 19:364–372
6. Knaus W, Draper E, Wagner D, Zimmerman JE (1985) Prognosis in acute organ system failure. Ann Surg 202:685–693
7. Estep TN, Bechtel MK, Bush SL, Miller TJ, Szeto S, Webb LE (1989) The purification of hemoglobin solutions by heating. In: Brewer G (ed) Progress in clinical and biological research. Alan R Liss, New York, pp 325–336
8. Estep TN, Bobka EW, Ebeling AA, Hai TT, Nelson DJ, Pankau RJ, Srnak A (1989) Novel aspects of diaspirin cross-linked hemoglobin synthesis and purification. Biomater Artif Organs 17:636 (Abstract)
9. Gulati A, Sharma AC, Burhop KE (1994) Effect of stroma-free hemoglobin and diaspirin cross-linked hemoglobin on the regional circulation and systemic hemodynamics. Life Sci 55:827–837
10. Gulati A, Singh G, Rebello S, Sharma AC (1995) Effect of diaspirin crosslinked and stroma-reduced hemoglobin on mean arterial pressure and endothelin-1 concentration in rats. Life Sci 56:1433–1442
11. Moore FA, Haenel JB, Moore EE, Whitehill TA (1992) Incommensurate oxygen consumption in response to maximal oxygen availability predicts postinjury multiple organ failure. J Trauma 33:58–65
12. Shoemaker WC, Appel PL, Kram HB, Waxman K, Lee TS (1988) Prospective trial of supranormal values of survivors as therapeutic goals in high-risk surgical patients. Chest 6:1776–1786
13. Rabinovici R, Neville LF, Rudolph AS, Feuerstein G (1995) Hemoglobin-based oxygen-carrying resuscitation fluids. Crit Care Med 23:801–804
14. Cumming PD, Wallace PD, Schorr JB, Dodd RY (1989) Exposure of patients to human immunodeficiency virus through transfusion of blood components that test antibody negative. N Engl J Med 321:941–946
15. Alter HJ, Purcell RH, Shih JW, Melpolder JC, Houghton M, Choo Q, Kuo G (1989) Detection of antibody to hepatitis C virus in prospectively followed transfusion recipients with acute and chronic non-A, non-B hepatitis. N Engl J Med 321:1494–1500
16. Bunn HF (1993) The use of hemoglobin as a blood substitute. Am J Hematol 42:112–117
17. Vassar MJ, Holcroft JW (1992) Use of hypertonic-hyperoncotic fluids for resuscitation of trauma patients. J Intensive Care 7:189–198
18. Bilello K, Schultz S, Powell C, Jaffin J, Cole F, Malcolm D (1994) Diaspirin crosslinked hemoglobin (DCLHb™): control of pressor effect with anti-hypertensive agents. Artif Cells Blood Substit Immobil Biotechnol 22:819–825
19. Frey L, Kesel K, Pruckner S, Pacheco A, Welte M, Messmer K (1994) Is sodium acetate dextran superior to sodium chloride dextran for small volume resuscitation from traumatic hemorrhagic shock? Crit Care Trauma 79:517–524
20. Mazzoni MC, Warnke KC, Arfors K, Skala TC (1994) Capillary hemodynamics in hemorrhagic shock and reperfusion: in vivo and model analysis. Am J Physiol 267:H1928–H1935
21. Przybelski RJ, Malcolm DS, Burris DG, Winslow RM (1991) Cross-linked hemoglobin solution as a resuscitative fluid after hemorrhage in the rat. J Lab Clin Med 117:143–151
22. Malcolm D, Kissinger D, Garrioch M (1992) Diaspirin cross-linked hemoglobin solution as a resuscitative fluid following severe hemorrhage in the rat. Biomater Artif Cells Immobilization Biotechnol 20:495–497

23. Powell CC, Schultz SC, Burris DG, Drucker WR, Malcolm DS (1995) Subcutaneous oxygen tension: A useful adjunct in assessment of perfusion status. Crit Care Med 23:867-773
24. Hess JR, Fadare SO, Tolentino LS, Bangal NR, Winslow RM (1989) The intravascular persistence of crosslinked human hemoglobin. In: Anonymous progress in clinical and biological research. Alan R Liss, New York, pp 351-357
25. Hess JR, Macdonald VW, Winslow RM (1992) Dehydration and shock: an animal model of hemorrhage and resuscitation of battlefield injury. Biomater Artif Cells Immobilization Biotechnol 20:499-502
26. Hess JR, Macdonald VW, Brinkley WW (1993) Systemic and pulmonary hypertension after resuscitation with cell-free hemoglobin. J Appl Physiol 74:1769-1778
27. Przybelski RJ, Kant GJ, Bounds MJ, Slayter MV, Winslow RM (1990) Rat maze performance after resuscitation with cross-linked hemoglobin solution. J Lab Clin Med 115:579-588
28. Schultz SC, Hamilton I, Malcolm DS (1993) Use of base deficit to compare resuscitation with lactated ringer's solution, haemaccel, whole blood, and diaspirin cross-linked hemoglobin following hemorrhage in rats. J Trauma 35:619-626
29. Schultz SC, Powell CC, Burris DG, Nguyen H, Jaffin J, Malcolm DS (1994) The efficacy of diaspirin crosslinked hemoglobin solution resuscitation in a model of uncontrolled hemorrhage. J Trauma 37:408-412
30. Gulati A, Sen AP, Sharma AC, Singh G (1997) Role of ET and NO in resuscitative effect of diaspirin cross-linked hemoglobin after hemorrhage in rat. Am J Physiol 273:H827-H836
31. Gulati A, Sen AP (1998) Dose-dependent effect of diaspirin crosslinked hemoglobin on regional blood circulation of severely hemorrhaged rats. Shock 9:65-73
32. Kumar A, Sen AP, Saxena PR, Gulati A (1997) Resuscitation with diaspirin crosslinked hemoglobin increases cerebral and renal blood perfusion in hemorrhaged rats. Artif Cells Blood Substit Immobil Biotechnol 25:85-94
33. Gulati A, Rebello S (1994) Role of adrenergic mechanisms in the pressor effect of diaspirin cross-linked hemoglobin. J Lab Clin Med 124:125-133
34. Gulati A, Sharma AC (1994) Prazosin blocks the pressor but not the regional circulatory effects of diaspirin crosslinked hemoglobin. Life Sci 55:121-130
35. Sharma AC, Gulati A (1995) Yohimbine modulates diaspirin crosslinked hemoglobin-induced systemic hemodynamics and regional circulatory effects. Crit Care Med 23:874-884
36. Gulati A, Sharma AC, Singh G (1996) Role of endothelin in the cardiovascular effects of diaspirin crosslinked and stroma reduced hemoglobin. Crit Care Med 24:137-147
37. Schultz SC, Grady B, Cole F, Hamilton I, Malcolm DS, Burhop K (1993) A role for endothelin and nitric oxide in the pressor response to diaspirin cross-linked hemoglobin. J Lab Clin Med 122:301-308
38. Sharma AC, Singh G, Gulati A (1995) Role of NO mechanism in cardiovascular effects of diaspirin cross-linked hemoglobin in anesthetized rats. Am J Physiol 269:H1379-H1388
39. Katsuyama SS, Cole DJ, Drummond JC, Bradley K (1994) Nitric oxide mediates the hypertensive response to a modified hemoglobin solution (DCLHb™) in rats. Artif Cells Blood Substit Immobil Biotechnol 22:1-7
40. Kida Y, Iwata S, Gyoutoku Y, Aikou A, Yamakawa T, Nishi K (1991) Vascular responsiveness to various vasoactive substances after exchange transfusion with pyridoxalated hemoglobin polyoxyethylene conjugate (PHP) solution in anesthetized rats. Artif Organs 15:5-14
41. Flint LM, Cryer HM, Simpson CJ, Harris PD (1984) Microcirculatory norepinephrine constrictor response in hemorrhagic shock. Surgery 96:240-247
42. Hutchins PM, Goldstone J, Wells R (1973) Effects of hemorrhagic shock on the microvasculature of skeletal muscle. Microvasc Res 5:131-140
43. Zingarelli B, Caputi AP, Di Rosa M (1994) Dexamethasone prevents vascular failure mediated by nitric oxide in hemorrhagic shock. Shock 2:210-215
44. Wennmalm A, Benthin G, Petersson A-S (1992) Dependence of the metabolism of nitric oxide (NO) in healthy human whole blood on the oxygenation of its red cell haemoglobin. Br J Pharmacol 106:507-508
45. Thiemermann C, Szabo C, Mitchell JA, Vane JR (1993) Vascular hyporeactivity to vasoconstrictor agents and hemodynamic decompensation in hemorrhagic shock is mediated by nitric oxide. Proc Natl Acad Sci USA 90:267-271

46. Thiemermann C (1994) The role of the L-arginine: nitric oxide pathway in circulatory shock. Adv Pharmacol 28:45–79
47. Harbrecht BG, Wu B, Watkins SC, Marshall HP, Jr., Peitzman AB, Billiar TR (1995) Inhibition of nitric oxide synthase during hemorrhagic shock increases hepatic injury. Shock 4: 332–337
48. Brown IP, Williams RL, McKirnan MD, Limjoco UR, Gray CG (1995) Nitric oxide synthesis inhibition does not improve the hemodynamic response to hemorrhagic shock in dehydrated conscious swine. Shock 3:292–298
49. Ventura S, Ludbrook J (1995) N-nitro-L-arginine methyl ester blocks the decompensatory phase of acute hypovolaemia in conscious rabbits by a brainstem mechanism. Eur J Pharmacol 277:265–269
50. Sen AP, Dong Y, Saxena PR, Gulati A (1998) Modulation of resuscitation effect of diaspirin cross-linked hemoglobin by L-NAME in rats. Shock 9:223–230
51. Vemulapalli S, Chiu PJS, Griscti K, Brown A, Kurowski S, Sybertz EJ (1994) Phosphoramidon does not inhibit endogenous endothelin-1 release stimulated by hemorrhage, cytokines and hypoxia in rats. Eur J Pharmacol 257:95–102
52. Zimmerman RS, Maymind M, Barbee RW (1994) Endothelin blockade lowers total peripheral resistance in hemorrhagic shock recovery. Hypertension 23:205–210
53. Chang H, Wu G-J, Wang S-M, Hung C (1993) Plasma endothelin level changes during hemorrhagic shock. J Trauma 35:825–833
54. Ohlstein EH, Storer BL (1992) Oxyhemoglobin stimulation of endothelin production in cultured endothelial cells. J Neurosurg 77:274–278
55. Gulati A, Sharma AC, Robbie G, Saxena PR (1995) Endothelin ET_A receptor antagonist, BQ-123, blocks the vasoconstriction induced by sarafotoxin 6b in the heart but not other vascular beds. Gen Pharmacol 26:183–193
56. Sharma AC, Singh G, Gulati A (1995) Role of nitric oxide mechanism in the cardiovascular effects of diaspirin crosslinked haemoglobin in anaesthetized rats. Am J Physiol 269: H1379–H1388

Blood Substitutes – Effects on the Microcirculation

W. J. Sibbald and A. Sielenkämper

Introduction

In addition to carrying oxygen (O_2), cell-free hemoglobin (Hb) solutions exhibit direct interactions with the circulation. In an 'unstressed' circulation, for example, Hb solutions augment mean arterial pressure (MAP) and systemic vascular resistance [1–3]. Interactions of Hb solutions with the regional circulations include an organ-specific redistribution of blood flow, particularly toward the splanchnic organs [3, 4]. Recent studies have proposed that the circulatory effect of Hb solutions may be mediated by scavenging nitric oxide (NO) [5–9], or interacting with endothelin (ET) [6, 8–10]. In contrast to the remarkable effects on the regional circulation, cell-free Hb solutions do not adversely impact cardiac output (CO) in healthy animals [3], nor *in vitro* myocardial contractility [11]. Hb solutions may therefore influence the regional and central levels of the circulation in different ways.

A next step in the evaluation of Hb solutions was defining their effects in models where the circulation is 'stressed', for example, in sepsis and trauma-induced hemorrhage. Infusing Hb solutions in animal models of hemorrhage was accompanied by recovery of both systemic perfusion pressures and surrogate markers of tissue hypoxia such as metabolic acidosis [12–14]. Infusing crosslinked Hb and pyridoxalated Hb polyoxyethylene (PHP) solutions in sepsis normalized the typical high CO, low systemic resistance profile of this syndrome [9, 15]. Finally, crosslinked Hb also improved splanchnic perfusion and reduced mortality in an animal model of sepsis [15].

Since microcirculatory dysfunction is a critical feature of the pathophysiology of shock and sepsis, it is timely that a critical analysis of the effects of cell-free Hb on the microcirculation be debated. Specific questions of contemporary interest include: (i) independent of an ability to carry O_2, is there a unique interaction of Hb solutions on the microcirculation which could explain the benefit observed in pre-clinical and clinical studies of shock and sepsis?; and, (ii) will Hb solutions find a clinical role as therapeutic adjuncts to resuscitate an injured microcirculation? In this chapter, we will discuss the effects of Hb solutions on the microcirculation, both under physiologic conditions and under conditions of critical illness. To support this review, a MedLine search was conducted to identify all relevant work describing the interaction of cell free Hb and the microcirculation, from January 1975 to December 1997. Literature retrieved was reviewed and

Table 1. Modified evidence-based guidelines to determine the effects of cell-free hemoglobins on the microcirculation

	Level of evidence
Prospective, randomized, blinded trials	Ia
Prospective, randomized, unblinded trials	Ib
Controlled, non-randomized trials	II
Retrospective studies	III
Book chapters, other scientific reports	IV

graded according to a modified schema, demonstrated in Table 1. An added objective of this review will be to speculate on mechanisms which may explain observed interactions of Hb preparations and the injured microcirculation.

Physiology

The microcirculation is a functionally independent entity which encompasses a vessel unit consisting of arterioles, venules, and capillaries, with diameters that range from 5 μm to 100 μm. The microcirculation is largely concerned with local adjustments of blood flow to support the changing nutritional needs of parenchymal cells, including the removal of metabolic by-products [16]. While a primary purpose of the microcirculation is to facilitate the tissues' nutritional needs, its endogenous vasomotor activity also influences control of systemic perfusion pressures and the inter-organ distribution of blood flow [16]. Microcirculatory blood flow is actively regulated by: (i) changes in vascular resistance and perfusion pressures originating from parent arterioles, and (ii) alterations of vascular tone within the capillary network. The latter includes changes in resistance of terminal arterioles (and possibly even active constriction of endothelial cells) which redistributes red blood cell (RBC) flow within the capillary networks [16, 17]. Blood flow within the microcirculation may also exhibit passive control, for example, when influenced by rheologic influences and network geometry (the latter may vary considerably between tissues) [18].

Microcirculatory blood flow is typically non-uniform. Both temporal heterogeneity (changes over time) and spatial heterogeneity (differences between vessels) of capillary flow is common. Capillary flow heterogeneity is lessened by metabolic stress and increasing RBC supply to the tissues [18,19]. Increased heterogeneity might therefore be expected when RBC supply to individual microcirculations is reduced.

Under resting conditions, the number of RBC perfused capillaries in most tissues is less than the number of no-flow (but anatomically existent) capillaries. It is therefore estimated that only 25–35% of available capillaries are perfused in ambient conditions. In 'stress' situations, however, capillaries can be recruited to maintain metabolic autoregulation. Another determinant of functional capillary density is the arterial perfusion pressure, such that capillary density falls under conditions of significant suppressions in pressure. The microcirculatory determinants of tissue O_2 availability include its large surface area and low O_2 gradients. Capillary oxygen tension (PO_2) is usually not higher than 30 mm Hg. If not located just within the diffusion field of an arteriole, each capillary supplies a defined tissue volume. This means that capillary flow cessation (e.g., decreased functional capillary density) may subject localized tissue units to hypoxic conditions. The normal heterogeneity of capillary blood flows is reflected by both spatial and temporal variability of Hb saturations in neighboring tissue units [20].

An important determinant of capillary perfusion is the vascular tone of terminal arterioles and their parent vessels. Since NO and endothelin are endogenous mediators which exhibit a significant impact on the regulation of vascular tone [10, 21], both will contribute to the regulation of capillary perfusion. NO and endothelin may be viewed as counterparts – NO mediates vasodilatation and endothelin exhibits vasoconstrictive activity.

Microcirculatory Dysfunction in Acute Illness

Hemorrhage

Hemorrhage acutely limits the circulation's ability to maintain tissue oxygenation, for two reasons; namely (1) intravascular volume is depressed and (2) O_2 content is lost. If more than 30% of the total blood volume is lost, hypotension, shock and metabolic acidosis develop. Microcirculatory dysfunction complicating hemorrhage may complicate both the initial volume depletion (ischemia) and the subsequent restoration of convective O_2 delivery (reperfusion).

Acute blood loss is accompanied by pre-capillary constriction because of neurohumoral activation, thus reducing capillary hydrostatic pressures. By thereby modifying the Starling forces, fluid is redistributed from the extravascular spaces to augment the intravascular fluid volume. When the limited capacity of this compensation is exhausted, cell ischemia may supervene, and result in anaerobic glycolysis and increased lactate production [22].

In the early 'no-flow' phases, hemorrhage is accompanied by depressed functional capillary density [23, 24], decreased RBC velocity [24], and intermittency of capillary perfusion [23]. Also noted is an increase in capillary vasomotion, perhaps representing a regulatory mechanism to counteract the decrease in capillary perfusion in hemorrhagic hypotension [23]. The resulting depression in capillary surface area and RBC flow are microvascular co-determinants in the development of hemorrhage-induced tissue hypoxia.

During this "no flow" period in hemorrhagic shock, cell "priming" occurs. This phenomenon, manifest only when the tissue is reperfused, results in the release of second messengers (intracellular calcium, cyclic adenosine monophosphate (cAMP), reactive O_2 species (ROS)) during the restoration of flow. The reperfusion phase is therefore characterized by a generalized inflammatory state, in which mediator generation facilitates leukocyte entrapment in the microcirculation and mediator release, all of which cause subsequent tissue injury [25].

Sepsis

Widespread inflammation in sepsis is facilitated by mediator excess. Hypotension occurs when the intravascular volume is significantly depressed, for example when venodilation and microvascular fluid loss is not accompanied by appropriate fluid resuscitation, and when myocardial depression limits the ability to maintain the CO.

Microcirculatory dysfunction is now recognized to be a significant component of the ubiquitous circulatory injury in sepsis. An increase in microvascular permeability, together with an increase in the normal heterogeneity of capillary RBC flow, create conditions which cause tissue injury. Microcirculatory flow alterations in sepsis may be explained by either remote or local consequences of the sepsis syndrome. Hypotension complicating excessive vasodilation or myocardial depression will depress microcirculatory RBC flow. At the regional levels of the circulation, depressed reactivity to normal neurohumoral mechanisms of vasoregulation will alter the inter-organ distribution of blood flows [26], thereby impacting on microvascular flows. At local levels, microcirculatory RBC flow abnormalities may also be the result of any of the following: excessive interstitial edema, endothelial swelling, and leukocyte or RBC entrapment. The consequence of all these factors is an excessive heterogeneity of capillary RBC flow, both spatially and temporally [27, 28].

These microcirculatory abnormalities contribute to the inability to maximally extract O_2 reported in sepsis [29]. What has not yet been demonstrated in sepsis is the mechanism of parenchymal cell injury accompanying this microcirculatory dysfunction.

Effects of Cell-Free Hemoglobins on the Unstressed Microcirculation

We were able to identify only three *in vivo* studies which described the effects of cell-free Hb on the intact microcirculation (Table 2). One of the more frequently cited is Tsai study et al's [30] on the effects of an $\alpha\alpha$-Hb-preparation and dextran on the skin microcirculation, determined after isovolemic exchange transfusion. After hemodilution to 50% of the initial hematocrit (Hct), microvascular O_2 transport capacity (the product of O_2 transport capacity [RBC plus Hb], functional capillary density, and capillary RBC velocity) was no different when comparing $\alpha\alpha$-Hb and dextran interventions. However, it appeared that functional capillary density decreased gradually with Hb exchange transfusion while RBC velocity increased, until the Hct fell to < 50% of initial values. The authors [30] proposed that a depression in capillary density with the intervention was an (expected) autoregulatory response of the microcirculation to an increase in O_2 availability in the presence of cell-free Hb. This data is graded as level II evidence.

Recently, a controlled study [24] (level II evidence) evaluated both moderate isovolemic exchange infusion and hypervolemic infusion of crosslinked Hb on striated skin muscle in hamsters. Both interventions were followed by arteriolar

Table 2. Effects of cell-free hemoglobins on intact microcirculations

	Studies	Level of evidence
Direct observations		
Increased RBC velocity, moderately decreased capillary density	Nolte et al. [24], Tsai et al.[30]	II
Leukocyte – endothelium interaction and permeability unchanged, short-lasting arteriolar constriction	Nolte et al. [24]	II
Indirect observations		
Increased vascular endothelial stress (aortic endothelial cells)	Motterlini et al. [32]	II
More homogeneous distribution of tissue oxygen tensions	Nolte et al. [33]	II

constriction (short-lasting) and a modest decrease in capillary density, while RBC velocity (a strong determinant of O_2 delivery (DO_2) to the tissues [31]), increased by 50%. The Hb infusion did not accentuate leukocyte-endothelium interaction or modify microvascular permeability [24]. These latter observations are important since earlier *in vitro* studies (level II) had suggested that exposure to cell-free Hb solutions induced oxidative stress in vascular endothelial cells from porcine aorta [32].

Finally, recent findings on microvascular tissue O_2 transport after treatment with crosslinked Hb support the results of the *in vivo* microcirculation studies. In a non-randomized study [33] (level II), where local tissue PO_2 in the striated skin muscle of the hamster was analyzed using a Clark-type electrode, mean tissue PO_2 decreased slightly following Hb infusion. However, infusing the Hb solution was followed by a more homogeneous distribution of tissue PO_2.

In summary, *in vivo* data does not demonstrate any deleterious interaction of modified cell-free Hb solutions on intact microcirculations in muscle and hamster cheek pouch. Whether this conclusion is generalizable to other organ microcirculations cannot be determined at this time.

Effects of Cell-Free Hemoglobins on the Microcirculation after Hemorrhage

Compared to resuscitation with other colloids or crystalloids, cell-free Hb preparations seem to be more effective and rapid in reversing the O_2 debt induced by acute hemorrhage in various animal models [8, 12, 13, 34]. Although there are many possible reasons to explain an apparent superiority of cell-free Hb in this setting, it is tempting to speculate that unique effects on the microcirculation may be contributory.

The effects of Hb solutions on the microcirculation in resuscitation from acute hemorrhage have been assessed only in the hamster skinfold preparation. While

Table 3. Effects of infusion of cell-free hemoglobins on the microcirculation after acute hemorrhage

	Studies	Level of evidence
Direct observations		
Increase in capillary density to the same extent than with colloid infusion, but less than with autologous blood infusion	Kerger et al. [31], Nolte et al. [24]	II
Recovery of arteriolar and/or venular RBC velocity	Kerger et al. [31], Nolte et al. [24]	II
Arteriolar and/or venular constriction	Kerger et al. [31]	II
No arteriolar or venular constriction	Nolte et al. [24]	II
Less leukocyte rolling and sticking compared to infusion of autologous blood, permeability unaffected	Nolte et al. [24]	II
Indirect observations		
Improved/more homogeneous tissue oxygen tensions as compared to colloid or Ringer's lactate infusion	Nolte et al. [33], Kerger et al. [31]	II

this model is suitable to study a variety of microvascular and oxygenation endpoints, it is not clear to what extent findings in this tissue can be generalized to the core organs. Of available studies, data have been obtained prospectively in all, but without evidence that treatment was randomized. Thus, all have been classified as level II evidence (Table 3).

When o-raffinose crosslinked and oligomerized Hb was administered after 2 h of hemorrhagic shock at half the volume of the initially shed blood, functional capillary density was quickly elevated (from $11.3 \pm 28.2\%$ to $51.2 \pm 22.1\%$), although it did not return to pre-shock levels [35]. While a similar effect was observed after the administration of both dextran and crystalloid, autologous blood restored capillary perfusion to a slightly greater extent. Although no differences for recovery of arteriolar and venular blood flow and RBC velocity were observed between the different interventions in this experiment, for animals treated with cell-free Hb and autologous blood, it appeared that tissue PO_2 increased to a greater extent than following the infusion of either dextran or crystalloid. This study also reveals that o-raffinose crosslinked and oligomerized Hb significantly reduced the diameter of both feeding arterioles and venules [35].

In another study [24], diaspirin crossliked Hb (DCLHb) was administered as replacement therapy after the removal of 50% of the total blood volume. This intervention restored venular RBC velocity (which had fallen to zero in shock) to 112% of baseline levels within one hour after treatment. Infusion of autologous blood yielded a similar result (post treatment RBC velocity was 86% of baseline). In comparison, an infusion of dextran 60 was followed by a recovery of RBC velocity to only 56% of baseline levels, perhaps because restoration of MAP was not as complete. While functional capillary density in the Hb-treated animals was restored as effectively as in the dextran-treated animals, the highest percentage of recovery was seen after infusing autologous blood. Leukocyte rolling and sticking was not altered by the Hb infusion, but increased when autologous blood was administered [24].

In the final study reviewed, colloid resuscitation after hemorrhage increased the microvascular tissue PO_2 in hamster striated skin muscle less than cross-linked Hb and autologous blood. Resuscitation with DCLHb was also followed by a more homogeneous distribution of tissue PO_2 levels, even when compared to blood [33].

In summary, experiments which have measured the effects of Hb solutions as resuscitating agents in hemorrhagic shock models demonstrate:
1) improved microcirculatory flow behavior, probably better than that achieved with colloid and perhaps not as great as that achieved with autologous blood;
2) no independent effect to alter any interaction between leukocytes, the microcirculation, and its endothelium, unlike that observed with autologous blood;
3) a more homogeneous distribution of tissue PO_2 level compared to colloid and blood.

These favorable effects of infusing Hb solution in hemorrhagic shock are consistent with the indirect evidence of a microcirculatory benefit of these solutions in hemorrhagic shock, for example, a reversal of metabolic acidosis [12, 14], an increase in systemic O_2 uptake (VO_2) [8], and improved tissue morphology [34].

Effects of Cell-Free Hemoglobin on the Septic Microcirculation

The interaction of Hb solutions and sepsis has only been the focus of experimental work over the last few years. Some studies have postulated a protection of Hb solution infusion against lethal endotoxemia after Hb pre-treatment [36, 37]. Other studies, however report an acceleration of early mortality [38]. In the septic circulation, however, there is evidence that Hb solutions may be of benefit.

In an ovine model in which a live *Pseudomonas aeruginosa* infusion was used to create a hyperdynamic circulatory state, a subsequent bolus infusion of oxalated pyridoxalated Hb plyoxyethylene conjugate increased the systemic vascular resistance and the MAP, while the cardiac index (CI) decreased [9]. Bolus infusion of DCLHb in rats with peritonitis created similar effects [15], and also demonstrated an improved perfusion of vital organs, especially the intestine, following intervention.

In a cecal ligation and perforation model of sepsis in rats, we determined the efficacy of DCLHb. Isovolemic hemodilution to create anemic hypoxia was continued until a directly measured decline in systemic VO_2 was confirmed. Table 4 summarizes the effects of hemodilution on O_2 transport variables and arterial lactates [39]. When systemic VO_2 was supply dependent, study animals were randomized to one of three interventions; namely an isovolemic exchange transfusion with about 50% of total blood volume of: (i) fresh packed RBCs; (ii) fresh

Table 4. Effect of isovolemic hemodilution (using rat plasma) to O_2 supply dependency (OSD) on O_2 transport variables and arterial lactate in septic rats (n = 48).

	Baseline	OSD
Systemic O_2 uptake (ml/min/100g)	2.79 ± 0.11	$1.51 \pm 0.04*$
Systemic O_2 delivery (ml/min/100g)	0.59 ± 0.37	$2.44 \pm 0.13*$
Systemic O_2 extraction ratio	0.34 ± 0.02	$0.69 \pm 0.04*$
Lactate (mmol/L)	1.3 ± 0.1	$8.2 \pm 0.5*$

* $p < 0.0001$ (from paired t-test)

packed RBCs diluted to a Hb content of 100 g/L; or (iii) DCLHb solution, the latter also formulated at a concentration of 100 g/l [39]. Infusion of all three solutions was followed by an immediate increase in systemic VO_2 (Fig. 1) and a concomitant fall in arterial lactate levels. The improved systemic VO_2 with DCLHb was not a consequence of a concomitant increase in systemic DO_2, but rather due to an improved systemic O_2 extraction (Fig. 2). From this level Ib study, we concluded that DCLHb exhibited a beneficial effect on the microcirculation, and that the improved O_2 extraction would have been the consequence of an increase in functional capillary density or decrease in heterogeneity of blood flow (Table 5).

In follow-up experiments (level Ib), we directly measured the effects of a bolus infusion of DCLHb (600 mg/kg) on the microcirculation, using intravital microscopy on the terminal arterioles and capillary networks of the ileal mucosa in septic rats. We found that DCLHb was followed by a statistically significant (15%) increase in both functional capillary density and terminal arteriolar RBC velocity (unpublished data), thereby providing an explanation for the effects on tissue O_2 extraction previously described. The systemic vascular resistance and MAP increased at the same time, thus suggesting the possibility that hemodynamic effects of the Hb solution may have explained the improved microcirculatory blood flow.

In a clinical phase II trial [40] (level II) to investigate the effects of 100–500 ml of a 10% solution of DCLHb on hemodynamics in critically ill patients, arte-

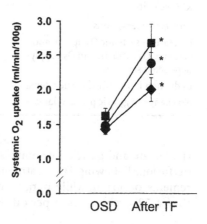

Fig. 1. Effect of transfusion (TF) of fresh RBCs (*squares*), fresh diluted RBCs (*circles*), and diaspirin crosslinked hemoglobin (*diamonds*) on systemic O_2 uptake in O_2 supply-dependent septic rats (n = 12 per group). Infusing fresh RBCs and DCLHb increased systemic O_2 uptake; * $p < 0.001$ for transfusion effect

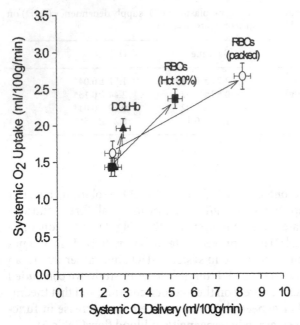

Fig. 2. Changes in the systemic O_2 uptake/delivery relationship (arrows) following resuscitation from O_2 supply-dependency using isovolemic exchange transfusion with fresh RBC preparations and diaspirin crosslinked hemoglobin (n = 12 septic rats per group). Rats treated with fresh RBCs exhibited an increase in O_2 uptake and O_2 delivery. The improved O_2 uptake following diaspirin crosslinked hemoglobin infusion was explained by an increase in O_2 extraction ratio from 0.62 ± 0.07 to 0.76 ± 0.11 (significance for transfusion effect within the group and between group effect as compared to the RBC groups)

Table 5. Effects of infusion of cell-free hemoglobins on the microcirculation in sepsis

	Studies	Level of evidence
Direct observations		
15% increase in capillary density and RBC velocity	Sielenkämper (unpublished)	Ib
Indirect observations		
Increase in systemic O_2 uptake and systemic O_2 extraction in O_2 supply-dependent septic rats	Sielenkämper et al. [39]	Ib
Reduction in intestinal tissue edema	Mourelatos et al. [15]	IV
No change in gastric pHi and lactate	Reah et al. [40]	II

rial lactate and gastric intramucosal pH (pHi) were used as an index of tissue perfusion. Following Hb treatment, a 75% reduction in norepinephrine requirements occurred, while parameters of tissue perfusion remained unchanged over a 72 h observation period. However, this study was small, the group of

patients was heterogeneous with many of them not meeting the current definition of sepsis, and finally gastric tonometry was utilized only in 7 out of 14 patients [40].

In summary, there is evidence that DCLHb improves microcirculatory flow abnormalities in sepsis. In terms of the effects of Hb solutions on microvascular
permeability, we were able to find only one qualitative observation, namely, that
intestinal edema appeared to be radically diminished after DCLHb treatment of
septic animals (level IV evidence) [15].

Comments

Cell-free Hb solutions are characterized by different properties which may, to a
varying degree and also dependent on the conditions under which they are infused, influence flow and O_2 transport in the microvascular networks. These
properties include interaction with NO and ET, colloidal effects, a right-shifted O_2
dissociation curve, and other Hb specific effects which in part depend on the biochemical properties of individual Hb preparations.

Most Hbs bind NO, an endogenous mediator which contributes to regulating
vascular tone, and which may be dependent on a dynamic interaction with RBC
Hb to support the maintenance of homeostasis [21]. An increase in binding of
NO during the infusion of cell-free Hb is followed by vasoconstriction and increased MAP, both in animals [1–3] and humans [41]. It is therefore not surprising that an improved arterial pressure with modified cell-free Hb is accompanied
by improved microvascular flow after both hemorrhage [24, 35] and sepsis (unpublished data) and that this is then accompanied by improved tissue oxygenation in both types of illness [33, 35, 39]. However, it is uncertain if the improved
microvascular perfusion which accompanies Hb solutions is solely the effect of
improved perfusing pressures under such conditions, or whether NO scavenging
at the level of the microcirculation provide an added reason for improved microcirculatory flows.

The colloidal effects of cell-free Hb results from their protein character. It is
likely that their efficacy as resuscitation fluids in hemorrhage are partly explained by their colloidal effects (in addition to their O_2 carrying properties and
vascular effects). When given as a topload infusion in subjects with normal arterial Hb concentration, Hb preparations may cause additional hemodilution.
However, compared to infusion with another colloid, Hb infusion may cause less
hemodilution and, therefore, prevent the increased heterogeneity of microvascular perfusion, which occurs in protracted hemodilution [19].

A further feature of some Hb solutions is a rightward shift of their O_2 dissociation curve, compared to human blood [39, 42, 43]. A higher P_{50} of Hb solution
may increase O_2 offloading in the microcirculation, and, therefore, explain the
improved tissue oxygenation observed when these Hb preparations are infused
after hemodilution [43] and in sepsis [39]. However, there is no clear evidence as
yet that right-shifting the O_2 dissociation curve is important in modifying an
acute tissue O_2 debt.

Although most of the available information shows that appropriate use of cell-free Hb improves the microcirculatory flow and tissue oxygenation when compromised in shock, a recent *in vitro* study suggested that infusing cell-free Hb induces increased activity of endothelial heme oxygenase, a microsomal stress protein. This may indicate the possibility of increased O_2 radical formation and oxidative stress in the microcirculation [32]. Although these data appear to be in disagreement with the aforementioned evidence of improved peripheral tissue blood flow and oxygenation, one cannot exclude that oxidative stress may be induced by Hb infusion despite an overall positive effect on both the convective and diffusive O_2 transport to the tissues.

An alternative explanation for the observation that cell-free Hb provides specific benefits for tissue oxygenation is its characteristic distribution in the plasma compartment, outside the red blood cell. Especially in anemia, improved O_2 extraction after Hb infusion (Fig. 2) may be related to a more homogeneous intravascular distribution of the Hb as compared to RBCs. As explained before, anemia is a situation where RBC flow to the individual capillaries is reduced and perfusion is very heterogeneous [19]. Thus, extreme hemodilution might be a situation in which cell-free Hbs are highly efficacious because of Hb presence in RBC-free plasma gaps or in capillaries without RBC supply (Fig. 3). Recently, evidence for this hypothesis was presented using a bovine Hb [43].

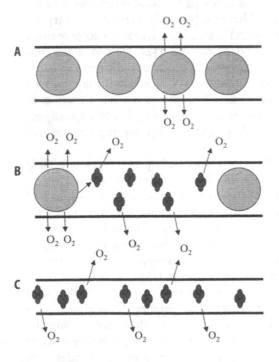

Fig. 3. Schematic diagram on the effects of cell-free hemoglobin on O_2 transport within the microcirculation. **A** Normal situation; O_2 transport occurs from the red cell across the capillary membrane. **B** Hemodilution with large plasma gaps and presence of cell-free hemoglobin; O_2 may be transported directly from the red cell to the tissues or may be delivered from cell-free hemoglobin, cell-free hemoglobin may also function as a carrier vehicle for initially red-cell located O_2. **C** Capillary without red blood cell flow; presence of cell-free hemoglobin in such capillaries may improve microregional O_2 delivery

Conclusions

Hb solutions improve microcirculatory blood flows in animal models of diseases characterized by hypotension and tissue ischemia, such as hemorrhage and sepsis. However, no firm conclusions can be drawn at this point, since the evidence is limited both quantitatively (low number of studies) and qualitatively (only a few studies provide level I evidence). The observed beneficial effects on RBC microvascular flows are consistent with an improved tissue oxygenation, but it remains to be elucidated if this phenomenon is explained by the vascular effects of the Hb solutions, or specific effects, for example, intravascular distribution of the cell-free Hb or an altered O_2 dissociation curve.

References

1. Kida Y, Maeda M, Iwata S, Goto K, Nishi K (1995) Effects of pyridoxalated hemoglobin poly-oxyethylene conjugate and other hemoglobin related substances on arterial blood pressure in anesthetized and conscious rats. Artif Organs 19:117–128
2. Rabinovici R, Rudolph AS, Feuerstein G (1989) Characterization of hemodynamic, hematologic, and biochemical responses to administration of liposome-encapsulated hemoglobin in the conscious, freely moving rat. Circ Shock 29:115–132
3. Sharma AC, Gulati A (1994) Effect of diaspirin cross-linked hemoglobin and norepinephrine on systemic hemodynamics and regional circulation in rats. J Lab Clin Med 123:299–308
4. Gulati A, Sharma AC, Burhop KE (1994) Effect of stroma-free hemoglobin and diaspirin cross-linked hemoglobin on the regional circulation and systemic hemodynamics. Life Sci 55:827–837
5. Hart JL, Ledvina M, Muldoon M (1997) Actions of diaspirin cross-linked hemoglobin on isolated rat and dog vessels. J Lab Clin Med 129:356–363
6. Schultz CS, Grady B, Cole F, Hamilton I, Burhop K, Malcolm DS (1993) A role for endothelin and nitric oxide in the pressor response to diaspirin cross-linked hemoglobin. J Lab Clin Med 122:301–308
7. Sharma AC, Singh G, Gulati A (1995) Role of NO mechanism in cardiovascular effects of diaspirin cross-linked hemoglobin in anesthetized rats. Am J Physiol 269:H1379–H1388
8. Gulati A, Sen AP, Sharma AC, Singh G (1997) Role of ET and NO in resuscitative effect of diaspirin cross-linked hemoglobin after hemorrhage in rat. Am J Physiol 273:H827–H836
9. Bone HG, Schenarts PJ, Booke M, et al (1997) Oxalated pyridoxalated hemoglobin polyoxyethylene conjugate normalizes the hyperdynamic circulation in septic sheep. Crit Care Med 25:1010–1018
10. Gulati A, Sharma AC, Singh G (1996) Role of endothelin in the cardiovascular effects of diaspirin crosslinked and stroma reduced hemoglobin. Crit Care Med 24:137–147
11. Yamakawa T, Miyauchi Y, Nishi K (1990) Effects of pyridoxalated hemoglobin polyoxyethylene conjugate and stroma-free hemoglobin on cardiac function in isolated rat heart. Artif Organs 14:208–217
12. Schultz SC, Hamilton IN, Malcolm DS (1993) Use of base deficit to compare resuscitation with lactated ringer's solution, haemaccel, whole blood, and diaspirin cross-linked hemoglobin following hemorrhage in rats. J Trauma 35:619–624
13. Schultz SC, Powell CC, Burris DG, Nguyen H, Jaffin J, Malcolm DS (1995) The efficacy of diaspirin crosslinked hemoglobin solution resuscitation in a model of uncontrolled hemorrhage. J Trauma 37:408–412

14. Sprung J, Mackenzie CF, Barnas GM, et al (1995) Oxygen transport and cardiovascular effects of resuscitation from severe hemorrhagic shock using hemoglobin solutions. Crit Care Med 23:1540–1553
15. Mourelatos MG, Enzer N, Ferguson JL, Rypins EB, Burhop KE, Law WJ (1996) The effects of diaspirin cross-linked hemoglobin in sepsis. Shock 5:141–148
16. Zweifach BW (1994) Vitalism revisited – an historical perspective of microcirculatory concepts. Int J Microcirc 14:122–131
17. Tsai AG, Friesenecker B, Intaglietta M (1995) Capillary flow impairment and functional capillary density. Int J Microcirc 15:238–243
18. Ellis CG, Wrigley SM, Groom AC (1994) Heterogeneity of red blood cell perfusion in capillary networks supplied by a singe arteriole in resting skeletal muscle. Circ Res 75:357–368
19. Tyml K, Cheng L (1995) Heterogeneity of red blood cell velocity in skeletal muscle decreases with increased flow. Microcirculation 2:181–193
20. Caspary L, Thum J, Creutzig A, Lubbers DW, Alexander K (1995) Quantitative reflection spectrophotometry: spatial and temporal variation of Hb oxygenation in human skin. Int J Microcirc 15:131–136
21. Jia L, Bonaventura C, Bonaventura J, Stamler JS (1996) S-nitrosohaemoglobin – a dynamic activity of blood involved in vascular control. Nature 380:221–226
22. Sielenkämper AW, Sibbald WJ (1998) Pathophysiology of hypotension. In: Singer, Webb A, Shapiro, Suter P (eds) Oxford textbook of critical care. Oxford University Press, Oxford (in press)
23. Vollmar B, Preissler G, Menger D (1994) Hemorrhagic hypotension induces arteriolar vasomotion and intermittent capillary perfusion in rat pancreas. Am J Physiol 267:H1936–H1940
24. Nolte D, Botzlar A, Pickelmann S, Bouskela E, Messmer K (1997) Effects of diaspirin-cross-linked-hemoglobin (DCLHb) on the microcirculation of striated skin muscle in the hamster: A study on safety and toxicity. J Lab Clin Med 130:314–327
25. Waxman K (1996) Shock: Ischemia, reperfusion, and inflammation. New Horizons 4:153–160
26. Martin CM, Yaghi A, Sibbald WJ, McCormack D, Paterson NAM (1993) Differential impairment of vascular reactivity of small pulmonary and systemic arteries in hyperdynamic sepsis. Am Rev Respir Dis 148:164–172
27. Lam C, Tyml K, Martin C, Sibbald W (1994) Microvascular perfusion is impaired in a rat model of normotensive sepsis. J Clin Invest 94:2077–2083
28. Farquhar I, Martin CM, Lam C, Potter R, Ellis CG, Sibbald WJ (1996) Decreased capillary density in vivo in bowel mucosa of rats with normotensive sepsis. Surg Res 60:22–29
29. Nelson DP, Samsel RW, Wood LDH, Schumacker PT (1988) Pathological supply dependence of systemic and intestinal O2 uptake during endotoxemia. J Appl Physiol 64:2410–2419
30. Tsai AG, Kerger H, Intaglietta M (1995) Microcirculatory consequences of blood substitution with aa-hemoglobin. In: Winslow RM, Vandegriff KD, Intaglietta M (eds) Blood substitutes – Physiological basis of efficacy. Birkhauser, Boston, Basel, Berlin, pp 155–174
31. Kerger H, Torres IP, Rivas M, Winslow RM, Intaglietta M (1995) Systemic and subcutaneous microvascular oxygen tension in conscious Syrian golden hamsters. Am J Physiol 37:H802–H810
32. Motterlini R, Foresti R, Vandegriff K, Intaglietta M, Winslow RM (1995) Oxidative-stress response in vascular endothelial cells exposed to acellular hemoglobin solutions. Am J Physiol 269:H648–H655
33. Nolte D, Steinhauser P, Pickelmann S, Berger S, Hartl R, Messmer K (1997) Effects of diaspirin-crosslinked-hemoglobin (DCLHb) on local tissue oxygen tension in striated skin muscle: An efficacy study in the hamster. J Lab Clin Med 130:328–338
34. Siegel JH, Fabian M, Smith JA, Constantino D (1997) Use of recombinant hemoglobin solution in reversing lethal hemorrhagic hypovolemic oxygen debt shock. J Trauma 42:199–212
35. Kerger H, Tsai AG, Saltzman DJ, Winslow RM, Intaglietta M (1997) Fluid resuscitation with O2 vs. non-O2 carriers after 2 h of hemorrhagic shock in conscious hamsters. Am J Physiol 272:H525–H537

36. Otterbein L, Chin BY, Otterbein SL, Lowe VC, Fessler HE, Choi AMK (1997) Mechanism of hemoglobin-induced protection against lethal endotoxemia in rats: a ferritin-independent pathway. Am J Physiol 272:L268–L275
37. Otterbein L, Sylvester SL, Choi AMK (1995) Hemoglobin provides protection against lethal endotoxemia in rats: the role of heme oxygenase-1. Am J Respir Cell Mol Biol 13:595–601
38. Aranow JS, Zhuang J, Wang H, Larkin V, Smith M, Fink MP (1996) A selective inhibitor of inducible nitric oxide synthase prolongs survival in a rat model of bacterial peritonitis: comparison with two nonselective strategies. Shock 5:116–121
39. Sielenkämper AW, Chin-Yee IH, Martin CM, Sibbald WJ (1997) Diaspirin crosslinked hemoglobin improves systemic oxygen uptake in oxygen supply-dependent septic rats. Am J Respir Crit Care Med 156:1066–1072
40. Reah G, Bodenham AR, Mallick A, Daily EK, Przybelski RJ (1997) Initial evaluation of diaspirin cross-linked hemoglobin (DCLHb) as a vasopressor in critically ill patients. Crit Care Med 25:1480–1488
41. Przybelski RJ, Daily EK, Kisicki JC, Mattia-Goldberg C, Bounds MJ, Colburn WA (1996) Phase I study of the safety and pharmacologic effects of diaspirin cross-linked hemoglobin solution. Crit Care Med 24:1993–2000
42. Chatterjee R, Welty LV, Walder RY, et al (1986) Isolation and characterization of a new hemoglobin derivative cross-linked between the a chains (lysine $99a_1$, lysine $99a_2$). J Biol Chem 21:9929–9937
43. Standl T, Horn P, Wilhelm S, et al (1996) Bovine haemoglobin is more potent than autologous red blood cells in restoring muscular tissue oxygenation after profound isovolemic haemodilution in dogs. Can J Anesth 43:714–723

Perfluorocarbons as Oxygen Carriers

M. Lamy, M. Mathy-Hartert, and G. Deby-Dupont

Introduction

At the same time that the clinical need for blood and blood products has increased, brought about, in part, by an increase in high blood loss surgery, attempts to find solutions capable of replacing hemoglobin (Hb) for the transport of oxygen (O_2) have become more and more serious. The risks of homologous blood transfusion (transmission of cytomegalovirus, hepatitis B and C, and human immunodeficiency virus (HIV), etc. ...), even if statistically limited and potentially susceptible to further reduction, have also driven the search for blood substitutes. Two major pathways have been followed in this search, that of modified Hb solutions and that of perfluorocarbon (PFC) solutions. These can be used in acute situations as blood substitutes, or as adjuncts to elective perioperative hemodilution, to allow reductions in hematocrit (Hct) beyond values usually accepted as tolerable [1, 2].

The PFCs, which are diametrically opposed to the Hb molecule in terms of chemical structure and reactivity, were developed during the Second World War. Their total chemical and biochemical inertness made these compounds indispensable for the manipulation of the uranium derivatives used in the fabrication of the first atomic bomb. But it was the initial experiments of Clark and Gollan in 1966 [3] that brought attention to the capacity of PFC to dissolve O_2; their famous demonstration of a rat immersed in a solution of PFC saturated in O_2 at atmospheric pressure, breathing normally remains a key step in the history of the biomedical use of PFC [3, 4]. A simplistic belief that these substances would soon provide a useful blood substitute arose from these experiments. As is often the case, initial unbridled enthusiasm rapidly encountered obstacles, associated with the novelty of this class of molecules, such as excessive retention within the body and insufficient stability of the emulsions, in addition to certain side effects. These highlighted the need to better understand the mechanisms of O_2 transport by PFC solutions, as well as to prepare PFC-rich emulsions to ensure optimal oxygenation [4]. Thirty years later, the first PFC-rich emulsions are undergoing phase II clinical trials, and it is reasonable to expect the start of phase III clinical trials in 1998, as well as marketing of these products in the near future.

Characteristics of Pure Perfluorocabons

The PFCs are low molecular weight organic compounds (usually from 400 to 500 daltons) (Table 1). They are linear or cyclic hydrocarbons occasionally containing O_2 or nitrogen atoms, and in which all the hydrogen atoms of the carbon chain have been replaced by fluorine atoms. The carbon-fluorine bond is strong, and relatively non-polarizable; the process of hyperfluorination leads to total chemical inertness, and a complete lack of metabolism *in vivo*. The PFCs are the most compressible, the most inert, the most hydrophobic, and the most dense liquids known. They are transparent fluids, with a low surface tension; certain PFCs (such as perflubron) have a positive spreading coefficient. Their densities are between 1.8 and 2 (i.e., twice that of water), and they are immiscible in water. They are stable, can be stored at room temperature, and can be sterilized without damage. In addition to their chemical stability, they possess a property that is indispensable for use as blood substitutes, the ability to dissolve gases (such as O_2 and carbon dioxide (CO_2)) without covalent bonds, proportionally to their applied partial pressure. This property explains the linear solubility curves for O_2 in PFCs (Fig. 1), compared to the sigmoid curve for oxyhemoglobin saturation. The slope of the solubility curve becomes steeper as the concentration of PFC increases. Because O_2 is transported without chemical bonding, its unloading, for example at the tissues, is considerably facilitated. The presence of fluorine atoms also gives the PFCs useful properties for diagnostic testing using nuclear magnetic resonance imaging (NMR). It is their high density, and not their immiscibility, that makes their utilization as pure solutions in the intravascular space impossible. Fortunately, they can be emulsified, allowing them to be used in aqueous media [5, 6].

Numerous PFCs, with differing structures, have been synthesized and used either in pure solution or as emulsions. The first was a branched cyclic ether, followed by a tertiary amine (n-tripropylamine), a series of ethers, by the bicyclic PFCs (perfluorodecalin), and finally by linear molecules with eight to ten carbon chains (perfluorooctyl bromide, perfluorooctylethane, perfluorodichlorooctane) [4, 5]. These substances differ by their stability in emulsion, by the physiologic response they induce, and by the rapidity of their excretion from the body. The elimination of PFCs takes place by pulmonary excretion after passage through the reticulo-endothelial system (especially of the liver and spleen). The retention

Table 1. Physico-chemical characteristics of perfluorocarbons

- Perfluorinated carbon chain with molecular weight 450 to 550 daltons
- Linear or cyclic structure
- Chemical and biochemical inertness
- Non-inflammable, colorless
- Low vapor pressure, almost odorless
- Non-conductive, insoluble in aqueous media
- Density approaching 2 g/ml, positive dispersion coefficient (perflubron)
- Solubility of gas proportional to applied partial pressure

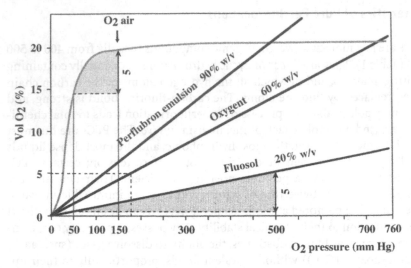

Fig. 1. Oxygen transport and delivery of different perfluorocarbon emulsions: comparison with hemoglobin

time within the body increases exponentially as a function of the molecular weight, with the exception of PFCs containing a lipophilic extremity (e.g., the bromide atom in perflubron) [5].

The synthesis of PFCs for biomedical use was initially performed either by electrochemical fluorination or by metal fluoride compounds, both of which are relatively crude techniques which lead to the formation of numerous potentially toxic byproducts and require complex purification steps. Currently, these syntheses are carried out using elective processes which have better yields and produce lower levels of impurities (consequently reducing the complexity of the purification). The potential biomedical applications of perfluorocarbons can be divided into five categories [6–8]:

1) used in pure form, for liquid ventilation, intraluminal oxygenation of the intestine, in ophthalmology, and for medical imaging
2) used as emulsions in aqueous media as blood substitutes for O_2 transport
3) used as inverse phase emulsions (water droplets dispersed in the PFC) or as gels for the distribution of bioactive molecules by the pulmonary route
4) used as amphiphilic aggregates, which form supramolecular structures (tubules, vesicles, ribbons, fibers, etc.) and as gels, as vectors for active medicinal agents
5) used as hybrid molecules combining a hydrogenated chain with a perfluorinated chain, as stabilizing links for the preparation of third generation PFC emulsions.

Characteristics of Perfluorocarbon Emulsions

The properties of PFC emulsions depend on both the components of the emulsion, but also on the proportion of the various components and on the sizes of the emulsion particles. The latter parameter is particularly important because it influences the stability of the emulsion, the surface area available for gas exchange, the viscosity, and the intravascular half-life (determined by the process of phagocytosis), and therefore the *in vivo* toxicity or side effects. There is a correlation between the size of the particles and the toxicity of the emulsions; the acute toxicity increases rapidly for emulsions containing particles with a size greater than 0.4 μm. In second generation emulsions, the mean size of the particles is approximately 0.25 μm, with none larger than 0.6 μm. These emulsions are generally milky-white in appearance, and become transparent when the particles are smaller than 0.1 μm. The surface charge of the particles is also important, because this determines the rapidity of phagocytosis and the interactions with platelets (which are charged negatively). The interactions could potentially lead to formation of microthrombi [4, 5].

The two surfactants whose use has proved pratical in the preparation of emulsions are Pluronic F-68 (polyethylene oxide-polypropylene oxide block-polymer), and egg yolk phospholipids. Although it is not acutely toxic, Pluronic F-68 is no longer used clinically because it appears to be responsible for certain side effects, such as complement activation, which can lead to an inflammatory reaction [9]. The emulsions are prepared using ultrasonication or high-pressure homogenization. Sonication appears to be partially destructive, and liberates free fluoride ions, which alters the composition of the emulsion, and could increase the risk of toxicity.

The characteristics of the ideal emulsion for use as a blood substitutes are the following: the absence of incompatibility; the absence of risk of transmission of infectious diseases; long duration of conservation; easy access (in terms of avoiding the difficulties of, for example, blood collection and processing); absence of metabolism and more particularly non-reactivity with O_2; no binding with O_2; allowing easy tissue unloading, viscosity and rheologic parameters similar to those of blood, permitting the particles to flow through swollen and/or blocked capillaries, where red blood cells might not pass.

The solubility of O_2 in PFC emulsions is proportional to the partial pressure (PO_2) (Fig. 1). The mechanisms of transport and delivery are therefore entirely different from those of erythrocytes. The oxyhemoglobin saturation curve for erythrocytes is sigmoid, with a relatively early plateau (for a PO_2 of approximately 150 mm Hg), while a fall in PO_2 from 150 to 50 mm Hg leads to unloading of 25% of the bound O_2. To obtain similar efficiency when PFC emulsions are used as blood substitutes, experimental animals must breathe an atmosphere enriched in O_2 (Fig. 1), and the same conditions would be fulfilled for use of the emulsions in humans [5, 8, 10].

First Generation Emulsions: The Past

The first PFC-based emulsions were prepared in 1967 using plasma, with large size particles (2–3 µm). They contained 20% of FX-80, a cyclic perfluorocarbon (3M) [4]. In 1968 a second emulsion (FC-47, 3M) composed mainly of a linear PFC (tri-n-butylamine) emulsified with Pluronic F-68 as a surfactant, was used successfully to replace the entire blood volume of a rat, with survival for several hours [11]. The first emulsion authorized by the Food and Drug Administration (FDA) for injection in humans (for percutaneous transluminal coronary angioplasty, PTCA) was the Japanese emulsion Fluosol® (Green Cross Corp., Osaka, Japan) (Table 2). This product is a 20% w/v (approximately 10% v/v) emulsion containing two PFCs, perfluorodecalin and perfluorotripropylamine (in a 70:30 ratio), emulsified by Pluronic F-68 and by egg yolk lecithin [12]. Its use showed that transport and delivery of O_2, without major toxic effects, was possible. It also revealed the shortfalls and weaknesses of this first generation emulsion, and led to a better understanding of the improvements necessary for the second generation. The major shortcomings of Fluosol were the long tissue retention of one of its components, its limited intravascular half-life (which, when taken together with the low percentage of PFC limited the amount of O_2 transported),

Table 2. Main characteristics of perfluorocarbon (PFC) emulsions

First generation

- PFC mixture (cyclic and linear)
- Low concentration of PFC → low oxygen transport
- Emulsification with egg yolk phospholipids and/or other emulsifiers (polyoxyethylene – polyoxypropylene polymer type)
- Inflammatory side effects, long-term tissue retention, difficult to use, limited conservation at room temperature
- Archetypal emulsion: Fluosol^{DA} (Green Cross Corporation)
  20% w/v (perfluorodecaline – perfluorotripropylamine 70/30)
  3.9% w/v Pluronic F-68 / egg-yolk phospholipids / glycerol (2.7/0.4/0.8)

Second generation

- One linear PFC, lipophilic molecule
- Higher PFC concentration (± 60 % w/v) → better O_2 transport
- Emulsification with egg-yolk phospholipids
- No inflammatory side effects, reduced tissue retention, ready-to-use, long-term conservation at room temperature
- Archetypal emulsion: Oxygent™ (Alliance Pharmaceutical)
  60% w/v perflubron (perfluorooctylbromide)
  4% w/v egg yolk phospholipids

Third generation

Current generation, result of new research:

Archetypal emulsion:
- Linear PFC, lipophilic molecule (perflubron)
- High concentration 90% w/v
- High stabilization with mixed hydrocarbon/fluorocarbon molecules = molecular dowels
- Emulsification with egg yolk phospholipids and molecular dowels (2/1.4% w/v)

and its unsatisfactory stability. This problem necessitated conditioning Fluosol as three separate preparations (a primary emulsion which was frozen, and two secondary solutions), which were then mixed and oxygenated just prior to use. Fluosol also had certain side effects, such as inhibition of white blood cells and complement activation, attributed to the surfactant used to fabricate the emulsion [5, 9, 13].

Second Generation Emulsions: The Present

Since the use of Fluosol, considerable progress has been realized, allowing the production of more concentrated emulsions containing better tolerated surfactants. The archetypal second generation emulsion is Oxygent™ (Alliance Pharmaceutical Corp., San Diego, CA). This product is based on the use of perfluorooctyl bromide, better known by its generic name of perflubron, which is a linear PFC containing eight carbon atoms. A single terminal bromine atom lends lipophilicity and limits its tissue persistence. The important physico-chemical properties are shown in Table 3, compared to water [5,8]. Oxygent™ has a concentration of 60% w/v, and uses egg-yolk phospholipids as emulsifying agents [14]. The particles have a mean diameter of 0.16 to 0.18 μm. It dissolves 28 ml O_2/100 g at 37 °C and 750 mm Hg. It can be stored at refrigerated temperature for up to two years.

Oxyfluor™ (Hemagen-Baxter) is another second generation product [6]. This is a 56% w/v emulsion, based around perfluorodichlorooctane (PFDCO, a lipophilic PFC with a molecular weight of 471 and a density of 1.76), with egg-yolk phospholipids and safflower oil as surfactants. At equilibrium with 100% O_2 at 37°C, it dissolves 17.2% O_2 by volume. It is stable at room temperature for over one year.

The two emulsions have similar properties of O_2 transport and delivery, stability, and viscosity.

The main progress of the second generation emulsions is an important increase in the emulsion concentration, enormously enhancing the O_2-carrying capacity and eliminating the dilution of patient's blood at time of administration.

Table 3. Physico-chemical properties of perflubron, compared to those of water

	Water	Perflubron ($C_8H_{17}Br$)
Molecular weight (daltons)	18	465
Density (g/cm³ at 25 °C)	1.0	1.93
Viscosity (Cstokes at 25 °C)	1.0	1.1
Vapor pressure (mm Hg at 37 °C)	47	11
Surface tension (dyne/cm at 25 °C)	72	18
O_2 solubility at 37°C (ml O_2/100 ml liquid)	3	53
CO_2 solubility at 37°C (ml CO_2/100 ml liquid)	57	210

Another progress of these emulsions is their stability, obtained by using a crucial amount of egg yolk phospholipids and better emulsification techniques (high-pressure homogenization, microfluidization) [15]. The second generation emulsions are easy to use (formulated "ready-for-use") in buffered saline with physiological osmolarity, viscosity, and pH values), and have no acute toxicity or major side effects. Their administration is not associated with hemodynamic effects or with a decrease in cardiac output (CO), and they do not activate complement. The small size of the particles allows them to become concentrated in the thin layer of plasma between the red blood cells and the vascular wall (near-wall particle excess phenomenon) and to easily perfuse all the capillaries of the microcirculation. During states of local vasoconstriction and ischemia, during which erythrocytes no longer circulate, the plasma can continue to flow, while transporting O_2 and guaranteeing O_2 delivery (DO_2), especially as these molecules unload O_2 twice as rapidly as Hb [16]. These emulsions are therefore ideal for assuring tissue perfusion, even when the dose administered would appear insufficient to significantly increase total arterial blood content (CaO_2).

Third Generation Emulsions: The Future

These emulsions currently in early preclinical development are based on emulsification of a PFC by a phospholipid, but they also contain linear molecules with both hydrocarbon/fluorocarbon properties, which serve to stabilize the emulsion. The earlier, classical formulation combines PFCs and the hydrocarbon chains of phospholipids which have very little affinity for each other. The third generation emulsions contain mixed-property molecules, which act as dowels, the hydrocarbon end anchored on one side in the oily chains of the phospholipid film, and the fluorinated end anchored on the other side in the PFC itself. This allows preparation of concentrated emulsions (up to 90% w/v) with particles with a mean size of 0.22 μm, which are stable for at least six months at 40°C (accelerated aging conditions). A maximal effect is noted at equimolar mixtures of PFC and these dowels [8, 17, 18]. A typical formulation of a third generation emulsion is the following: perflubron/egg yolk phospholipids/mixed fluorinated-hydrogenated diblock as molecular dowels (90/2/1.4% w/v), dispersed in phosphate buffer, with tocopherol and EDTA as antioxidants, and emulsified by microfluidization. This emulsion can be diluted in aqueous media without becoming unstable, even in the presence of calcium (which can destabilize earlier emulsion formulations). We have used this third generation emulsion to test cytotoxicity after dilution in complex cell culture media without loss of stability [19].

Uses of Pure Perfluorocarbons

Liquid Ventilation

Because PFCs dissolve large volumes of gas, are highly fluid, and have low surface tension, they are well suited for use during liquid ventilation to improve oxygenation during acute respiratory distress syndrome (ARDS). The low surface tension allows them to cover the alveolar surface uniformly; this also explains why these molecules have been explored as a means of distributing pharmaceutical drugs to the lung.

Studies of liquid ventilation have used perflubron (LiquiVent™, Alliance Pharmaceutical Corp., San Diego, CA), an excellent O_2 (50 ml/dl) and CO_2 (210 ml/dl) transporter which is eliminated by evaporation and is only marginally absorbed through the alveolus. Two techniques are used, total liquid ventilation or partial liquid ventilation (PLV or PAGE, perfluorocarbon associated gas exchange). During total liquid ventilation, the lungs are fully filled with the PFC, and are ventilated with a flow-limited, time-cycled liquid ventilator with tidal volumes of liquid [20]. PLV is accomplished by instilling a volume of PFC close to that of the functional residual capacity, and ensuring gas exchange by means of classical mechanical ventilation, using gas tidal volumes of 10 to 15 ml/kg [21]. This technique does not, therefore, require special equipment, but does require periodic reinjections of PFC, to replace losses due to evaporation. When instilled in the lung, the PFC penetrates into collapsed alveoli, improving oxygenation and increasing pulmonary compliance by reductions of surface tension. Studies have been successful in the premature lamb, the sheep, the dog, the rabbit, and the baboon using animal models of ARDS [20, 22-27], and using isolated lungs [28]. These have shown increased oxygenation (improved arterial saturation) and CO_2 removal, and usually improved pulmonary mechanics. The first successful use of warmed and oxygenated PFC for total liquid ventilation, using tidal volumes instilled and removed by gravity, was reported in the premature newborn in 1990 [29]. Clinical studies in six pediatric patients aged from eight weeks to 5 1/2 years suffering from ARDS sufficiently severe as to necessitate extracorporeal life support (ECLS) showed that PLV, started after two to nine days of ECLS with a total cumulative dose of PFC of 45.2 ml/kg, brought about an improvement in oxygenation in the first four days of the treatment, with improvement in lung compliance. These six patients survived, but the authors reported two pneumothoraces potentially attributable to the PFC [30].

PLV, with compensation for losses to evaporation, is being studied in the adult with ARDS. In a recent study, PLV was used for one to seven days (38 ml/kg mean total cumulative dose), and was associated with 50% survival, an improvement in compliance, a fall in physiologic shunt, and improved gas exchange [31]. The authors report two complications potentially attributable to PLV, one pneumothorax, and one mucus plug.

From the studies conducted to date, we can conclude that the product can be administered safely, that it distributes within the lung under the influence of gravity (it occupies more than 2/3 of the lung of the adult with ARDS), and that its administration leads to improved gas exchange (and therefore oxygenation), compliance, and decreased surface tension, countering a tendency to "inflate" the lung [20, 25, 32–34]. Its pulmonary clearance would appear to be approximately three weeks [32]. The intrapulmonary use of PFCs would also appear to have a beneficial effect on alveolar macrophages, by reducing their inflammatory response [35]. Clinical studies using LiquiVent are now being conducted using a multicenter protocol, and the usual difficulties with this type of undertaking are being encountered, especially when mortality rates are used as the final end-points.

Intraluminal Oxygenation of the Intestine

Severe changes in the intestinal mucosa are encountered in situations of ische-mia-reperfusion, which are often seen clinically (necrotizing enterocolitis, partial mesenteric arterial insufficiency). A crucial therapeutic option would be rapid delivery of O_2 *in situ*. Oxygenated PFCs, delivered via the intestinal lumen could fulfill this therapeutic role, and have been successfully tested in animal models of intestinal ischemia-reperfusion. Use during the ischemic phase preserves the structure of villi and crypts, and protects intestinal function, as evidenced by reductions in translocation of toxic elements such as bacteria and endotoxin [36, 37]. No human clinical studies have yet been reported of the use of PFCs for intestinal oxygenation in situations of ischemia-reperfusion.

Use in Medical Imaging

When liquid PFC is ingested, it darkens the image of the bowel in magnetic resonance imaging (MRI) (by lack of signal due to the absence of hydrogen atom) and facilitates the distinction of the gastro-intestinal (GI) tract from adjacent tissues. Its low viscosity and high density lead to rapid passage through the intestine with full imaging possible 20 to 40 minutes after oral administration. The clinical use for GI imaging of liquid perflubron (Imagent GI®) was approved by the FDA several years ago [8, 25]. The presence of a bromine atom in perflubron makes it radio-opaque and renders it useful for X-ray imaging of the bronchial tree and alveoli, and for GI tract imaging when bowel obstruction is suspected [8, 17, 32].

Organ Transplantation

One of the principal hindrances in transplantation surgery is the time limit imposed by organ conservation for organs such as the heart, the intestine, and the pancreas. Cold ischemia leads to metabolic modifications which are worsened upon reperfusion, but which could be avoided by assuring continous oxygenation of the organ after harvesting. Oxygenated PFCs have been used in this manner for cardiac, pulmonary, pancreatic, and hepatic preservation in animal models [38, 39]. The pancreas was treated either by total immersion in the liquid, or by a two-layer technique (the organ placed on the PFC, and covered by University of Wisconsin solution) at 4 °C with excellent results. Even after 90 minutes of warm ischemia or 96 hours of cold conservation, successful engraftment was seen in 80 to 90% of cases; this correlated with preserved tissue levels of adenosine triphosphate (ATP) [39].

Use in Ophthalmology

The high density of PFCs allows their use in ophthalmology, to reposition and splint detached or torn retina [40]. This use of PFCs is quite recent, and the results published to date are fragmentary but promising.

Use of Perfluorocarbon Emulsions

The clinical use of emulsions of PFCs are essentially those of perioperative hemodilution, resuscitation from hemorrhagic shock, and those of the treatment of ischemic problems where emulsions serve as a temporary vector for O_2, delaying or avoiding the administration of blood [1, 5, 6, 8, 13, 17, 25].

Perioperative Hemodilution and Resuscitation

First generation emulsions: Starting in 1970, numerous publications reported successful use of 12 to 25% emulsions of PFC as partial or complete blood substitutes in various animal species [4, 5]. These studies definitively showed the absence of acute toxicity and ability of these emulsions to transport O_2. Certain experiments using total exsanguination of the rat demonstrated that oxygenated emulsions allow sufficient O_2 transport to yield 100% survival for at least 20 hours in an atmosphere of 90% O_2 /10% carbon monoxide. Under these extreme experimental conditions, the animal was devoid of erythrocytes, and newly formed red blood cells were immediately "poisoned" by the carbon monoxide, so they could not transport O_2. The PFC was thus the only possible vector for DO_2 in these animals.

Fluosol, the most common first generation emulsion, was used clinically in the U.S.A. to treat severe anemia in surgical patients who refused blood transfusion for religious reasons [41–43]. The emulsion was administered to a maximum dose of 5 g PFC/kg, which provided a "transient boost" to the CaO_2 but were ineffective in severe anemia and unnecessary in moderate anemia [42]. The first clinical study summarizing results from 186 patients treated with Fluosol in 26 hospitals in Japan was published in 1982 [44]. This study concluded that the emulsion was safe, had a beneficial effect as a plasma expander, and that it contributed to DO_2. An overview of the clinical studies with Fluosol in Japan (401 patients, from 1979 to 1982) was presented in 1985 [45]. In 1989, Fluosol (Alpha Therapeutics Corporation, Los Angeles, CA) was approved in the United States by the FDA for use during PTCA, a typical clinical situation uniformly associated with localized myocardial ischemia [46]. Despite numerous publications showing beneficial effects of Fluosol during PTCA (up to a maximum dose of 1.14 g/kg), the clinical utility of this intervention remains controversial [5, 46]. Because technical advances now allow PTCA with autoperfusion catheters which prevent ischemia, the use of Fluosol is no longer necessary; the product has been withdrawn from the market.

Fluosol has been used to treat cerebral ischemia following subarachnoid hemorrhage, with demonstrated increases in blood flow, but no conclusive results can be drawn as to its efficacy [5, 44, 47]. It has also been used in acute myocardial infarction and in anticancer therapy (brain and lung tumors) [5, 44]. As a conclusion based on the reported human data, it would appear that Fluosol DA is difficult to use from a practical point of view, is devoid of toxicity for the patient, but has an intravascular half-life too short, and too low a concentration to be efficacious [10, 48]

Second generation: Several emulsions have been, and continue to be tested in animals, especially in hemorrhagic shock models [49–51]. In the dog, an emulsion based on PFDCO (Oxyfluor: Hemagen) was associated with 100% survival, compared with 63% in a group resuscitated with lactated Ringer's solution, with improved tissue oxygenation and increased DO_2 in the PFC group [49].

In humans, use of second generation emulsions has been considered in the clinical situations of anemia, trauma, high blood loss surgery, perioperative hemodilution, ischemia, and in organ conservation for transplantation. To date, more than one dozen studies have been performed in humans using perflubron-based emulsions, particularly with Oxygent™ (Table 4). These studies have enrolled more than 500 subjects in phases I and II [50]. Administration of these emulsions in phase I studies to more than 200 volunteers and surgical patients demonstrated the absence of hemodynamic effects (including vasoconstriction), an increase in CO related to the hemodilution, no effect on bleeding time, coagulation, and immune function. These initial preclinical and clinical studies have shown that a PFC dose of 1.35 g/kg can support DO_2 despite ongoing blood loss. Certain transitory side effects have been noted for the highest doses administered (1.8 g PFC/kg), such as an elevation in temperature of 1 to 1.5 °C in the first four to six hours following infusion, and a modest decrease in the platelet count, without bleeding complications, over the first two to three days after administration. Pharmacokinetic studies have confirmed that the plasma half-life is related to the dose of perflubron, and increases from 6.1 ± 1.9 h at a dose of 1.2 g PFC/kg to 9.4 ± 2.2 h at a dose of 1.8 g PFC/kg. Multicenter, phase II, randomized, controlled, single-blind studies have been completed in about 250 orthopedic, urologic, and gynecologic surgery patients. As of the beginning of 1998, initial results indicate an absence of toxic effects on hemodynamic, hematologic, and biochemical parameters. Several phase II studies in cardiac surgery with extracorporeal circulation are in their final stages [51].

Table 4. Summary of human studies with Oxygent™

Study phase	Patients	n	Objective	Status
I	Healthy volunteers	110	a	Completed
I	Surgical	100	a	Completed
II	General surgery:			
	– Orthopedic	144	b	Completed
	– Gynecologic and urologic	108	b	Completed
II	Cardiopulmonary bypass (CPB)	36 + 27	c	Completed (?)
III	CPB, ?	?	d	Planned

a: safety
b: global improvement of oxygenation and/or reversal of transfusion trigger
c: neurological problems (gas emboli) and/or minimal hematocrit
d: blood substitute, therapy of tissue hypoxia

The use of second generation emulsions seems to be particularly promising during perioperative hemodilution. Three main strategies have been developed in this context to avoid the risks associated with transfusion of homologous blood: preoperative donation; acute normovolemic hemodilution (ANH), and intra- and postoperative autologous blood salvage using red cell recovery devices. These techniques alones, are often insufficient. The concomitant use of PFC emulsions would allow reductions of the patient's Hct below currently accepted thresholds during ANH while maintaining or improving tissue oxygenation. With this goal in mind, phase III studies will begin soon in situations requiring protection from tissue ischemia (e.g., myocardial ischemia, transient anemia following high blood-loss surgery, or cerebral protection from gas emboli, for example during open heart surgery), and in situations where allogeneic blood transfusion avoidance is desirable [8, 52, 53].

Organ Transplantation

The perfluorocarbon emulsions of the first generation have been used for preservation of many organs (heart, lung, liver, pancreas, kidney) as infusion before transplantation to avoid reperfusion damage, as single flush before cold storage or as preservation medium with or without perfusion. A good protection of the energy potential and functional activity of the transplant was often observed, and associated with a better oxygenation, reducing free radical damage [54]. Second generation emulsions have been used for preservation of pulmonary transplants, either as a flush into the pulmonary artery prior to classical cold preservation, or as an autoperfusion by a working heart-lung preparation. In these models, the morphologic and functional alterations in the transplant were clearly inferior to those seen when other conservation fluids (EuroCollins, autologous blood, stroma-free Hb) were used. This avoided the onset of increased pulmonary vascular resistance, but did not increase the viability of the graft [55, 56]. Hypothermia is used to depress metabolism during organ storage, but may represent a limiting factor in organ preservation. To prevent this hypothermia, Oxygent™ was perfused at 37 °C or used at 25 °C for static storage in canine kidney autografts with promising results [57]. Another limiting factor in transplantation surgery is the shortage of the donor pool of heartbeating cadavers. Warm ischemic damage hinders attempts to expand the organ donor pool into nonheartbeating cadavers. Oxygent™ supplemented perfusate has already been evaluated, with promising results, for canine kidney salvage postmortem [58]. Studies are now on the way with a concentrated third generation emulsion (stabilized with molecular dowels) for intestine preservation in hypothermia (unpublished data), and for organ block preservation in normothermia [59].

Medical Imaging and Radiotherapy

Concentrated emulsions of perflubron are potentially useful blood pool contrast agents for use in computed tomography, especially for the liver and spleen, where the particles of the emulsion are preferentially phagocytosed. This may provide a highly sensitive technique for the detection of metastasic lesions. These emulsions could also serve to increase DO_2 to tumors, in order to increase their sensitivity to radiotherapy. Hyperfluorination, which implies an absence of hydrogen atoms in the perflubron molecule, makes it useful as a negative contrast medium for MRI (abdomen and plevis). The use of ^{19}F could also be useful for MRI, but the signal from this atom is weaker than that of hydrogen, and the molecular environment hinders the intrepretation of this signal. This use for perflubron has, nonetheless, been considered for the study of tissue oxygenation and tumor blood flow. The compressibility of perflubron also makes it useful for the ultrasonic evaluation of cardiac and vascular flows, in infarcted zones, and possibly even for lymphography [16]. Various clinical applications have been contemplated and phase III clinical trials have just commenced with Imagent, a second generation microbubble contrast agent, for enhancement of ultrasound images to aid in the evaluation of cardiac function and blood flow abnormalities.

Beneficial and Harmful Secondary Effects

As their vapor pressure is not very high (which decreases the possiblity of gas embolism and pulmonary edema), because of the meticulous purification of PFCs and of the ingredients used in the formulation of the emulsions, and because of the rigorous control of the size of the particles of the emulsion, acute toxicity is not seen with the formulations currently in clinical development. Secondary effects have, however, been described during use of pure PFCs and emulsions.

The use of pure PFC solutions for liquid ventilation exposes the patient to the risk of side effects, the most important of which is intravascular passage of the

PFC. This is particularly true for severely injured lungs. Animal studies suggest that the passage of PFC into the bloodstream is negligible and that its elimination is effected by evaporation within 24 to 48 hours after stopping the treatment [6, 10]. The long-term persistence of PFCs in pulmonary tissue (traces have been detected up to two years after treatment) described by Calderwood et al. in 1975 [60] would no longer appear to be a problem with use of PFOB. On the other hand, phagocytosis by alveolar macrophages is seen (demonstrated cytologically), and the possibility of a pathway involving dissolution in lipid, deposition in fat, re-uptake by the bloodstream, and ending with elimination by the lung does exist [4]. There does not seem to be direct absorption by the tissues or into bone.

The use of PFCs for liquid ventilation is also associated with numerous beneficial side effects, notably as concerns the inflammatory reaction. PLV in the rabbit has provided a positive stimulus for the metabolism of surfactant phospholipids, by increasing the synthesis and secretion of phosphatidylcholine [61]. In a sheep model, total liquid ventilation followed by PLV, was followed by a reduction in intra-alveolar hemorrhage, edema, and inflammatory infiltration into the lung [26], and a reduction in alveolar debris and intra-pulmonary inflammatory response when compared to gaseous ventilation [20, 24, 26, 31]. These anti-inflammatory properties have been attributed to the perflubron itself, because when used in vitro, it reduces the production of reactive O_2 species (ROS) by alveolar macrophages [62] and may trap the NO produced by these cells without altering their capacity to synthesize and liberate this mediator. Perflubron also decreases the production of cytokines by endotoxin stimulated macrophages [63]. When human neutrophils are exposed to perfluorocabon, they produce less detectable hydrogen peroxide (H_2O_2) and have lower chemotactic response [64]. Perflubron reduces the infiltration and degranulation of neutrophils (as measured by the presence of myelopcroxidase) in the lung during inflammation induced by administration of cobra venom factor. It would also appear to protect human alveolar cells in culture during oxidative stress [65]. We have shown that perflubron does not penetrate into cultured human alveolar epithelial cells (A 549 line) and that it protects these cells from activated neutrophils (unpublished data). Finally, a potentially interesting use for PFCs is related to their ability to penetrate and recruit alveoli; these compounds could be used during liquid ventilation to administer antibiotics, with production of high local concentrations and minimal vascular uptake. This could reduce the various toxicities associated with certain antibiotics (renal toxicity, for example). A study of this application has been carried out using gentamycin.

As for emulsions, among the undesirable and potentially harmful side effects already described for the first generation product Fluosol, are activation of complement and phagocytic cells and adherence of leukocytes, but these effects are principally due to the surfactant used (Pluronic F-68), and are no longer seen with second generation emulsions using newer surfactants [9, 66]. For first generation emulsions, reversible lung hyperinflation (after four to seven days) has been noted, but this phenomenon is no longer seen with subsequent products [5, 67].

A potential limitation on the dose of emulsified PFCs is the elimination capacity by the reticulo-endothelial system. This could possibly lead to hepatic engorgement and a temporary impairment of immune defense mechanisms. This, of course, could be quite dangerous, especially in situations where infection is present or threatened. The small particle size of second generation emulsions considerably decreased this risk. The search for PFCs in various tissues such as lung, liver, spleen, etc., has shown neither high levels of accumulation nor excessive persistence.

On the other hand, among the beneficial biological effects, are the anti-inflammatory effects of these emulsions. They appear to reduce the erythrocyte aggregability and hemolysis and the platelet activation induced by "heart assist devices", and to protect the erythrocytes against oxidative hemolysis and lipid peroxidation. They also inhibit the infiltration of ischemic muscle by leukocytes and decrease the chemiluminescence produced by neutrophils stimulated by phorbol myristate acetate [68]. Until now, there are no reported toxic or side effects that could result from oxidation of the phospholipidic surfactant or from in vivo production of lysophosphatides. Typical ingredients (such as tocopherol) are often added to the emulsion to prevent this lipid oxidation [15].

We have studied the effect of a third generation PFC emulsion on neutrophil activation, and shown that the production of ROS by these cells (measured overall by induced chemiluminescence) is attenuated in the presence of the emulsion. It is not currently possible to determine if these effects are the result of a direct action of the components of the emulsion on the neutrophil-produced O_2 species, or rather on the cellular metabolic processes via phagocytosis of the emulsion particles themselves. We studied the effect of a 90% solution (w/v) of perflubron stabilized by molecular dowels on cultured human endothelial cells, with an eye to investigate the future use of third generation emulsions for the preservation of perfused isolated organs at 4°C, room-temperature, or at 37°C. We looked for signs of possible cytotoxicity [19]. The emulsion was diluted in the cell culture medium, and was placed in contact with the cells for variable time periods (up to 48 hours). We compared the effects of the diluted emulsion with those of two

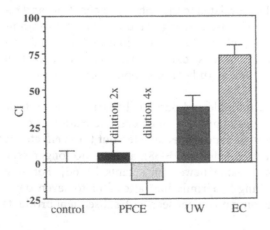

Fig. 2. Cytotoxicity of a third generation perfluorocarbon emulsion (PFCE) on cultured human umbilical vein endothelial cells (at 37°C): comparison with University of Wisconsin (UW) and EuroCollins solutions (EC). Cytotoxicity was estimated by the release of pre-incorporated ^{51}Cr.

widely used clinical conservation fluids, EuroCollins (EC) and University of Wisconsin (UW) solution. We felt that in subsequent investigations, we would dilute the PFC emulsion with these liquids. We observed no cytotoxicity with the emulsion diluted 2-, 3-, or 4-fold in the culture media, regardless of the duration of contact and/or temperature. On the other hand, both EC and UW showed cytotoxicity at room temperature and at 37 °C, related to the high potassium concentration of these two solutions (Fig. 2). Microscopic examination (both visual and electronic) revealed no morphologic changes (size and shape) or alterations of organelles (normal aspect of membranes, of the mitochondria, of the endoplasmic reticulum, normally sized vacuoles in normal numbers, and no changes in the nucleus). Density gradient analysis of endothelial cells showed no increase in cellular weight caused by "phagocytosis" of the emulsion (Fig. 3).

Conclusions

The PFCs are unquestionably products whose clinical use is promising as a temporary treatment to prevent tissue hypoxia, allowing maintenance of tissue oxygenation. Their excellent O_2 transport properties and their total chemical inert-

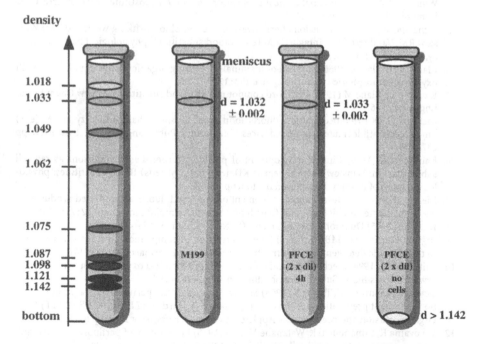

Fig. 3. Density gradient analysis of endothelial cells after incubation (4 h, 37 °C) with a third generation perfluorocarbon emulsion
Left: density gradient markers; M199: endothelial cells cultured in normal conditions (M199 medium); PFCE 4 h: endothelial cells incubated with perfluorocarbon emulsion; PFCE no cells: control with emulsion alone

ness allow their use without fear of acute toxicity due to reaction with O_2. They do, however, show some risk of side effects, particularly problems associated with hepatic overload and/or modulation of the inflammatory reaction if used at very high doses. These side effects are analogous to those seen during use of modified Hb solutions and may well limit the maximal clinical dose that can be administered safely. Their use as emulsions appears to be especially indicated in situations of acute hemorrhage caused by trauma, GI bleeding, high blood-loss surgery, and for perioperative hemodilution. During states where tissue ischemia is at risk (brain, heart), PFC emulsions may be useful, especially for the prevention of cerebral ischemia during cardiopulmonary bypass for cardiac surgery. In this situation, air microbubbles are felt to be a source of cerebral tissue hypoxia. Finally, it would appear that the use of emulsions for the conservation of harvested organs for transplantation may be a future application which may allow reductions in ischemic damage to the organ. When used pure, PFCs are interesting compounds for various states of localized ischemia, such as pulmonary injury, intestinal injury, in medical imaging, and in ophthalmology.

References

1. Winslow RM (1992) Potential clinical applications for blood substitutes. Biomat Artif Cells Immobil Biotechnol 20:205–217
2. Tomasulo P (1995) Transfusion alternatives: impact on blood banking worldwide. In: Winslow RM, Vandegriff KD, Intaglietta M (eds) Blood substitutes: physiological basis of efficacy, Birkhäuser, Boston, pp 1–19
3. Clark LC, Gollan R (1966) Survival of mammals breathing organic liquids equilibrated with oxygen at atmospheric pressure. Science 152:1755–1756
4. Riess JG, Le Blanc M (1978) Perfluoro compounds as blood substitutes. Angew Chem Int Ed Engl 17:621–634
5. Riess JG (1990) Hemocompatible fluorocabon emulsions. In: Sharma CP, Szycker M (eds) Blood compatible materials and devices, Technomic Publishing Co Inc, Lancaster, pp 237–270
6. Kaufman JR (1995) Clinical development of perfluorocarbon-based emulsions as red cell substitutes. In: Winslow RM, Vandegriff KD, Intaglietta M (eds) Blood substitutes: physiological basis of efficacy, Birkhäuser, Boston, pp 53–74
7. Riess JG (1994) The design and development of improved fluorocarbon-based products for use in medicine and biology. Artif Cells Blood Substit Immobil Biotechnol 22:215–234
8. Riess JG (1995) Du fluor dans nos artères (!). New J Chem 19:891–909
9. Ingram DA, Forman MB, Murray JJ (1993) Activation of complement by fluosol attributable to the pluronic detergent micelle structure. J Cardiovasc Pharmacol 22:456–461
10. Faithfull NS (1994) Mechanisms and efficacy of fluorochemical oxygen transport and delivery. Artif Cells Blood Substit Immobil Biotechnol 22:181–197
11. Geyer RP, Monroe RG, Taylor K (1968) Survival of rats totally perfused with a perfluorocarbon-detergent preparation. In: Norman JV, Folkman J, Hardison LE, Ridolf LF, Veith FJ (eds) Organ perfusion and preservation, Appleton-Century-Crofts, New York, pp 85–95
12. Yokoyama K, Yamanouchi K, Watanabe M, et al (1975) Preparation of perfluorodecalin emulsion; an approach to the red cell substitute. Fed Proc 34:1478–1483
13. Lowe KC (1991) Synthetic oxygen transport fluids based on perfluorochemicals: applications in medicine and biology. Vox Sang 60:129–140
14. Riess JG (1991) Fluorocarbon-based in vivo oxygen transport and delivery systems. Vox Sang 61:225–239

15. Riess JG, Krafft MP (1992) Elaboration of fluorocarbon emulsions with improved oxygen carrying capabilities. Adv Exp Med Biol 371:465–472
16. Faithfull NS (1992) Oxygen delivery from fluorocarbon emulsions – aspects of convective and diffusive transport. Biomat Artif Cells Immobil Biotechnol 20:797–804
17. Riess JG (1994) Highly fluorinated systems for oxygen transport, diagnosis and drug delivery. Colloids and Surface A: Physicochem Eng Asp 84:33–48
18. Cornelus C, Krafft MP, Riess J (1994) Improved control over particle sizes and stability of concentrated fluorocarbon emulsions by using mixed fluorocarbon/hydrocarbon molecular dowels. Artif Cells Blood Substit Immobil Biotechnol 22:1183–1191
19. Mathy-Hartert M, Krafft MP, Deby C, Deby-Dupont G, Meurisse M, Lamy M, Riess JG (1997) Effects of perfluorocarbon emulsions on cultured human endothelial cells. Artif Cells Blood Substit Immobil Biotechnol 25:563–575
20. Hirschl RB, Merz SI, Montoya JP (1995) Development and application of a simplified liquid ventilator. Crit Care Med 23:157–163
21. Fuhrman BP, Paczan PR, DeFrancisis M (1991) Perfluorocarbon associated gas exchange. Crit Care Med 19:712–722
22. Leach CL, Fuhrman BP, Morin FC, Rath MG (1993) Perfluorocarbon associated gas exchange (partial liquid ventilation) in respiratory distress syndrome: A prospective, randomized, controlled study. Crit Care Med 21:1270–1278
23. Tütuncü AS, Akpir K, Mulder P, Erdmann W, Lachmann B (1993) Intratracheal perfluorocarbon administration as an aid in the ventilatory management of respiratory distress syndrome. Anesthesiology 79:1089–1093
24. Tütuncü AS, Faithfull NS, Lachmann B (1993) Comparison of ventilatory support with intratracheal perfluorocarbon administration and conventional mechanical ventilation in animals with acute respiratory failure. Am Rev Respir Dis 148:785–792
25. Faithfull NS (1994) The role of perfluorochemicals in surgery and the ICU. In: Vincent J-L (ed) Yearbook of intensive care and emergency medicine, Springer-Verlag, Berlin, pp 264–275
26. Hirschl RB, Tooley R, Parent A, Johnson K, Bartlett RH (1996) Evaluation of gas exchange, pulmonary compliance, and lung injury during total and partial liquid ventilation in the acute respiratory distress syndrome. Crit Care Med 24:1001–1008
27. Overbeck MC, Pranikoff T, Yadao CM, Hirschl RB (1996) Efficacy of perfluorocarbon partial liquid ventilation in a large animal model of acute respiratory failure. Crit Care Med 24:1208–1214
28. Tooley R, Hirschl RB, Parent A, Bartlett RH (1996) Total liquid ventilation with perfluorocarbons increases pulmonary endexpiratory volume and compliance in the setting of lung atelectasis. Crit Care Med 24:268–273
29. Greenspan JS, Wolfson MR, Rubenstein SD, Shaffer TH (1990) Liquid ventilation of human preterm neonates. J Pediatr 117:106–111
30. Gauger PG, Pranikoff T, Schreiner RJ, Moler FW, Hirschl RB (1996) Initial experience with partial liquid ventilation in pediatric patients with the acute respiratory distress syndrome. Crit Care Med 24:16–22
31. Hirschl RB, Pranikoff T, Wise C, et al (1996) Initial experience with partial liquid ventilation in adult patients with the acute respiratory distress syndrome. JAMA 275:383–389
32. Kazerooni EA, Pranikoff T, Cascade PN, Hirschl RB (1996) Partial liquid ventilation with perflubron during extracorporeal life support in adults: radiographic appearance. Radiology 198:137–142
33. Tütuncü AS, Lachmann B (1994) Perfluorocarbons as an alternative respiratory medium. In: Reinhart K, Eyrich K, Sprung C (eds) Sepsis. Current perspectives in pathophysiology and therapy, Springer Verlag, Berlin, pp 549–563
34. Eanes R (1995) On the horizon: liquid ventilation. J Obstet Gynecol Neonat Nurs 24:119–124
35. Smith TH, Steinhorm DM, Thusu K, Fuhrman P, Dandona P (1995) A liquid perfluorochemical decreases the in vitro production of reactive oxygen species by alveolar macrophages. Crit Care Med 23:1533–1539
36. Haglund U (1993) Therapeutic potential of intraluminal oxygenation. Crit Care Med 21:S69–S71

37. O'Donnell KA, Caty MG, Zheng S, Rossman JE, Azizkhan RG (1997) Oxygenated intraluminal perfluorocarbon protects intestinal mucosa from ischemia/reperfusion injury. J Pediatr Surg 32:361–365
38. Lehtola A, Harjula A, Heikkilä L, et al (1990) Single lung allotransplantation in pigs. Transplantation 49:1066–1074
39. Kuroda Y, Morita A, Fujino Y, Tanioka Y, Ku Y, Saitoh Y (1993) Successful extended preservation of ischemically damaged pancreas by the two-layer (University of Wisconsin solution/perfluorochemical) cold storage method. Transplantation 56:1087–1090
40. Peyman GA, Schulman JA, Sullivan B (1995) Perfluorocarbon liquids in ophthalmology. Surv Ophthalmol 39:375–395
41. Tremper KK, Friedman AE, Levine EM, Lapin R, Camarillo D (1982) The preoperative treatment of severely anemic patients with a perfluorochemical oxygen-transport fluid, Fluosol-DA. N Engl J Med 307:277–283
42. Gould SA, Rosen AL, Sehgal LR, et al (1986) Fluosol-DA as a red-cell substitute in acute anemia. N Engl J Med 314:1653–1656
43. Spence RK, McCoy S, Costabile J, et al (1990) Fluosol DA-20 in the treatment of severe anemia: randomized controlled study of 46 patients. Crit Care Med 18:1227–1230
44. Mitsuno TM, Ohyanagi H, Naito R (1982) Clinical studies of a perfluorochemical whole blood substitute (FLuosol-DA). Summary of 186 cases. Ann Surg 195:60–69
45. Mitsuno, Ohyanagi H (1985) Present status of clinical studies of Fluosol-DA (20%) in Japan. Int Anesthesiol Clin 23:169–184
46. Forman MB, Perry JM, Hadley Wilson B, et al (1991) Demonstration of myocardial reperfusion injury in humans: results of a pilot study utilizing acute coronary angioplasty with perfluorochemical in anterior myocardial infarction. J Am Coll Cardiol 18:911–918
47. Swann KW, Ropper AH, Zervas NT (1983) Initial results of a clinical trial of Fluosol-DA 20% in acute cerebral ischemia. Progr Clin Biol Res 122:399–406
48. Spence RK, Norcross ED, Costabile J, et al (1994) Perfluorocarbons as blood substitutes: the early years. Experience with Fluosol DA-20% in the 1980s. Artif Cells Blood Substit Immobil Biotechnol 22:955–963
49. Goodin TH, Grossbard EB, Kaufman RJ, et al (1994) A perfluorochemical emulsion for prehospital resuscitation of experimental hemorrhagic shock: a prospective, randomized, controlled study. Crit Care Med 22:680–689
50. Keipert PE (1998) Perfluorocarbon emulsions: future alternatives to transfusion. In: Chang TMS (eds) Blood substitutes: principles, methods, products and clinical trials, Karger Landes System, pp 127–156
51. Cochran RP, Kunzelman KS, Vocelka CR, Akimoto H, Thomas R, Soltow LO, Spiess BD (1997) Perfluorocarbon emulsion in the cardiopulmonary bypass prime reduces neurologic injury. Ann Thorac Surg 63:1326–1332
52. Holman WL, McGiffin DC, Vicente WV, Spruell RD, Pacifico AD (1994) Use of current generation perfluorocarbon emulsions in cardiac surgery. Artif Cells Blood Substit Immobil Biotechnol 22:979–990
53. Spiess BO, Cochran RP (1996) Perfluorocarbon emulsions and cardiopulmonary bypass: a technique for the future. J Cardiothorac Vasc Anesth 10:83–89
54. Bando K, Teramoto S, Tago M, Seno S, Murakami T, Nawa S, Senoo Y (1988) Oxygenated perfluorocarbon, recombinant human superoxide dismutase, and catalase ameliorate free radical induced myocardial injury during preservation and transplantation. Thorac Cardiovasc Surg 96:930–938
55. Kaplan E, Diehl JT, Peterson MB, et al (1990) Extended ex vivo preservation of the heart and lungs. J Thorac Cardiovasc Surg 100:687–698
56. Zhao L, Smith JR, Eyer CL (1995) Effects of a 100% perfluorooctylbromide emulsion on ischemia/reperfusion injury following cardioplegia. Artif Cells Blood Substit Immobil Biotechnol 23:513–531
57. Brasile L, DelVecchio P, Amyot K, Haisch C, Clarke J (1994) Organ preservation without extreme hypothermia using an Oxygent™ supplemented perfusate. Artif Cells Blood Substit Immobil Biotechnol 22:1463–1468

58. Brasile L, DelVecchio P, Rudofsky U, Haisch C, Clarke J (1994) Postmortem organ salvage using an Oxygent™ supplemented perfusate. Artif Cells Blood Substit Immobil Biotechnol 22:1469–1475

59. Voiglio EJ, Zarif L, Gorry FC, Krafft MP, Margonari J, Martin X, Riess J, Dubernard MF (1996) Aerobic preservation of organs using a new perflubron/lecithin emulsion stabilized by molecular dowels. J Surg Res 63:439–446

60. Calderwood HW, Ruiz BC, Tham MK, Modell JH, Saga SA, Hood CI (1975) Residual levels and biochemical changes after ventilation with perfluorinated liquid. J Appl Physiol 39: 603–607

61. Steinhorn DM, Leach CL, Fuhrman BP, Holm BA (1996) Partial liquid ventilation enhances surfactant phospholipid production. Crit Care Med 24:1252–1256

62. Smith TM, Steinhorn DM, Thusuk K, et al (1995) A liquid perfluorochemical decreases the in vitro production of reactive oxygen species by alveolar macrophages. Crit Care Med 23:1533–1539

63. Thomassen MJ, Buhrow LT, Wiedemann HP (1997) Perflubron decreases inflammatory cytokine production by human alveolar macrophages. Crit Care Med 25:2045–2047

64. Rossman JE, Caty MG, Rich GA, Karamanoukian HL, Azizkhan RG (1996) Neutrophil activation and chemotaxis after in vitro treatment with perfluorocarbon. J Pediat Surg 31: 1145–1150

65. Varani J, Hirschl RB, Dame MM, Johnson K (1996) Perfluorocarbon protects lung epithelial cells from neutrophil-mediated injury in an in vitro model of liquid ventilation therapy. Shock 6:339–344

66. McDonagh PF, Wilson DS (1995) The initial response of blood leucocytes to incubation with perfluorocarbon blood substitute emulsions. Artif Cells Blood Substit Immobil Biotechnol 23:439–447

67. Flaim SI (1994) Pharmacokinetics and side effects of perfluorocarbon-based blood substitutes. Artif Cells Blood Substit Immobil Biotechnol 22:1043–1054

68. Edwards CM, Lowe KC, Rohlke W, Geister U, Reuter P, Meinert H (1997) Effects of a novel perfluorocarbon emulsion on neutrophil chemiluminescence in human whole blood. Artif Cells Blood Substit Immobil Biotechnol 25:255–260

Serum-Free Hemoglobin Increases Tumor Necrosis Factor Synthesis and Lipopolysaccharide Lethality

K. J. Tracey

Introduction

"The pestilential poison is driven by the heart into the liver and the rest of the body to spoil such weak and ignoble members with a harmful inflammation. ..."
Athanasius Kircher (1680)

Father Kircher's description of plague is timely and compelling, because the clinical picture of sepsis and septic shock syndrome is little changed in 318 years. His concept of a toxin circulating in association with infection was prescient, though it required some 200 years to bring scientific focus on the active principle released from Gram negative bacterial cultures. Molecular identification of bacterial "poisons" did not occur until the mid-twentieth century, with the recognition that bacterial lipopolysaccharide (LPS) causes massive derangements in mammalian homeostasis. Invasive infections in the intensive care units and emergency departments of our modern hospitals are thankfully not associated with widespread outbreaks of plague, but the signs and symptoms of overwhelming sepsis and septic shock syndrome continue to leave an indelible impression on those charged with the care of these patients.

Tumor Necrosis Factor Mediates LPS Lethality

What has changed quite recently, is our understanding of the pathogenic mechanisms underlying sepsis and septic shock syndrome. From studies of LPS-mediated toxicity, it has become clear that many pathologic and metabolic responses are not mediated by LPS directly, but as a result of LPS stimulation of monocytes/macrophages. Stimulated macrophages secrete biological mediators including tumor necrosis factor (TNF), interleukin-1 (IL-1), nitric oxide (NO), and others, which signal specific metabolic, hemodynamic, and cytotoxic responses locally and systemically. TNF, a 17 kD cytokine, occupies a pivotal mediator role, because it is one of the earliest cytokines produced during invasive infection, and its appearance stimulates the release of numerous downstream mediators. This host response has been termed the pro-inflammatory mediator cascade. In controlled, physiological amounts, the net effects of TNF and the mediator cascade are beneficial, because it activates defense mechanisms to enhance the clearance of pathogens, and promotes wound healing. When over-produced however, TNF triggers lethal shock and tissue injury. This injurious toxicity of TNF was initially reported in rats [1] and dogs [2], but has subsequently been observed in diverse mammalian species, from mouse to man.

The uncontrolled release of TNF represents a highly unusual circumstance in nature, because the mammalian host has evolved a series of strict regulatory mechanisms that prevent the inappropriate overexpression of TNF. Stimulation of macrophages by LPS occurs following receptor-ligand interaction between LPS and CD14 present on the macrophage surface. Macrophages are minimally responsive to highly purifed LPS under serum free conditions, but a liver-derived serum factor termed LPS-binding protein (LBP) forms complexes with LPS. The LPS-LBP complex is the most potent known macrophage stimulating agent [3]. Within minutes after LPS-LBP binding to macrophage CD14 there is transcriptional and translational activation of the TNF gene, followed by the release of cytotoxic quantities of TNF.

Nature has provided some feedback-protective mechanisms to reduce the damaging effects of overabundant TNF release. For instance, TNF activates several "protective" or counter-regulatory pathways that feedback-inhibit additional TNF production. TNF release induces the activity of proteolytic enzymes which cleave TNF receptors present on most cells. These cleaved fragments bind TNF and neutralize its bioactivity, thereby serving a protective role against the cytototoxicity of TNF. TNF also causes the release of glucocorticoid hormones, which effectively suppress TNF transcription by preventing the translocation of nuclear factor-kappa B (NF-KB) to the nucleus [4]. This counter-regulatory mechanism has been evoked to explain the widespread anti-inflammatory activities of glucocorticoid agents in a variety of clinical states in which macrophages are activated and TNF is released (e.g., rheumatoid arthritis, inflammatory bowel disease, and allograft rejection).

In the middle of this century Hume and Egdahl [5] removed the pituitary gland from animals (hypophysectomy), and demonstrated that pituitary-derived factors are required to stimulate the "fight or flight" response to injury and invasion. Interest in the neuroendocrine-immune response subsequently became widespread, in part because of the ubiquitous role of this system in host defense. Early investigators realized that hypophysectomized animals are exquisitely sensitive to LPS lethality, because lethality is observed in hypophysectomized animals treated with 1000-fold lower doses of LPS as compared to controls. The more recent realization that TNF is a pivotal mediator of LPS lethality, and that glucocorticoids occupy an important endogenous regulatory mechanism to suppress TNF synthesis, prompted investigation into the interactions of TNF and glucocorticoids in mediating LPS lethality following hypophysectomy. Serum TNF levels are significantly increased in endotoxemic hypophysectomized rats as compared to controls, and this increased production correlates with diminished serum corticosterone levels [6]. Anti-TNF antibodies, which effectively protect normal animals from endotoxin lethality, also protect hypophysectomized animals from endotoxin lethality. When these observations were considered together, it was widely presumed that the absence of glucocorticoids following hypophysectomy allowed uncontrolled systemic TNF release, which in turn accounted for the increased sensitivity of hypophysectomized animals to LPS.

For several reasons we considered this explanation unsatisfactory. First, thousands of patients have been subjected to hypophysectomy for treatment of diabetic retinopathy, breast cancer, or pituitary tumor, but clinical recognition of overwhelming sepsis as an important complication is lacking. Second, although glucocorticoids can be used to restore protection of hypophysectomized animals from LPS, the doses required to achieve this protection are supra-physiological [6]. Finally, administration of hydrazine has been demonstrated to confer protection against LPS toxicity in normal mice [7]. Although this protective effect is dependent upon an intact pituitary gland, hydrazine has no significant stimulating effect on corticosterone release. For these reasons we considered an alternative possibility: that hypophysectomy induces the release of a serum factor which increases macrophage sensitivity to LPS, resulting in increased TNF release.

Serum Free Hemoglobin increases TNF Synthesis

We reasoned that it would be possible to detect the appearance of a "positive-acting" factor by adding serum from hypophysectomized rats to LPS-stimulated murine macrophage-like RAW cells, and comparing the release of TNF to macrophages stimulated in the presence of control serum. In agreement with our hypothesis, we observed a significant increase of TNF production after stimulation with LPS in the presence of hypophysectomized rat serum (Table 1). Thus, hypophysectomy induced the appearance of a serum activity which increased macrophage sensitivity to LPS. Using this observation as a bioassay, we fractionated pooled hypophysectomized serum by ultrafiltration, anion exchange chromatography, and gel filtration, and identified the purified activity as a 65 kD protein. We were very surprised when the results of amino terminal microsequencing revealed the identity of the active protein as hemoglobin (Hb) (unpublished observations). To confirm the identity of Hb as a mediator of enhanced LPS sensitivity in macrophages, we measured TNF release in macrophages stimulated with low levels of LPS (1 ng/ml) in the presence of Hb. Purified Hb enhanced LPS sensitivity by more than 1000-fold, and this effect was completely inhibited by addition

Table 1. Hemoglobin is a hypophysectomy induced serum factor that increases TNF release in LPS-stimulated macrophages

- Hypophysectomy serum enhances LPS-stimulated macrophage TNF release.
- Fractionation and purification of this activity reveals a 65 kD protein.
- Amino acid sequence confirms identity as hemoglobin.
- Serum free hemoglobin levels significantly increased in hypophysectomized serum as compared to controls.
- Purified hemoglobin increases TNF synthesis by 1000-fold in LPS-stimulated macrophages.
- Anti-hemoglobin antibodies prevent enhanced TNF release.
- Purified hemoglobin increases LPS lethality in animals.

of anti-Hb antibodies. Finally, we returned to the hypophysectomized serum samples and measured serum free Hb levels to demonstrate that levels were significantly increased. Thus, hypophysectomy induces an increase of serum free Hb levels which accounts for a 1000-fold increased sensitivity of LPS-stimulated macrophages in releasing TNF.

It was previously known that red cell deformability is reduced in hypophysectomized rodents, which combined with derangements of sodium and fluid homeostasis from diabetes insipidus, may well underlie the increases in serum free Hb we observed. White and coworkers [8] demonstrated the importance of free Hb in mediating LPS lethality. In their studies, co-administration of albumin or Hb with 14.5 nanograms of LPS was not lethal to mice, although they observed significant toxicity in the Hb treated animals. At 1000-fold higher doses of LPS, Hb caused 100% lethality, whereas albumin co-treatment caused only limited toxicity, suggesting that Hb increased LPS toxicity by at least 1000-fold [8]. More recently, Levin and colleagues [9, 10] observed increased lethality after co-treatment with Hb and LPS, a finding they attributed to saturable binding of Hb to LPS (Kd = 3.1×10^8) which increases LPS sensitivity in macrophages.

Clinical Relevance

Several intriguing clinical possibilities are suggested by these results. It is reasonable to speculate that free Hb contaminating packed red blood cells may be biologically active, because LPS is ubiquitous in clinical samples and the resultant Hb/LPS complexes will activate TNF release. It is plausible that this mechanism may account for some pyrogenic and inflammatory reactions to blood transfusion, because TNF and other pro-inflammatory cytokines mediate fever and systemic inflammatory responses. Contrariwise, an excess of free Hb might bind LPS and reduce its pathogenic effects, like an excess of soluble CD14 inhibits LPS stimulation of macrophages. It is also useful to consider whether the pro-inflammatory activities of Hb act to confound outcome assessment in clinical trials for sepsis. Hemolysis occurs frequently during the host response to infection, surgery, burn injury, and other critical illnesses, but the effects of serum free Hb on the immune and cytokine response in these states is unknown. Recent clinical results of administering haptoglobin to patients during cardiac surgery demonstrated protection against renal injury, but it is unknown if the observed protection was mediated by altered renal Hb clearance, or through suppression of cytokine release.

Conclusion

Animal models of endotoxin lethality continue to help improve our understanding of the host response to infection and injury. Hypophysectomy has been widely used to sensitize animals to LPS, and to identify the biological effects of classical hormones and cytokines in the host stress response. We were at first surprised by the finding that Hb is the hypophysectomy-induced serum factor that increases TNF synthesis. On further consideration however, the inflammatory mediator cascade has already proved to be more complicated than most investigators initially presumed, because ubiquitous proteins share diverse and overlapping biological activities. By recognizing the potential role of Hb in stimulating some activation of this cascade, it may now be possible to derive an improved understanding of how the "protective" cytokine cascade can occasionally become "deranged," or deadly.

References

1. Tracey, KJ, Beutler B, Lowry SF, et al (1986) Shock and tissue injury induced by recombinant human cachectin. Science 234:470–474
2. Tracey KJ, Lowry SF, Fahey III TF, et al (1987) Cachectin/tumor necrosis factor induces lethal shock and stress hormone responses in the dog. Surg Gynecol Obstet 164:415–422
3. Schumann RR, Leong SR, Flaggs GW, et al (1990) Structure and function of lipopolysaccharide binding protein. Science 249:1429–1431
4. Auphan N, DiDonato JA, Rosette C, Helmberg A, Karin M (1995) Immunosuppression by glucocorticoids: inhibition of NF-kappa B activity through induction of I kappa B synthesis. Science 270:286–290
5. Humet DM, Egdahl RH (1959) The Importance of the brain in the endocrine response to injury. Ann Surg 150:697
6. Zuckerman SH, Shellhaas J, Butler LD (1989) Differential regulation of lipopolysaccharide-induced interleukin 1 and tumor necrosis factor synthesis: effects of endogenous and exogenous glucocorticoids and the role of the pituitary-adrenal axis. Eur Immunol 19:301–305
7. Silverstein R, Turley BR, Christoffersen CA, Johnson DC, Morrison DC (1991) Hydrazine sulfate protects D-galactosamine-sensitized mice against endotoxin and tumor necrosis factor/cachectin lethality: Evidence of a role for the pituitary. J Exp Med 173:357–365
8. White CT, Murray AJ, Smith DJ, Greene JR, Bolin RB (1986) Synergistic toxicity of endotoxin and hemoglobin. J Lab Clin Med 108:132–137
9. Kaca W, Roth RI, Levin J (1994) Hemoglobin, a newly recognized lipopolysaccharide (LPS)-binding protein that enhances LPS biologic activity. J Biochem 269:25078–25084
10. Su D, Roth RL, Yoshida M, Levin J (1997) Hemoglobin increases mortality from bacterial endotoxin. Infect Immun 65:1258–1266

Enhancement of Tissue Oxygenation by Intracellular Introduction of Inositol Hexaphosphate by Flow Electroporation of Red Blood Cells

L. Einck and J. W. Holaday

Introduction

Inadequate tissue oxygenation accompanies many acute and chronic medical conditions, including congestive heart failure, myocardial infarction, peripheral vascular disease, sickle cell anemia, stroke, shock and severe blood loss. Surgical procedures are also restricted by the need to conserve blood flow and maintain tissue oxygenation. The complications of inadequate tissue oxygenation range from the discomfort and pain associated with intermittent claudication, to death of tissues vital for function of essential organs, resulting in disability or death of the patient.

We are developing an instrument that will enhance the ability of red blood cells to deliver oxygen (O_2) to organs and tissues. An electroporation device and a disposable flow chamber are used to replace the natural allosteric effector molecule in red blood cell (RBC) hemoglobin (Hb), 2,3-diphosphoglycerate (DPG) with inositol hexaphosphate (phytic acid, IHP). The resulting IHP-treated blood exhibits a profound right shift of the normal O_2 dissociation curve and increases deposition of O_2 in tissues two- to threefold greater than untreated blood. Hematological parameters of the RBC are not altered by this procedure, and the enhanced O_2 delivery (DO_2) capacity of IHP-treated blood may last for the life span of a human RBC (on average 90–120 days). This enhanced DO_2 capacity does not require mechanical augmentation (e.g., a ventilator) or the delivery of purified gaseous O_2 to the patient, and the release of O_2 in tissues is physiologically regulated, resulting in decreased cardiac work. The electroporation device and chamber can be incorporated into existing apheresis instrument technologies and procedures. Ultimate applications of this therapeutic procedure to acute and chronic cardiorespiratory diseases are discussed below.

Oxygen Release from Hemoglobin

The normal Hb complex in a RBC is composed of four nearly identical Hb chains, two α and two β, each of which can combine with one O_2 molecule. As successive chains in the complex pick up an O_2 in the lung, where the partial pressure of O_2 (PO_2) is high, the ability of the next chain to pick up O_2 is enhanced. The usual level of Hb oxygenation in the lungs, with a PO_2 of 100 mm Hg, is 97% (close to

100 percent capacity, or one O_2 molecule for each chain). As blood leaves the lung and circulates throughout the body, O_2 is released and is taken up by peripheral tissues. The difference in PO_2 between the lungs (100 mm Hg) and the tissue (40 mm Hg) establishes the maximum amount of O_2 which can be delivered by a red blood cell. The normal release of O_2 in tissues is 27% at approximately 40 mm Hg in venous blood (or approximately one O_2 molecule released from each 4-chain Hb complex) [1].

The release of O_2 in tissues (where PO_2 is significantly lower than in the lung) is enhanced by a change in the binding affinity of O_2 for its Hb chain. The 'right shift' of the O_2 release curve is controlled by several allosteric mechanisms: Bohr-effect, DPG, and carbon dioxide (CO_2)-binding [2]. Several physiologic parameters also strongly influence the DO_2 capacity of mammalian Hb: temperature (less at low, greater at high), pH (less at high, greater at low), and intracellular concentration of DPG (less at low, greater at high).

Attachment of an allosteric effector molecule to the Hb alters the steric relationship of each Hb chain to the others. The normal allosteric effector is DPG, a product of glucose metabolism and a highly charged anion (Fig. 1) that binds to a pocket created by the four Hb chains. Changes in Hb affinity for O_2 reflect the physical relationship between the chains: Hb chains that are physically closer (the relaxed or R state) have greater O_2 affinity; Hb chains that are physically farther apart (tense or T state) have lower O_2 affinity. DPG, because of its size and relationship to each chain in the allosteric pocket, causes the chains to be in a T state. One molecule of O_2 is released from the 4-chain Hb complex and the O_2 release curve shifts to the right (Fig. 2). DPG binding has a low affinity and is reversible, and binding and release of DPG occurs as many as a hundred million times in the life of a red blood cell.

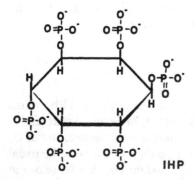

2,3-DPG

IHP

Fig. 1. Molecular structure of allosteric effectors 2,3-DPG and IHP

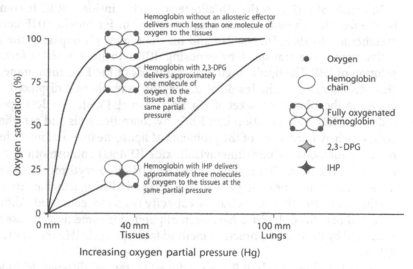

Fig. 2. Comparison of Hb oxygen dissociation curve in the presence or absence of the allosteric inhibitors DPG and IHP

IHP as an Allosteric Effector to Increase Tissue Oxygenation

What is IHP?

Unlike mammals, birds and reptiles use a different and much larger molecule, inositol pentaphosphate, to cause a steric shift in the relationship of the four Hb chains. This interaction results in the release of up to 75% of bound O_2 and is one of several physiologic adaptations that allows birds to supply muscles with the enormous amounts of O_2 required for flight. In 1985, Dr. Claude Nicolau and his colleagues [3] at the Centre de Biophysique Moléculaire at Orleans, France, discovered how to insert a molecule similar in structure to inositol pentaphosphate, inositol hexaphosphate (IHP; Fig. 1), into the RBC. Like DPG and inositol pentaphosphate, IHP inserts into the allosteric cleft of the Hb complex and modifies the Hb chain relationships to facilitate O_2 release. Similar to inositol pentaphosphate, IHP increases the O_2 released by Hb at 37 °C by 2.8 fold, for an average release of 2–3 O_2 molecules compared to 1 released with DPG. The affinity of IHP for Hb is greater than 1000 times that of DPG, and, under physiological conditions, IHP can permanently replace DPG from its Hb allosteric binding site [4].

IHP, or phytic acid, is the sugar alcohol inositol (an important constituent of certain lipids) substituted with 6 phosphate groups (Fig. 1). A related sugar, the magnesium/calcium salt of phytic acid, is called phytin and is an abundant extracellular supporting material in higher plants. Neither phytic acid nor phytin are produced by mammalian cells; however, inositol phosphates are metabolized in some tissues.

Insertion of IHP into the Hb allosteric pocket inside a RBC is complicated by the fact that there is no transport mechanism for moving IHP across RBC membranes. In 1985, Dr. Nicolau and his colleagues [3] bypassed the need for active membrane transport by exposing RBCs to lipid vesicles formed in a solution of IHP. The lipids fused with the lipids of the RBC membrane, and the IHP was liberated on the inside of the erythrocyte where it displaced DPG and bound to the allosteric pocket of Hb. Ropars et al. [5, 6], also developed a procedure for IHP incorporation into RBCs by controlled lysis and resealing of the cells, which avoided some of the problems of liposome interactions. Other incorporation methods include dimethylsulfoxide (DMSO) and osmotic shock treatment of red cells. By all methods of inserting IHP into erythrocytes, treated cells have circulation times, shape, and life spans indistinguishable from normal erythrocytes, and their O_2 releasing capacity is greatly enhanced. Although the potential benefits of IHP-Hb have been apparent for some time, its use has been restricted by the lack of a practical method for large-scale IHP incorporation into RBCs.

Animal studies with IHP-RBCs produced by several different techniques described above demonstrate enhanced O_2 release in piglets [7], baboons [8, 9], and dogs [10] with therapeutically relevant right shifts of the O_2 release curve. *In vitro*, the effect of IHP-treated RBCs on cardiac control mechanisms has also been tested in isolated heart models [11–14]. Most importantly, however, infusion of IHP-treated erythrocytes into experimental animals increased deposition of O_2 in tissues, increased tissue PO_2, and decreased cardiac output (CO), all desirable clinical parameters in cardiac malfunction [3, 15–18]. IHP-erythrocyte treatment of animals with a reduced blood supply to the heart (as occurs in heart attacks) dramatically reduces tissue destruction and concomitant mortality rates [19]. Nonetheless, these methods of IHP incorporation, although they prove the potential benefits, are limited by low yields and cumbersome procedures that are not amenable to scale-up for clinical applications.

Tissue Oxygenation Physiology and the Effects of IHP

DO_2 to tissues is well-regulated and involves multiple organ systems (e.g., heart, lung, vasculature, bone marrow etc.). It will not be possible in this chapter to fully review the complex physiology of these integrated, homeostatic systems which work together in response to enormous environmental variations to provide O_2 within a rather narrow physiologic window, and keep up with the tissues' metabolic demands. We will review some salient points below, with reference to the role IHP may play in augmenting these homeostatic systems.

Oxygen which is released from the Hb:IHP or Hb:2,3-DPG is identical; therefore, the physiology of O_2 unloading at the RBC/plasma/endothelial cell interface functions normally. However, in hypoxic tissue which has been inadequately served, there will be more O_2 released into the plasma following treatment with IHP-RBCs. This will increase the plasma O_2 concentration, which will steepen the O_2 gradient and increase O_2 diffusion into tissues.

Physiologically, the initial homeostatic response to adequate tissue oxygenation is arteriole vasoconstriction. An IHP treated RBC patient is unlikely to be significantly affected in this aspect. That is, the arterioles in patients will respond appropriately to maintain appropriate O_2 levels in tissue.

Significant advances in understanding O_2 unloading in arterioles were made from experiments with unencapsulated, cross-linked, Hb preparations. It has been observed for many years that these preparations have a significant pressor effect; that is, they induce vasoconstriction. In order to increase the efficacy of these preparations, the Hb in these preparations is usually cross-linked in such a way to induce a significant right shift. However, recent work summarized by Tsai et al. [20], has demonstrated that right-shifted Hb releases O_2 too soon; in the arterioles, rather than the capillary bed. This results in arteriole vasoconstriction and the observed pressor effect. However, Vandegriff and Windslow [21] report that when the Hb is encapsulated, as in RBCs or liposomes, the O_2 release is slower because O_2 must diffuse out of the vesicle to the site of consumption.

Extensive analysis of transit times through the vascular bed as well as plasma O_2 saturation levels suggest that IHP-treated RBCs, unlike Hb preparations described above, will deliver O_2 physiologically in the capillary bed and in greater amount than untreated RBCs. Thus, any observed pressor effect is due to satiation of tissue O_2 needs. That is, the arterioles in patients infused with IHP-treated RBCs will respond appropriately to maintain appropriate O_2 levels in tissue.

Moving from the tissue to the whole body level, when local vasoconstriction occurs throughout the body as the metabolic needs of the tissues are met, compensatory cardiac mechanisms come into play, resulting in decreased cardiac work. This physiologic feedback effect would suggest that the enhanced tissue oxygenation produced by infusion of IHP-treated RBCs would result in reduced CO by decreasing stroke volume and rate. In fact, this has been established in pigs given the equivalent of one unit of IHP-treated blood (1/8 total blood volume) [18].

The Electroporation Process

Although effective in limited animal studies, as reviewed above, previous methods to incorporate IHP into RBCs suffered from major problems. These techniques were inefficient, recovery was poor, and cell yield and incorporation was inconsistent from experiment to experiment [3, 22]. None of the techniques described above are suitable for practical application at a clinical or commercial scale.

Working collaboratively with Dr. Claude Nicolau at the Center for Blood Research, Harvard Medical School, EntreMed has developed a novel, reproducible, and practical method for inserting IHP into erythrocytes with high yield and sufficient volume to improve tissue oxygenation. The novel technique requires electroporation of cells, e.g., passage of RBCs through a high electrical field to make pores in the membrane (Fig. 3).

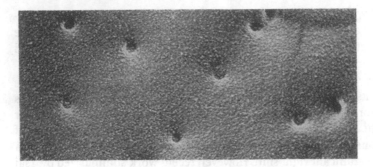

Fig. 3. Scanning electron microscopy (SEM) of transient pores produced by electroporation, 40 nanoseconds after the electrical pulse (Reproduced with the permission of the publisher)

This procedure requires a device that incorporates a red cell separation function with a flow electroporation device in a stand-alone instrument. Prototype instruments combine standard apheresis technology for RBC separation, collection and washing with a proprietary, disposable flow electroporation cell suitable for clinical use and mass production (Fig. 4). The instrument has demonstrated reproducible right shifts adequate for therapeutic efficacy (Fig. 5). Specifically, a

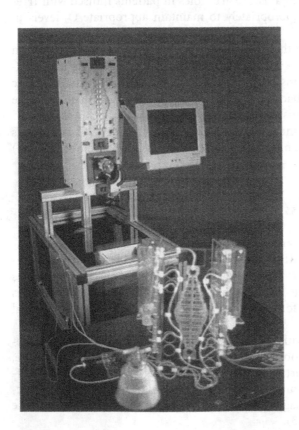

Fig. 4. Cell permeation instrument and disposable flow electroporation cell

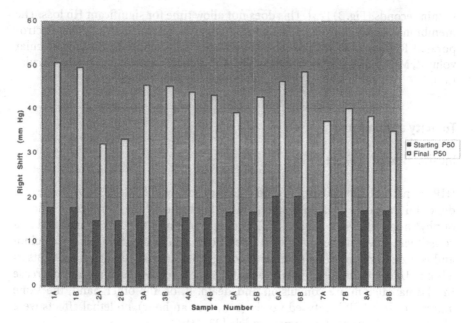

Fig. 5. Eight units of stored human blood were run in parallel in two prototype instruments (A & B), resulting in significant right shifts in oxygen delivery

unit of RBC collected by centrifugation and mixed with an IHP solution is passed through a flow electroporation chamber using a peristaltic pump. A high voltage electrical current periodically passed across the chamber temporarily permeabilizes the RBCs and enhances transport of the IHP molecules into the cells where the IHP displaces 2,3-DPG and binds to the Hb. Excess IHP is removed by standard centrifuge washing steps with a saline solution. IHP-treated RBCs are collected into a standard blood bag and recombined with the other blood components, or placed in a storage solution as packed red cells. Processing a unit of blood for IHP incorporation requires 2–3 hours. The right shift obtained from these electroporated IHP cells indicates nearly 100% IHP incorporation with an acceptable yield (> 85% of the apheresed red cells).

Eight units of stored donor blood were divided and run independently in two separate prototype instruments (Fig. 5). The mean corpuscular Hb (MCH) loss across eight runs with two separate instruments was acceptably low, averaging less than 10%. The incorporation of electroporated molecules is uniform across the red cell population as shown by the incorporation of FITC-dextran (data not shown). IHP-treated blood demonstrated an average P50 of 42 mm Hg ±5.8 following electroporation when compared to the red cells used as starting material.

Specifically relating to the process of flow electroporation, the procedure itself appears to have a very transient effect on the RBCs. The conditions used in the flow electroporation device generate pores that are approximately 80–120 nm in diameter as measured by electron microscopy and open in milliseconds and close within seconds (Fig. 3) [23]. This does not allow time for significant Hb loss. The membranes appear to reform without change in their properties. The electroporated RBCs appear to have a slightly larger cell volume (mean corpuscular volume, MCV), and it is as yet unknown if this characteristic persists in circulation.

Toxicity and Safety

Inositol Hexaphosphate (IHP)

IHP is a natural antioxidant [24] and a dietary anti-neoplastic [25–29]. Some evidence for the safety of IHP is demonstrated by studies of the therapeutic efficacy of phytin for other uses [30, 31]. IHP is completely non-toxic when ingested as a constituent of vegetable material. It does, however, chelate extracellular calcium and is toxic in mammals if administered intravenously in very large amounts as a bolus. Under these conditions, the biological consequences of a rapid decrease in plasma calcium are convulsion and death. If, on the other hand, the same amount of free IHP is infused slowly (e.g., over an hour), no lethal effects were observed in experimental animal models [32, 33].

Animal studies suggest that the IHP-Hb complex in IHP-containing red blood cells is very stable. Dr. Nicolau and his colleagues noted no toxicity in their studies in any animal model (personal communication). Preliminary acute toxicity studies, where IHP-Hb complexes were injected into the peritoneum of mice, showed no adverse effects (data not shown), indicating that the peritoneal macrophages (which presumably remove the protein from the peritoneum) were able to metabolize and excrete the IHP:protein complex. The safety of the product (IHP-treated RBCs) produced by the electroporation technique must still be examined, both in regular preclinical toxicology studies and in a Phase I trial in humans.

IHP-Treated Human Blood

The hematologic characteristics (size, deformability, Hb content) of the electroporated IHP red cells are identical to the starting cells, except for a small increase in cell volume. Preliminary data indicate that these cells have a similar appearance and shelf life to a standard unit of packed RBCs, and are available for administration to either the donor (in the form of an autologous transfusion) or to an allogeneic recipient.

The primary goal of our Phase I clinical trial is to evaluate the potential toxicity associated with electroporation of IHP by examining the circulatory life span of RBCs. If the life span is comparable to transfused red cells, it can be assumed that the electroporated cells have not been compromised in any significant way, and that the properties of the cells have not been modified in such a way as to alert either the macrophages, which scavenge RBCs, or the B-cell dependent immune surveillance system, which recognizes foreign antigens and mounts an antibody response.

To achieve a therapeutic result, we envision that one or two units of blood would be drawn from the patient, processed for IHP incorporation as described above, and either reinfused to the donor or stored for future use. The complete safety profile following infusion of IHP-treated RBCs remains unknown pending clinical trials with volumes of transfused material adequate to achieve an increase in tissue oxygenation. Until that clinical experience, the potential safety of the IHP-RBC transfusion can only be evaluated on a theoretical basis. The physiology of DO_2 to tissue is regulated by many homeostatic mechanisms. The RBCs containing IHP will deliver substantially more O_2 to tissue per unit Hb than the remainder of the blood. Nevertheless, the volume of blood delivered to tissue will continue to be controlled by adjustments in vasoconstriction and CO such that the therapeutic benefit of increased DO_2 will be restricted to tissues that are ischemic and/or hypoxic.

The most analogous therapy which may indicate the potential benefits of IHP treated blood is routinely used in the patient population for which only the most conservative procedures are generally used, the neonate. Fetal Hb (Hb-F) is "left shifted" relative to adult Hb and does not interact well with 2,3-DPG. The P50 of fetal blood is approximately 18 torr compared to fresh adult blood which is 27 torr [34]. This phenomenon has been proposed as explaining in part why the proportionately small neonatal transfusion volume of adult donor blood was so effective (Dr. L.A. Chambers 1995 American Association of Blood Banks Meeting). Transfusion of a neonate with fresh adult RBCs is somewhat analogous to transfusion of an adult with IHP-treated RBCs. In both situations, RBCs with a right shift resulting in a low P50 are transporting more O_2 to hypoxic/ischemic tissue.

Effects of Enhanced Tissue Oxygenation

Control of tissue oxygenation occurs at multiple levels as briefly reviewed in the introduction and extensively reviewed recently [35]. The interrelationship between O_2 content of the blood and blood delivery (Q, 1/min) are well known. When the DO_2 exceeds tissue demands, the CO adjusts to maintain the appropriate DO_2 level. This physiological adjustment will manifest itself as a transient pressor effect. Such a hemodynamic response to hyperoxia has been observed in dogs and pigs with IHP-treated RBCs where CO fell and total peripheral resistance increased [18, 36].

The best known example of toxicity associated with excess tissue oxygenation is reperfusion injury. Reperfusion is associated with enhanced creatine kinase release, reduced blood flow, and increased lipid peroxidation following resumption of blood flow to ischemic tissue. Rao et al. [37] have demonstrated that intravenous injection of IHP, acting as an antioxidant, reduces ischemic heart reperfusion injury.

Endothelial-derived nitric oxide (NO) induces vasodilation. Free Hb has been implicated in NO scavenging induced vasoconstriction [38]. However, such vasoconstriction has not been observed with RBC transfusions which suggests that intact cells reduce the contact of Hb with the endothelial cell and hence do not inactivate NO [39].

The kidney deserves special attention relative to blood transfusion due to the significant blood flow and the toxicity observed with RBC substitutes. The kidney is the most efficient autoregulatory organ in the body and regulates blood flow across wide ranges of systemic blood pressure, utilizing both myogenic and tubuloglomerular feedback systems, the latter of which relates reabsorption to filtration rate. The kidney has derived mechanisms to protect itself from oversupply of O_2 including vasodilation and tubuloglomerular feedback. In addition, a countercurrent exchange mechanism exists, where, the close proximity of the arteriolar and venular capillaries shunts excess O_2 away from the tissues. The kidney appears to tolerate a wide range of PO_2 levels [40] such as would occur with exposure to IHP-treated blood.

In summary, available data indicate that the enhanced tissue DO_2 achieved by IHP-treated blood will be physiologically regulated, and will not be limited by the problems reviewed above. The tissue will regulate the amount of O_2 delivered according to homeostatic physiology; O_2 toxicity, NO release, and nephrotoxic effects are not anticipated. The major result will likely be 'abnormal' cardiovascular variables, such as decreased heart rate and stroke volume. Nonetheless, these 'abnormal' cardiovascular variables are expected consequences of the enhanced tissue oxygenation produced by IHP-treated blood.

Alternative Therapies

There is no comparable therapy as a method for making existing blood more efficient in releasing O_2 into tissues. Currently, packed RBCs (which contain substantial protein and cellular contamination), washed RBCs (which are protein depleted) or leukodepleted RBCs are used acutely to increase blood Hb. Only relatively small right shifts of the O_2-binding curves could be obtained by incubating human RBCs with glycolytic intermediates. This resulted in a temporary accumulation of intracellular DPG in response to specific stimulation of glycolysis, and no lasting improvement in patient health [41]. Recombinant human erythropoietin has been approved for some types of chronic anemia. Erythropoietin can increase the numbers of RBCs in circulation over weeks and months and improve tissue oxygenation only in patients with inadequate numbers of RBCs.

Brief Review of Blood Substitutes

Several groups are engineering stroma-free or recombinant Hb, or perfluorocarbons as a replacement for human blood. These products are designed to replace blood lost in acute traumatic injury or surgery, yet they have a very short therapeutic effect since they are metabolized and/or excreted within hours of administration. Issues of cost relative to benefit and the availability of starting materials for the preparation of Hb-based products will have to be evaluated [42]. Many of these product candidates are currently in early clinical trials, and data on the safety of the most recent improvements are not yet available. Nephrotoxicity and hypertension were observed to result from the administration of artificial Hb products. Unlike these efforts, 'we are not making better blood, we're making blood better'™ by incorporating IHP into Hb.

Clinical Considerations

Clinical Experience to Date

The physiologic effect of potentially therapeutic levels of IHP-treated RBCs (approximately one unit) in humans has not been examined in a clinical setting. However, IHP-RBCs produced by osmotic shock have been observed to have a long circulatory life in patients [43]. Preliminary clinical trials were conducted with two groups of six volunteers using IHP-RBCs prepared by osmotic shock or pulse. The pulse is induced by equilibrating a RBC suspension with DMSO and then rapidly diluting with an isotonic IHP solution. The yield produced by this process was very limited. Nonetheless, the post transfusion life span of those cells that survived 24 hours was similar to that of a normal RBC, with an average life of 90 days. Transfusion of IHP-RBCs prepared by osmotic shock into two patients with sickle cell disease resulted in a decrease in morphological sickling at low PO_2 but no increase in cell life span [44].

Therapeutic Effect of IHP-RBCs

As presently envisioned, the presence of IHP-RBCs will provide a physician with the opportunity to give a patient a "dual compartment" red cell compliment. An average normovolemic adult human has a total blood volume of approximately 6 L. In a patient with a therapeutic dose of IHP-RBCs (estimated to be about one unit), at least 5 L of the patient's RBCs will respond to tissue demands and synthesize 2,3-DPG to adjust the right shift. The other portion, 1–2 units or 0.5–1 L of RBCs, will contain Hb:IHP complexes and be permanently right shifted. Patients with inadequate tissue oxygenation respond by right shifting the blood to compensate as much as necessary or possible. When tissue demands are met, the 2,3-DPG levels in their blood will slowly decrease. All other control mechanisms for DO_2 will remain active.

Extrapolation from exchange transfusion experiments in piglets would suggest that one unit (500cc) of IHP-RBCs (P50 = 50 Torr) would result in a modest shift in a patient's P50 from 26.5 Torr to 31–32 Torr. Such a right shift has been shown to reduce CO by approximately 20–25% and increase the avDO$_2$ by 40–50% (Claude Nicolau, personal communication). Increased delivery of O_2 to ischemic tissue would be substantial. It is unclear at this time, especially in patients without tissue oxygenation deficiencies, whether the rest of the blood which does not contain IHP would further decrease its DPG content since oxygenation is being well maintained by their more efficient IHP-treated counterparts. Nevertheless, it is clear that if a portion of the RBCs are right shifted, that portion may provide a disproportionately larger share of the O_2 delivered.

Potential Clinical Uses of IHP-Treated Blood

The "Transfusion Trigger"

The opportunity to provide increased O_2 to inadequately perfused tissue, reduce demands on the cardiovascular system, or provide hemodynamic support while minimizing "donor exposure" is a compelling reason to consider the use of IHP-RBCs. Nevertheless, use of IHP blood is governed by the same guidelines used for all transfused blood products.

The practice of transfusion medicine has undergone a major re-evaluation in the last decade as the criteria used for determining appropriate therapy following the experience of significant blood-born transmission of the human immunodeficiency virus (HIV) and hepatitis viruses. The new guidelines for the use of red cell transfusions have not been tested by traditional 'blinded' clinical trials and instead have been determined by committee. These recommendations are made at all levels from the hospital to guidelines issued from national meetings. The implications are significant. The United States National Institutes of Health Consensus Development Conference focused primarily on the risks associated with transfusion. A new target or "transfusion trigger" was proposed. And, most significantly, the conference directed the physician's attention toward assessment of clinical need and symptoms rather than numbers alone. There could be no better recommendation as guidance for the use of IHP blood.

The "normal" cardiovascular and blood values typically measured to assess a patient's hemodynamic status will be shifted in patients with right-shifted blood. For example, the hematocrit (Hct) or Hb will inadequately represent the potential O_2 carrying capacity of the blood. The O_2 extraction ratio (O_2ER), often used to determine the adequacy of oxygenation, will be much lower than expected relative to actual tissue oxygenation. The CO, as measured by stroke volume and rate, will not correlate with overall hemodynamic performance. The use of IHP blood will therefore not only provide the physician with additional therapeutic utility, but will also pose additional factors to consider for optimum care.

Acute Transfusions

Over 17 million units of blood products were used in the US in 1993 to treat medical and surgical emergencies (anual report, American association of blood banks). Hospital trauma patients and patients with a number of clinical syndromes experience anemia caused by insufficient numbers of RBCs or Hb in their blood. Inadequate oxygenation of tissues and subsequent pathologic complications can be averted by transfusion with one or more units of packed red cells. Unfortunately, cells that are stored in blood banks rapidly lose the allosteric effector, DPG. According to Schwartz, et al. [45], although DPG levels in transfused blood return "... to normal within 6–24 hours, restoration may be delayed in the critically ill and massively transfused patient who is least able to tolerate increased microvascular resistance to flow and depression of tissue oxygenation". The thousand-fold higher affinity of IHP for the allosteric pocket of Hb suggests that its loss as an allosteric effector may be delayed over that of DPG. Thus, IHP blood may be ready to effectively carry and release O_2 to tissues at the moment of transfusion, not 6–24 h later.

More importantly, since IHP-treated RBCs transport 2–3 times as much O_2 to tissues as untreated RBCs, a physician may require fewer units of IHP-treated RBCs to achieve a clinically beneficial effect. Use of this product with enhanced DO_2 may expose patients to fewer units of heterologous blood, decrease exposure to viral diseases from blood donors, minimize immune function disturbances secondary to transfusions and reduce iron overload in chronic anemia. IHP-treated RBCs can be prepared in blood processing centers with exactly the same process presently used to prepare washed RBCs, except for the inclusion of a electroporation/IHP incorporation step.

Autologous Infusion and Surgery

In non-emergency situations, e.g., elective surgery, it is advantageous to completely avoid the use of heterologous blood donors and instead use autologous blood stored for later use. The amount of blood which can be drawn and stored prior to surgery, however, can limit the use of autologous blood. If autologous blood is enhanced for O_2 release by IHP, less blood may be required and allogeneic transfusion avoided.

IHP treatment of RBCs in the surgical room may also be extremely useful as an adjuvant to hemodilution during surgery. To avoid transfusions with quantities of stored DPG-deficient blood, surgeons supplement blood volume by hemodilution, a variant of autologous infusion where blood is withdrawn from a patient prior to surgery and replaced by saline, colloids or crystalloids. After the surgery is completed, the stored autologous blood is transfused back into the patient. IHP-treated blood processed during the surgical procedure might facilitate recovery by the patient and eliminate the need for a heterologous transfusion.

Cardiovascular Insufficiency

Many cardiovascular diseases, including congestive heart failure and myocardial infarction, are characterized by an insufficient supply of O_2 in the blood that bathes the tissues. Each of these diseases may benefit from the improved O_2 releasing capacity of IHP-treated blood. Since tissue oxygenation is tightly regulated by physiologic mechanisms, the result of a more efficient DO_2 to peripheral tissues by IHP-erythrocytes is a down regulation of blood flow until physiologic levels of oxygenation are achieved. To sustain this homeostatic balance of blood delivery and oxygenation of tissues, the body decreases the strength of cardiac muscle contraction. A more efficient delivery of O_2 to tissue ultimately results in a drop in pulse rate and cardiac stroke volume, each of which can have enormous benefit in extending the viability of the heart tissue and patient quality of life in, for example, congestive heart failure or myocardial infarction.

Stroke, central nervous system trauma, angina, and peripheral vascular disease (intermittent claudication) are also examples of disorders characterized by inadequate blood flow in response to tissue demands that may benefit from IHP-treated blood infusion. For peripheral vascular diseases, as IHP-treated RBCs deliver more O_2 per unit volume, the right shifted blood will be therapeutic, and possibly provide a mechanism for restoring organ function by allowing improved diet and exercise without pain to reverse the debilitating effects of the vascular disease process.

Shock

A reduced P50 has been observed in critically ill patients [46]. In a study of high-risk surgical patients, it was observed that there are increased metabolic requirements after surgical trauma and that the changes in cardiac index (CI) and DO_2 represent compensatory increases in circulatory functions stimulated by increased metabolic needs [47]. The right shift may therefore be a protective response or it may simply be a response to accumulated O_2 debt [48]. O_2 debt has been observed in severely traumatized patients and has a negative correlation with survival [49]. In a prospective trial of supranormal values of CI, DO_2, and O_2 VO_2, it was concluded that attaining supranormal circulatory values improves survival and decreases morbidity in the severely traumatized patient [50]. Such supranormal values may be achieved by fluid optimization and vasoactive drugs which may not always be in the patient's best interest [51]. Efforts have been made to understand the relationship between tissue hypoxia and shock; however, global measures of DO_2 and VO_2 may be inadequate and measures of tissue oxygenation such as gastric intramucosal pH (pHi) may be necessary to evaluate the cascade of multiple system organ failure [52–54]. The use of IHP-RBCs to provide enhanced tissue oxygenation without undue cardiac stress may prove to be very useful in the critical care setting to reverse the accumulation of O_2 debt.

Sickle Cell Anemia

Sickling is caused by deoxygenation of Hb S. Autologous transfusion of IHP RBCs prepared by osmotic shock into two patients with sickle cell disease resulted in a decrease in morphological sickling at low PO_2 but no increase in cell life span [43, 44]. Critical factors in the sickling phenomena are Hb concentration and deoxygenation [55]. The use of IHP-RBCs containing Hb-S and prepared by the osmotic shock method may have influenced both of these factors, simultaneously decreasing Hb concentration inside the RBCs and increasing the propensity of the Hb to deoxygenate.

Nevertheless a potential for use of IHP-RBCs for sickle cell anemia remains. Transfusion of IHP-RBCs containing normal Hb may provide a patient with a volume of blood with a profound right shift. This population of RBCs will deoxygenate more readily, provide substantial tissue oxygenation and not sickle. This will allow a greater portion of the patient's own Hb-S to remain oxygenated and therefore not sickle. The therapeutic potential of this approach will require examination by clinical trial.

Chronic Obstructive Pulmonary Disease

Chronic obstructive pulmonary disease (COPD) is characterized by improper lung function that translates into problems of O_2 loading. Although the treatment of RBCs with IHP facilitates the unloading of O_2, it is anticipated that the systemic hypoxia associated with COPD may be improved by IHP treatment. Thus, diseases like emphysema and chronic bronchitis may be partially ameliorated by this technology.

Adjunct to Chemotherapy and Radiotherapy

Cancer treatment may be enhanced with IHP therapy. Radiation therapy of cancer depends upon the formation of O_2 free radicals which impair the viability of rapidly growing tumor cells. Solid tumors, however, are poorly vascularized, and little O_2 carrying blood reaches the interior of the tumor mass. There is significant interest in oncology in augmenting the DO_2 into the tumor by using short-term therapy with synthetic Hb. IHP-treated autologous RBCs, however, which can deliver up to three times as much O_2 as normal cells but have an equivalent life span, may provide an alternative adjunctive therapy with fewer long-term complications compared to free Hb.

Conclusion

We are developing an instrument and method which will shift the O_2 affinity of Hb using flow electroporation to introduce IHP into human RBCs. These RBCs will enhance DO_2 to inadequately oxygenated tissue and reduce CO. EntreMed's enhancement of DO_2 product has shown no toxicity in experimental animals or in limited clinical trials in humans. Furthermore, IHP-treated blood may reduce the number of units of blood transfused, and thereby limit exposure to contaminating blood-borne pathogens, a growing clinical concern. Such RBCs will be therapeutic for a number of disease indications including cardiovascular disease, peripheral vascular disease, shock, stroke, sickle cell anemia and other diseases of inadequate tissue oxygenation. The machine uses a disposable centrifuge bowl and electroporation chamber and is readily compatible with current practice. We anticipate initiation of phase I clinical trials within the near future.

References

1. Benesch RE, Edalji R, Benesch, R (1977) Reciprocal interaction of hemoglobin with oxygen and protons. The influence of allosteric polyanions. Biochemistry 16:2594–2597
2. Pennell RB (1974) In: D McN Surgenor (Ed) The red blood cell, Vol I. Academic Press, New York, pp 93–146
3. Nicolau C, Teisseire BP, Ropars C, Vallez MO, Herigault RA (1985) Incorporation of allosteric effectors of hemoglobin in red blood cells. Physiological effects. Bibl Haematol 51: 92–107
4. Neya S, Funasaki N (1986) Quaternary equilibrium analysis of the imidazole methemoglobin bound with inositol hexaphosphate. Biochim Biophys Acta 872:141–146
5. Ropars C, Chassaigne M, Villereal MC, Avenard G, Harel C, Nicolau C (1985) Resealed red blood cells as a new blood transfusion product. Bibl Haematol 51:82–91
6. Stucker O, Laurent D, Duvelleroy M, Ropars C, Teisseire B (1985) Incorporation of inositol hexaphosphate in stored erythrocytes: Effect on tissue oxygenation. Life Support Syst 1:458–461
7. Deleuze PH, Bailleul C, Shiiya N, et al (1992) Enhanced O2 transportation during cardiopulmonary bypass in piglets by the use of inositol hexaphosphate loaded red blood cells. Int J Artif Organs 15:239–242
8. Di Mauro P, Langer M, Prato P, et al (1992) A baboon model to test physiological and adverse effects of human red cells loaded with inositol hexaphosphate (IHP). Adv Exp Med Biol 326:333–340
9. Franco RS, Weiner M, Wagner K, Martelo OJ, Ragno G, Pivacek LE, Valeri CR (1988) The 24-hour posttransfusion survival and lifespan of autologous baboon red cells treated with inositol hexaphosphate-polyethylene glycol or inositol hexaphosphate-adenosine triphosphate-polyethylene glycol to decrease oxygen affinity. Vox Sang 55:90–96
10. Liard JF, Kunert MP (1993) Hemodynamic changes induced by low blood oxygen affinity in dogs. Am J Physiol 264:R396–R401
11. Baron JF, Vicaut E, Stucker O, Villereal MC, Ropars C, Teisseire B, Duvelleroy M (1988) Cardiac effects of phytic acid induced high P50 with free and limited coronary blood flow. Biomater Artif Cells Artif Organs 16:871–885
12. Baron JF, Vicaut E, Stucker O, Villereal MC, Ropars C, Teisseire B, Duvelleroy M (1988) Effects of inositol hexaphosphate induced high P50 on an isolated rabbit heart with free and limited coronary blood flow. Biomater Artif Cells Artif Organs 16:359–361
13. Stucker O, Vicaut E, Villereal MC, Ropars C, Teisseire BP, Duvelleroy MA (1985) Coronary response to large decreases of hemoglobin-O_2 affinity in isolated rat heart. Am J Physiol 249:H1224–H1227
14. Stucker O, Vicaut E, Trouve R, Teisseire B, Duvelleroy M (1986) Effects of low hemoglobin affinity on coronary blood flow in the isolated rat heart. Adv Exp Med Biol 200: 333–338
15. Teisseire B, Ropars C, Villereal MC, Nicolau C (1987) Long-term physiological effects of enhanced O_2 release by inositol hexaphosphate-loaded erythrocytes. Proc Natl Acad Sci USA 84:6894–6898
16. Bailleul C, Borrelly-Villereal MC, Chassaigne M, Ropars C (1989) Modification of partial pressure of oxygen (P50) in mammalian red blood cells by incorporation of an allosteric effector of hemoglobin. Biotechnol Appl Biochem 11:31–40

17. Villereal MC, Ropars C, Hurel C, et al (1987) Oxygen transport to tissue modified by entrapment of an allosteric effector of haemoglobin in erythrocytes. Folia Haematol Int Mag Klin Morphol Blutforsch 114:488–492
18. Teisseire BP, Ropars C, Vallez MO, Herigault RA, Nicolau C (1985) Physiological effects of high-P50 erythrocyte transfusion on piglets. J Appl Physiol 58:1810–1817
19. Stucker O, Vicaut E, Villereal MC, Ropars C, Teisseire BP, Duvelleroy MA (1985) Coronary response to large decreases of hemoglobin-O_2 affinity in isolated rat heart. Am J Physiol 249:H1224–1227
20. Tsai AG, Kerger H, Intaglietta M (1995) Microcirculatory consequences of blood substitution with aa-hemoglobin. In: Winslow RM, Vandegriff KD, Intaglietta M (eds) Blood substitutes: physiological basis of efficacy. Birkhäuser, Boston, pp 155–174
21. Vandegriff KD, Windslow RM (1995) A theoretical analysis of oxygen transport: A new strategy for the design of hemoglobin-based red cell substitutes. In: Winslow RM, Vandegriff KD, Intaglietta, M (eds) Blood Substitutes: Physiological basis of efficacy. Birkhäuser, Boston, pp 143–154
22. Weiner M (1983) Right shifting of Hb-O_2 dissociation in viable red cells by liposomal technique. Biol Cell 47:65–70
23. Chang DC, Reese TS (1990) Changes in membrane structure induced by electroporation as revealed by rapid-freezing electron microscopy. Biophys J 58:1–12
24. Graf E, Eaton JW (1990) Antioxidant functions of phytic acid. Free Radic Biol Med 8: 61–69
25. Graf E, Eaton JW (1993) Suppression of colonic cancer by dietary phytic acid. Nutr Cancer 19:11–19
26. Hirose M, Ozaki K, Takaba K, Fukushima S, Shirai T, Ito N (1991) Modifying effects of the naturally occurring antioxidants gamma-oryzanol, phytic acid, tannic acid and n-tritriacontane-16, 18-dione in a rat wide-spectrum organ carcinogenesis model. Carcinogenesis 12:1917–1921
27. Vucenik I, Tomazic VJ, Fabian D, Shamsuddin AM (1992) Antitumor activity of phytic acid (inositol hexaphosphate) in murine transplanted and metastatic fibrosarcoma, a pilot study. Cancer Lett 65:9–13
28. Thompson LU, Zhang L (1991) Phytic acid and minerals: effect on early markers of risk for mammary and colon carcinogenesis. Carcinogenesis 12:2041–2045
29. Shamsuddin AM, Ullah A, Chakravarthy AK (1989) Inositol and inositol hexaphosphate suppress cell proliferation and tumor formation in CD-1 mice. Carcinogenesis 10:1461–1463
30. Iashvili BP, Baluda VP, Lukhoyanova TI, Kozelskaya LV, Katsitadze NG, Kamkamidze MV, Robakidze TA (1986) The effects of administration of drugs influencing haemostasis during treatment of patients with burns. Burns Incl Therm Inj 12:184–187
31. Khakimov Z, Mavlianov BR, Rakhmanov A, Mavlianov IR (1992) The effect of phytin, benzonal and their combination administered prophylactically on the pharmacodynamics of drugs metabolized in the liver in hypokinesia. Eksp Klin Farmakol 55:58–60
32. Gersonde K, Weiner M (1982) The influence of infusion rate on the acute intravenous toxicity of phytic acid; A calcium-binding agent. Toxicology 22:279–286
33. Rao PS, Liu XK, Das DK, Weinstein GS, Tyras DH (1991) Protection of ischemic heart from reperfusion injury by myo-inositol hexaphosphate, a natural antioxidant. Ann Thorac Surg 52:908–912
34. Strauss RG (1996) Neonatal erythropoiesis and red blood cell transfusions. In: Petz LD, Swisher SN, Kleinman S, Spence RK, Strauss RG (eds) Clinical practice of transfusion medicine, 3rd edition. Churchill Livingstone, New York, pp 633–645
35. Windslow RM (1995) A physiological basis for the transfusion trigger. In: Winslow RM, Vandegriff KD, Intaglietta M (eds) Blood substitutes: physiological basis of efficacy. Birkhäuser, Boston, pp 25–41
36. Liard JF, Kunert MP (1993) Hemodynamic changes induced by low blood oxygen affinity in dogs. Am J Physiol 264:R396–R401
37. Rao PS, Liu XK, Das DK, Weinstein GS, Tyras DH (1991) Protection of ischemic heart from reperfusion injury by myo-inositol hexaphosphate, a natural antioxidant. Ann Thorac Surg 52:908–912

38. Ignarro LJ (1990) Biosynthesis of endothelium-derived nitric oxide. In: George, R, Cho AK, Blachki TF (eds) Annual review pharmacology and toxicology. Annual Reviews Inc, Palo Alto, pp 525–560
39. Nakai K, Matsuda N, Amano M, et al (1994) Acellular and cellular hemoglobin solutions as vasoconstrictive factor. Artif Cells Blood Substit Immobil Biotechnol 22:559–564
40. Blantz RC, Evan AP, Gabbai FB (1995) Red cell substitutes in the kidney. In: Winslow RM, Vandegriff KD, Intaglietta M (eds) Blood substitutes: physiological basis of efficacy. Birkhäuser, Boston, pp 133–134
41. Valeri RC (1980) The red blood cell, Vol I. In: McN Surgenor D (ed) Academic Press, New York, pp 511–536
42. Spence RK (1996) In: Petz LD, Swisher SN, Kleinman S, Spense RK, Strauss RG (eds) Blood substitutes in clinical practice of transfusion medicine, 3rd edition.Churchill Livingstone, New York, pp 967–984
43. Franco R, Barker R, Mayfield G, Silberstein E, Weiner M (1990) The *in vivo* survival of human red cells with low oxygen affinity prepared by the osmotic pulse method of inositol hexaphosphate incorporation. Transfusion 30:196–200
44. Franco R, Barker-Gear R, Silberstein E, Mayfield G, Weiner M, Palascak J, Green R (1992) Sickle cells modified by an osmotic pulse in the presence of inositol hexaphosphate have decreased intracellular hemoglobin concentration and decreased *in vitro* sickling without prolonged *in vivo* survival. Adv Exp Med Biol 326:325–331
45. Schwartz SI, Shires GT, Spencer FC (1989) Principles of surgery, 5th edition. McGraw-Hill Book Company, New York
46. Myburgh Ja, Webb Rk, Worthley Li (1991) The P50 is reduced in critically ill patients. Intensive Care Medicine 17:355–358
47. Shoemaker WC, Appel PL, Kram HB (1993) Hemodynamic and oxygen transport responses in survivors and nonsurvivors of high-risk surgery. Crit Care Med 21:977–990
48. Mizock BA, Falk JL (1992) Lactic acidosis in critical illness. Crit Care Med 20:80-93
49. Bishop MH, Shoemaker WC, Appel PL, et al (1993) Relationship between supranormal circulatory values, time delays, and outcome in severely traumatized patients. Crit Care Med 21:56-63
50. Fleming A, Bishop M, Shoemaker W, et al (1992) Prospective trial of supranormal values as goals of resuscitation in severe trauma. Arch Surg 127:1175–1179
51. Timmins AC, Hayes M, Yau E, Watson JD, Hinds CJ (1992) The relationship between cardiac reserve and survival in critically ill patients receiving treatment aimed at achieving supranormal oxygen delivery and consumption. Postgrad Med J 68:S34-40
52. Gutierrez G (1991) Cellular energy metabolism during hypoxia. Crit Care Med 19:619–626
53. Gutierrez G, Bismar H, Dantzker DR, Silva N (1992) Comparison of gastric intramucosal pH with measures of oxygen transport and consumption in critically ill patients. Crit Care Med 20:451-457
54. Gutierrez G, Palizas F, Doglio G, et al (1992) Gastric intramucosal pH as a therapeutic index of tissue oxygenation in critically ill patients. Lancet 339:195–199
55. McManus ML, Churchwell KB, Strange K (1995) Regulation of cell volume in health and disease. N Engl J Med 333:1260–1266

Subject Index

Printing: Mercedes-Druck, Berlin
Binding: Buchbinderei Lüderitz & Bauer, Berlin